Applied Pharmaceutical Practice

Christopher A Langley

Senior Lecturer in Pharmacy Practice
Aston University School of Pharmacy,
Birmingham, UK

and

Dawn Belcher

Teaching Fellow, Pharmacy Practice,
Aston University School of Pharmacy,
Birmingham, UK

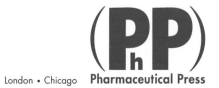

London • Chicago   **Pharmaceutical Press**

Published by the Pharmaceutical Press

An imprint of RPS Publishing

1 Lambeth High Street, London SE1 7JN, UK
100 South Atkinson Road, Suite 200, Grayslake, IL 60030–7820, USA

© Pharmaceutical Press 2009

(**P͟P**) is a trade mark of RPS Publishing

RPS Publishing is the publishing organisation of the
Royal Pharmaceutical Society of Great Britain

First published 2009

Typeset by Photoprint Typesetters, Torquay, Devon
Printed in Great Britain by Cambridge University Press, Cambridge

ISBN 978 0 85369 746 6

Applied Pharmaceutical Practice

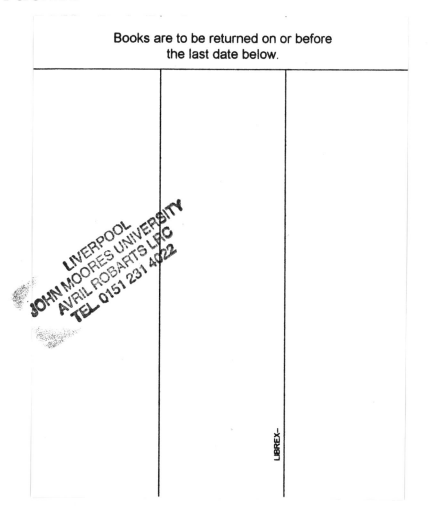

Books are to be returned on or before
the last date below.

LIBREX–

Contents

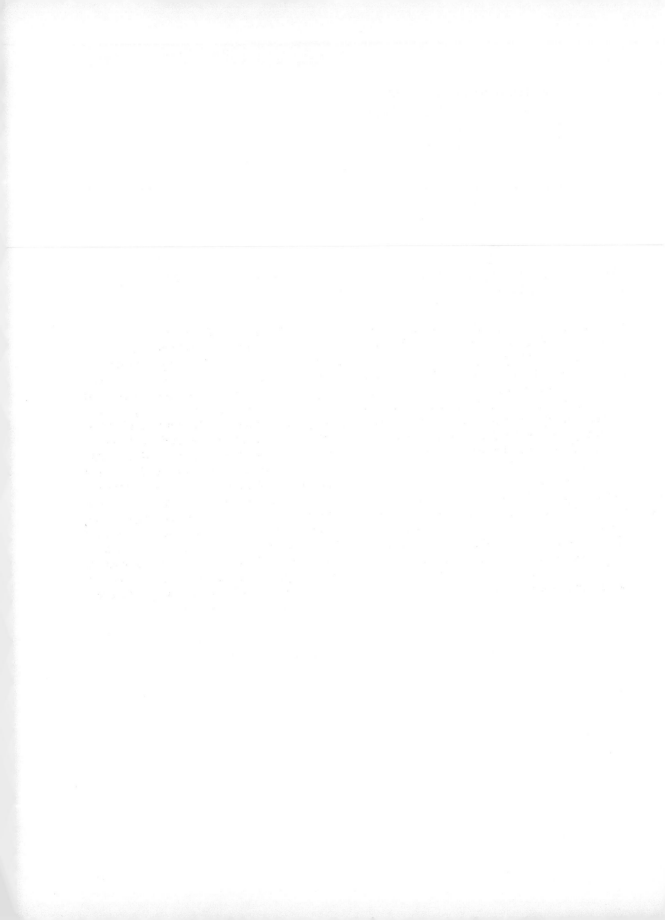

About the authors

Christopher A Langley BSc, PhD, MRPharmS, MRSC, FHEA

Chris Langley is a qualified pharmacist who graduated from Aston University in 1996 and then undertook his pre-registration training at St Peter's Hospital in Chertsey. Upon registration, he returned to Aston University to undertake a PhD within the Medicinal Chemistry Research Group before moving over full-time to Pharmacy Practice. He is currently employed as a senior lecturer in pharmacy practice, specialising in teaching the professional and legal aspects of the degree programme.

His research interests predominantly surround pharmacy education but he is also involved in research examining the role of the pharmacist with both primary and secondary care. This includes research into the pharmacist's role in public health and the reasons behind and possible solutions to the generation of waste medication.

Dawn Belcher BPharm, MRPharmS, FHEA

Dawn Belcher is a qualified pharmacist who graduated from the Welsh School of Pharmacy in 1977 and then undertook her pre-registration training with Boots the Chemist at their Wolverhampton store. After registration she worked as a relief manager and later as a pharmacy manager for Boots the Chemist until 1984. While raising a family she undertook locum duties for Boots the Chemist and in 1986 became an independent locum working for a small chain of pharmacies in the West Midlands, while also working for Lloyds Chemist.

In 1989 she began sessional teaching with the Pharmacy Practice group at Aston University which continued until she took a permanent post in 2001. She now enjoys teaching practical aspects of pharmacy practice while still keeping an association with Lloydspharmacy, where she is employed as a relief manager.

Preface

This text is designed to guide the student pharmacist or pharmacy technician through the main stages involved in pharmaceutical dispensing. The purpose of the book is to provide students with a core reference text to accompany the compulsory dispensing courses found in all undergraduate MPharm programmes and equivalent technical training courses.

Christopher A Langley
Dawn Belcher
Birmingham, United Kingdom
August, 2008

Abbreviations

ACBS   Advisory Committee on Borderline Substances
ACE   angiotensin converting enzyme
ADHD   attention deficit hyperactivity disorder
CD   controlled drug
CDA   completely denatured alcohol
CHI   community health index
CHIP   Chemicals (Hazard Information and Packaging for Supply) Regulations
CMP   clinical management plan
DEFRA   Department for Environment, Food and Rural Affairs
DPF   Dental Practitioners' Formulary
ESPS   Essential Small Pharmacies Scheme
ETP   electronic transmission of prescriptions
FHSAA   Family Health Services Appeal Authority
GMC   General Medical Council
GOC   General Optical Council
GP   general practitioner
GSL   general sale list
HIV   human immunodeficiency virus
HPC   Health Professions Council
HRT   hormone replacement therapy
HSW   Health Solutions Wales
IDA   industrial denatured alcohol
IMS   industrial methylated spirit
MAOIs   monoamine oxidase inhibitors
MDI   metered dose inhaler
MF   Measured and fitted
MHRA   Medicines and Healthcare products Regulatory Agency
MMS   mineralised methylated spirits
MURs   medicines use reviews
NCSO   no cheaper stock obtainable
NHS   National Health Service
NHSBSA   National Health Service Business Services Authority
NMC   Nursing and Midwifery Council
OP   original pack
OTC   over-the-counter
P   pharmacy medicine
PCO   Primary Care Organisation
PCT   Primary Care Trust

PGDs	Patient Group Directions
PIL	patient information leaflet
PIN	personal identification number
PMR	patient medication record
PO	pharmacy only
POD	patients' own drugs
POM	prescription-only medicine
PPD	Prescription Pricing Division
PSD	Practitioner Services Division
RPSGB	Royal Pharmaceutical Society of Great Britain
SLS	Selective List Scheme
SOPs	standard operating procedures
SPC	summary of Product Characteristics
TSDA	trade specific denatured alcohol
TTA	to take away
TTO	to take out
ZD	zero discount

1

Introduction, medicines classification and standard operating procedures

Upon completion of this chapter, you should be able to:

- understand the layout of this book and the broad contents of the different chapters
- describe the different categories of medicines classification
- use standard operating procedures (SOPs) and understand the role they play within pharmacy.

1.1 Introduction

The supply of medicines is a basic function of pharmacists and pharmacy technicians. With the advent of clinical pharmacy and the introduction of 'new roles' for pharmacists, the content of pharmaceutical education has altered to reflect these additions. However, the supply of medicines remains a key component of the role of pharmacy within modern healthcare and, therefore, it is vital that all pharmacists and pharmacy technicians are competent in medicines supply.

This text has been designed to guide the student pharmacist or pharmacy technician through the main stages involved in safe and effective medicines supply. The purpose of the book is to provide student pharmacists with a core reference text to accompany the compulsory dispensing courses found in all MPharm programmes. Additionally, it will be of equal value for student pharmacy technicians during their educational courses.

Key point 1.1

To gain the most from this text, it is suggested that the reader has access to either the print version or on-line version of a recent copy of both the *British National Formulary* and the respective *Drug Tariff* for their country (England and Wales, Northern Ireland or Scotland).

1.2 The layout of this book

To guide the reader through the different topics relating to medicines supply, this book has been divided into a number of different chapters.

Chapter 1 Introduction, medicines classification and standard operating procedures

This introduces the text and provides an outline of the key points behind medicines supply. It also covers the basic classification of medicines and the role of standard operating procedures.

Chapter 2 NHS supply in the community 1 – Prescription forms and prescribing

This introduces medicines supply in the community and covers the background details. National Health Service (NHS) prescription forms and the restrictions placed on different NHS prescribers in the community, including the role of the UK *Drug Tariffs*, are discussed.

Chapter 3 NHS supply in the community 2 – Prescribers and the dispensing process

This introduces the different NHS prescribers (for example, doctor, dentist, nurse, supplementary prescriber, etc.) within the community. Following on from this are details of the dispensing process to be followed when supplying medicines against NHS prescription forms, along with a collection of worked examples.

Chapter 4 NHS supply within hospitals

This addresses the supply of medicines via the NHS within hospitals.

Chapter 5 Non-NHS supply

This chapter covers similar material to Chapters 2 and 3, focusing on non-NHS supply, including the supply of medication against private prescription forms and the supply of medication via oral and written requisitions.

Chapter 6 Controlled drugs

This chapter uses some of the material already discussed in Chapters 2–5 and addresses the laws and regulations relating to the supply of controlled drugs, via both NHS and non-NHS routes.

Chapter 7 Emergency supply

This covers the key points behind the emergency supply of medicines by a pharmacist, both at the request of a prescriber and at the request of a patient.

Chapter 8 Patient counselling and communication 1 – The basics of patient communication

In this chapter the basics of patient communication are discussed, ensuring that pharmacists and pharmacy technicians are familiar with both verbal and non-verbal communication and are able to communicate effectively with patients and carers.

Chapter 9 Patient counselling and communication 2 – Product-specific counselling points

This provides specific detail of the important counselling points that need to be considered for specific dosage forms.

Chapter 10 Poisons and spirits

This covers the key points behind the supply of poisons and spirits from pharmacies.

1.3 Medicines classification

The Medicines Act 1968 defines three classes of medicinal products for human use. These are general sale list (GSL) medicines, pharmacy (P) medicines and prescription-only medicines (POM).

- **General sale list (GSL) medicines** (see Section 1.3.1) are medicines that can be purchased from a wide range of shops, general stores, supermarkets, newsagents, petrol stations, etc. Products classified as GSL are considered to be reasonably safe and therefore able to be sold without the supervision of a pharmacist.
- **Pharmacy (P) medicines** (see Section 1.3.2) may be sold from pharmacies under the supervision of a pharmacist. The pharmacist or the pharmacy technician/counter assistant

will ask a number of questions prior to making the sale to ensure that the medication is safe for the patient and will give advice as to the use of the product. Some medicines may only be sold when certain criteria have been met, for example, when supplying emergency hormonal contraception from a community pharmacy.

- **Prescription-only medicines (POMs)** (see Section 1.3.3) are usually obtained on the authorisation of a valid prescription form (either an NHS or a private prescription form) written by a recognised prescriber registered in the UK and presented at a registered pharmacy (although exceptions to this do exist, for example, dispensing doctors (see Section 2.3.1), in-patient hospital supply (see Section 4.2.1) and emergency supply at the request of a patient (see Sections 7.2 and 7.3)).

Traditionally, the prescriber would have been a doctor or a dentist, but recent changes to healthcare legislation and the introduction of supplementary and independent prescribers mean that many other healthcare professionals, such as nurses and pharmacists, are now also permitted to prescribe (see Section 3.2).

In addition to the above, the Misuse of Drugs Act 1971 and Misuse of Dugs Regulations 2001 concern medicines for human use that require extra controls. These medicines, termed 'controlled drugs' (or 'CDs'), are also classified using the Medicines Act classifications above, but there are stricter controls on their sale or supply (for further information see Chapter 6).

Key point 1.2

The Medicines Act 1968 defines three classes of medicinal products for human use:

- general sale list (GSL) medicines
- pharmacy (P) medicines
- prescription-only medicines (POMs).

1.3.1 General sale list (GSL) medicines

General sale list medicines are those for which all the active ingredients are listed in the Medicines (Products Other than Veterinary Drugs) (General Sales List) Order 1984.

Products categorised as GSL medicines have strict controls concerning their strength, use, pharmaceutical form and route of administration. The maximum dose or maximum daily dose will also be controlled for medicines for internal use. Another control that may be enforced is pack size, with a limit to the size of pack allowed as a GSL medicine. Examples of GSL medicines that have controlled pack sizes include:

- aspirin
- bisacodyl
- cetirizine
- clotrimazole
- ibuprofen
- loperamide
- loratadine
- paracetamol
- ranitidine.

Larger pack sizes of these medicines would render them P medicines (see Section 1.3.2) or in some cases POMs (see Section 1.3.3).

Paracetamol is an example of a medicine where the pack size makes a big difference to its legal classification. Table 1.1 lists the various pack sizes available.

There is no limit to the quantity of effervescent paracetamol that may be purchased at one time although the control through a pharmacy would be at the discretion of the pharmacist involved with the sale. While there is no legal requirement for general retailers (i.e. non-pharmacy) to limit the supply of paracetamol, the reason for the legislation was clearly explained (i.e. to reduce the number of intentional or accidental suicides using paracetamol) and many retailers introduced a code of practice or have programmed their tills to prevent multiple sales.

The following classes of medicinal products for human use are also not allowed to be classified as GSL medicines:

Table 1.1 Pack sizes and classification of paracetamol

Pack size (no. tablets or capsules)	Classification	Notes
Non-effervescent paracetamol tablets 500 mg or capsules 500 mg		
Up to 16	GSL	Maximum allowed to be purchased at any one time is 100 (i.e. six packs of 16)
17–32	GSL	But only allowed for sale through registered pharmacies (termed 'pharmacy only' or 'PO'), where the maximum that can be sold in packs of 16 or 32 is 100 (i.e. six packs of 16 or three packs of 32)
>32	POM	
Effervescent preparations of paracetamol 500 mg		
Up to 30	GSL	
>30	GSL	But only allowed for sale through registered pharmacies (termed 'pharmacy only' or 'PO')

- enemas
- eye drops
- eye ointments
- products containing aspirin or aloxiprin and intended for administration either wholly or mainly to children
- products for parenteral administration (a product given by injection, bypassing the enteral (gastro-intestinal) tract)
- products used as anthelmintics (a substance that expels or destroys intestinal worms)
- products used for irrigation of wounds, the bladder, vagina or rectum.

It should be noted that although the sale of GSL medicines from a pharmacy does not need to be under the supervision of a pharmacist, GSL medicines must still be sold under the 'personal control' of a pharmacist. The term 'personal control' comes from the Medicines Act 1968 and has never been interpreted in the courts. However, it is generally understood to mean that the pharmacist must be available on the premises. If the pharmacist is not available, no medicines (including GSL items) may be sold at all. For this reason, GSL medicines sold from pharmacies are often treated as pharmacy (P) medicines, which can only be sold from a pharmacy under the supervision of a pharmacist (see Section 1.3.2). Obviously, this restriction does not apply to GSL medicines sold from other (non-pharmacy) establishments.

> **Key point 1.3**
>
> General sale list (GSL) medicines can be purchased from a wide range of shops, general stores, supermarkets, newsagents, petrol stations, etc. Products classified as GSL are considered to be reasonably safe and therefore able to be sold without the supervision of a pharmacist.

1.3.2 Pharmacy (P) medicines

A pharmacy medicine is the definition given to medicinal products not included on the Prescription Only Medicines Order or the General Sale List or to products that are supplied outside the GSL package limit or maximum dosage limit. A few medicines are called pharmacy only (PO) medicines; these include medicines that would normally be included on the GSL but where the manufacturer has limited the supply of the medicines to pharmacies only (see Section 1.3.1). Examples include:

- Fybogel sachets
- Gaviscon Advance
- Rennie Duo preparations
- Robitussin Chesty Cough.

The Royal Pharmaceutical Society of Great Britain's Professional Standards and Guidance for the Sale and Supply of Medicines ((2) Supply of Over The Counter (OTC) Medicines) states that 'When purchasing medicines from pharmacies patients expect to be provided with high quality, relevant information in a manner they can easily understand.' With this in mind, whenever P medicines are sold from a pharmacy the sale must be made under the supervision of a pharmacist. All medicines counter assistants who regularly deal with requests for medicines must be trained. The training of assistants in pharmacies should be such that they will request information from the purchaser to ensure that the condition is suitable for self-medication and the product requested by the patient or suggested by the assistant is appropriate. Examples of suitable questions can be found in Section 8.2.1.

In addition, protocols must be in place to ensure that when necessary, patients are referred to the pharmacist for direct consultation. Patient groups particularly at risk are the very young or old and patients already taking other medications.

Key point 1.4

Pharmacy (P) medicines may be sold from pharmacies under the supervision of a pharmacist. The pharmacist, pharmacy technician or the pharmacy counter assistant will ask a number of questions prior to making the sale to ensure that the medication is safe for the patient and advice as to the use of the product will be provided.

Some medicines may only be sold when certain criteria have been met, for example, when supplying emergency hormonal contraception from a community pharmacy.

In addition, protocols must be in place to ensure that when necessary, patients are referred to the pharmacist for direct consultation. Patient groups particularly at risk are the very young or old and patients already taking other medications.

1.3.3 Prescription-only medicines (POMs)

These are medicines that are listed in the Prescription Only Medicines (Human Use) Order 1997. If the pack size of a POM is reduced it may be considered for licensing as a P or GSL medicine (see paracetamol example in Section 1.3.1). If a POM is intended for sale below a certain strength or dose then the medicine may be also considered to be a P medicine. An example of this is hyoscine butylbromide tablets 10 mg, which are normally classified as a POM but if packaged and labelled appropriately, a P classification is given. For P classification in this example, the packaging must state that a single dose must not exceed 20 mg and the daily dose must not exceed 80 mg and the pack must contain no more than 240 mg.

Medicines may also be exempted from POM classification if there are limitations on the use of the product. An example would be hydrocortisone cream 1% normally categorised as a POM but as a P medicine in packaging that limits the use of the cream to the treatment of allergic contact dermatitis, irritant dermatitis, insect bite reactions and mild to moderate eczema; it should be applied sparingly once or twice a day for a maximum of one week. The P form or 'over-the-counter' (OTC) form is only licensed for those indications and dosages listed above and further restriction to sales include unsuitability for OTC sale to treat:

- children under 10 years
- conditions on the face or anogenital area
- conditions where the skin is broken or infected, including cold sores, acne and athlete's foot
- pregnant women.

Medicines containing controlled drugs will generally be given a POM classification. Exemptions to this general rule include where the strength of the controlled drug included in the medication is below a certain value, when the medicine ingredient will be covered by Schedule 5 of the Misuse of Drugs Regulations 2001. Examples of these will be P medicines containing codeine, morphine or pholcodine. Further details of Schedule 5 medicines can be found in Chapter 6.

The reclassification of medicines from POM to P to GSL is an ongoing process in keeping with the NHS Plan where the intention is to increase the availability and patient choice of medicines. In 1983, loperamide was the first POM to have a P licence granted at the request of the manufacturer. Since then over 70 other medicines have been reclassified from POM to P.

Newly licensed POMs would not be considered for reclassification until the safety profile had been established. Drugs under intensive safety surveillance are indicated by a 'black triangle' in the *British National Formulary*, which generally continues for approximately two years, dependent on whether any issues related to safety are discovered.

Further declassification of 'new' P medicines to GSL has also occurred and examples include:

- aciclovir cream
- beclometasone nasal spray
- cetirizine tablets
- hyoscine butylbromide tablets
- loperamide capsules
- loratadine tablets
- nicotine replacement gum
- nicotine replacement patches
- ranitidine tablets.

Key point 1.5

Prescription-only medicines (POMs) are medicines that are listed in the Prescription Only Medicines (Human Use) Order 1997. They are usually obtained on the authorisation of a valid prescription form (either an NHS or a private prescription form) written by a recognised prescriber registered in the UK, presented at a registered pharmacy (although exceptions do exist).

Traditionally, the prescriber would have been a doctor or a dentist but under recent changes to healthcare legislation supplementary and independent prescribers have been introduced. This category includes many other healthcare professionals such as nurses and pharmacists.

1.4 Standard operating procedures

Standard operating procedures are often referred to as 'SOPs' and include all the written protocols and procedures in place within a pharmacy. They state the way the pharmacy expects tasks to be carried out to ensure a quality service is provided. They will include, for example, the questions that must be asked of a patient so that their needs can be correctly identified and appropriate action taken.

Key point 1.6

Standard operating procedures are often referred to as 'SOPs' and include all the written protocols and procedures in place within a pharmacy.

1.4.1 The history of standard operating procedures

Standard operating procedures have existed for the dispensing supply process in their current form since January 2005. They were put in place to ensure clinical governance of the dispensing procedure. 'Clinical governance' is the term used in the NHS and private healthcare system to describe a systematic approach to maintaining and improving the quality of patient care.

Because pharmacies differ so much, a single SOP could not be devised that would cover all pharmacies. Therefore each pharmacy has individually tailored SOPs for their working environment. Larger companies, with numerous pharmacies, may have single SOPs that cover all their premises. These were formally known as 'company policy'. It is considered good practice to have SOPs in place for all procedures carried out in the pharmacy.

What are the advantages of SOPs?

The advantages of SOPs are as follows:

1. They can assist with quality assurance, ensuring that patients receive a service that meets certain predefined standards.
2. They ensure consistency, which helps to maintain the level of service offered and therefore maintain good pharmaceutical practice at all times.
3. They help free up time for pharmacists, by enabling the delegation of certain tasks. This in turn enables pharmacists to engage in some of the new roles and provides enhanced roles for pharmacy technicians that recognise their specific expertise.
4. They set out clear lines of accountability, ensuring staff are aware of their own responsibilities.
5. They help locum and part-time staff understand the processes and running of the pharmacy.
6. They are useful templates for the training of new staff.
7. They provide additional information for the audit process.

1.4.2 The preparation of standard operating procedures

The Royal Pharmaceutical Society of Great Britain breaks down the preparation of a standard operating procedure into six stages:

1. **Objectives** – The purpose of the SOP.
2. **Scope** – What are the areas of work to be covered by the SOP? It is advisable that this should not be over complex.
3. **The stages of the process** – This is a description of how the task is carried out. It is important that this description is clear and unambiguous, preferably without the use of jargon.
4. **Responsibility** – Who is responsible for carrying out the procedure and who will ensure that staff members are suitably trained to carry out a procedure? In a working pharmacy this would also include contingency plans detailing what to do in cases of sickness or holiday leave, etc.
5. **Other useful information** – For example, details on how the SOP will be audited.

Auditing the processes will help to maintain standards and identify any areas where improvement could be made.
6. **Review** – Show how the process will be monitored to ensure that it remains up to date and relevant.

The new pharmacy contract for England and Wales

The new pharmacy contract (from April 2005) divides the activities that community pharmacies undertake into three tiers of service: essential services, advanced services and enhanced services. The essential services provided by a community pharmacy are compulsory and are the minimum required of a contractor as part of the pharmacy contract.

There are seven essential services identified in the contract:

1. dispensing
2. repeat dispensing
3. disposal of unwanted medicines
4. promotion of healthy lifestyles (public health)
5. signposting (provide information on where and how to access other health and social care providers)
6. support for self-care (help to minimise the inappropriate use of health and social care services)
7. clinical governance.

A similar contract exists within Scotland, with four core services: an acute medication service (AMS), a minor ailment service (MAS), chronic medication service (CMS) and a public health service (PHS). Additional services are to be agreed locally but on the basis of national (Scottish) specifications.

A pharmacy must have in place SOPs for all these activities. In addition other SOPs will be developed to aid the business. For example, an SOP covering OTC sales (sale of medicines and provision of advice), stock ordering and receipt of goods (ensuring stock received is what was ordered, is in date and does not have a short shelf-life, and is to be stored correctly), the receipt of telephone calls, etc., should be in place.

1.4.3 Examples of standard operating procedures

A detailed consideration of how to dispense NHS and non-NHS prescriptions can be found in the subsequent chapters of this book. However, consider an SOP for the dispensing of prescriptions (i.e. service number 1 from the list of essential services above). This can be broken down into a number of stages:

1. prescription reception
2. professional check
3. intervention and problem solving
4. label generation and collection of prescription item(s)
5. accuracy checking
6. handing out prescription item(s) to patients or their representatives
7. dealing with 'owings' when prescription forms are incompletely filled.

The list above covers the basic dispensing procedure and each stage will require a standard operating procedure. Figure 1.1 shows an example of a standard operating procedure for the reception of a prescription form within a community pharmacy.

In order to ensure that each SOP is being followed properly and that the SOP is functioning correctly, periodic audits of the processes covered by SOPs should be carried out. Figure 1.2 contains an example of a form for the audit of an SOP for the reception of a prescription form within a community pharmacy.

Exercise 1.1

Look at the questions in the audit in Figure 1.2. Which objectives are satisfied by adherence to these processes?

Exercise 1.2

Figure 1.3 contains an example of a standard operating procedure for the professional check of a dispensed prescription form within a community pharmacy. Using this information (and the example in Figure 1.2) fill out the audit question document in Figure 1.4 for the audit of prescription form returns from the Prescription Pricing Division (PPD) (see Section 3.3.8) with the questions you would ask.

Figure 1.5 contains an example of a clinical intervention form. This is a form used within a pharmacy to record any clinical interventions made. During the professional check of a prescription form, the pharmacist may note areas that require further action (for example, contacting the prescriber to confirm a dose, etc.). Once any appropriate action has been taken, a note of the action taken is made on a clinical intervention form. These forms can then also be used for audit purposes.

Exercise 1.3

Figure 1.6 contains an example of a standard operating procedure for the label generation and assembly of prescription items within a community pharmacy. Figure 1.7 contains an example of the corresponding audit form. Look at the questions in the audit. Which objectives are satisfied by adherence to these processes?

Figure 1.8 contains an example of a standard operating procedure for the check of prescription items within a community pharmacy and Figure 1.9 contains the corresponding audit form. These figures both make reference to a 'near miss' table. This is a form used to record dispensing errors that are identified during the checking procedure. By logging all errors, patterns can be identified and steps taken to prevent future errors. An example of a 'near miss' table can be found in Figure 1.10.

Exercise 1.4

Question 1: Figure 1.11 contains an example of a standard operating procedure for the handing out of prescription items within a community pharmacy. Using this information (and the example in Figure 1.2) fill out the audit question document in Figure 1.12 with the questions you would ask.

Question 2: Look at the questions in the audit. Which objectives are satisfied by adherence to these processes?

Exercise 1.5

This chapter has covered a number of examples of standard operating procedures and has shown how they are generated. Why not try making your own SOPs for your processes in dispensing classes? Or if you undertake any work or vacation placements, try to identify other areas where SOPs would be useful.

1.5 Chapter summary

This chapter has introduced the book and explained the contents of the subsequent chapters. In addition, basic medicines classification has been described, where medicines are classified into three categories: general sale list (GSL) medicines, pharmacy (P) medicines and prescription-only medicines (POMs). Finally, the purpose and construction of standard operating procedures (SOPs) has been introduced.

It is important that student pharmacists and pharmacy technicians understand the points covered in this chapter before moving on to any subsequent chapters.

STANDARD OPERATING PROCEDURE – DISPENSING
PRESCRIPTION FORM RECEPTION (NHS)

OBJECTIVES	To maintain good patient relations To ensure the prescription form presented relates to the named patient To ensure safe dispensing To ensure details on the reverse of a prescription form are correctly filled out, and any applicable fee is collected To ensure effective communication between patient and pharmacist
SCOPE	The reception of all NHS prescription forms brought into the pharmacy by patients or their representatives Prescription forms received in bulk (prescription form collection service) or those received by telephone call are excluded from this SOP
STAGES OF THE PROCESS	Greet patient in friendly manner Check name and address of the patient (rewriting it if handwritten and unclear) Check the reverse of the prescription form is filled out correctly If the prescription form is for a child, check the age or date of birth is specified Collect any prescription charge(s) and indicate this on the prescription form Indicate whether or not the patient or patient's representative is waiting or calling back and whether or not the patient or patient's representative has requested to see the pharmacist Pass the prescription form through to the dispensary for prompt processing
RESPONSIBILITY	All staff members working on the medicines counter
OTHER USEFUL INFORMATION	Audit carried out by pharmacist (or designated technician/supervisor) using the basic objectives and the stages of the process as a basis of the audit
REVIEW	Following audit, make time to review findings with all staff so that any deficiencies can be rectified and any points of good practice can be implemented within the whole group, not just on an individual basis

Figure 1.1 An example of a standard operating procedure for the reception of a prescription form within a community pharmacy.

STANDARD OPERATING PROCEDURE – DISPENSING
PRESCRIPTION FORM RECEPTION (NHS) – Audit

NAME OF AUDITOR: _____   DATE OF AUDIT: _____

AUDIT QUESTION	SATISFACTORY		AREAS OF NON-COMPLIANCE	RECOMMENDATIONS
	YES	NO		
1. Are patients/representatives greeted in a friendly manner?				
2. Is the identity of the patient checked (i.e. name and address)?				
3. Is the reverse side of the prescription form checked for signatures and completion?				
4. Is any applicable fee collected and noted on the prescription form?				
5. If the prescription form is for a child, is the age or date of birth checked?				
6. Is information transferred between patient and pharmacist (call back, waiting, request for advice)?				
7. Are prescription forms promptly passed to the dispensary?				

REVIEW DATE: _____   REVIEWED BY: _____

Figure 1.2   An example of an audit form for the audit of a standard operating procedure for the reception of a prescription form within a community pharmacy.

STANDARD OPERATING PROCEDURE – DISPENSING
PROFESSIONAL CHECK (NHS)

OBJECTIVES	To ensure that each prescription form is legally valid and is suitable and safe for the patient thus meeting all expected legal and professional standards To ensure the prescription item(s) are allowed to be prescribed on NHS prescription forms
SCOPE	Assessing all NHS prescription forms from any practitioner for validity, safety, legality and clinical suitability
STAGES OF THE PROCESS	Check prescription form includes all appropriate details: • Patient details • Drug name • Drug strength • Drug quantity • Date • Details of prescriber • Prescriber's signature Check the prescriber is allowed to prescribe item on an NHS prescription form Check the prescription form is still in date If for controlled drug check that the controlled drug requirements are met Check suitability of medication: • Is it suitable for the patient's condition? • Is the dose correct? • Any interactions with existing medication? • Are there any contraindications that may apply to this patient (e.g. pregnant patients, elderly, asthmatic, etc.)? • Are there any side-effects or particular precautions of which the patient should be made aware? • Check there is no evidence of non-concordance or inappropriate use or misuse by the patient
RESPONSIBILITY	Pharmacist
OTHER USEFUL INFORMATION	Any interventions should be entered in the clinical intervention form [see Figure 1.5] (and if possible, on the patient's PMR). The system should be audited regularly by the pharmacist in charge (peer audit if possible would be preferable as self audit is not always the most successful/accurate)
REVIEW	As a result of the audit review, discuss findings and update practices if necessary

Figure 1.3   An example of a standard operating procedure for the professional check of a dispensed prescription form within a community pharmacy.

STANDARD OPERATING PROCEDURE – DISPENSING
PROFESSIONAL CHECK (NHS) – Audit

NAME OF AUDITOR: _____ DATE OF AUDIT: _____

AUDIT QUESTION	SATISFACTORY		AREAS OF NON-COMPLIANCE	RECOMMENDATIONS
	YES	NO		
Review resubmissions (i.e. prescription forms returned from the Prescription Pricing Division*).				

REVIEW DATE: _____ REVIEWED BY: _____

Figure 1.4 A blank audit form for the audit of prescription form returns from the Prescription Pricing Division (PPD)* within a community pharmacy (*or equivalent – see Section 3.3.8).

STANDARD OPERATING PROCEDURE – DISPENSING
PROFESSIONAL CHECK (NHS)

CLINICAL INTERVENTION FORM

Date of Intervention:	
Pharmacist on Duty:	
Patient Name:	
Address:	
Date of Birth:	
Prescriber Name:	
Address:	
Details of Intervention:	
Action Taken:	
Response of Prescriber:	
Response of Patient: (if appropriate)	

Figure 1.5   An example of a clinical intervention form.

STANDARD OPERATING PROCEDURE – DISPENSING
LABEL GENERATION AND ASSEMBLY OF PRESCRIPTION ITEMS (NHS)

OBJECTIVES	To ensure prescription form details are accurately recorded on the PMR To produce labels that meet the legal and professional requirements To minimise the risk of error due to incorrect selection or incorrect labelling of prescription items To dispense products to a high professional standard in terms of accuracy and appearance
SCOPE	Generation of all labels for prescription medicines The assembly of all medications requested on a prescription form
STAGES OF THE PROCESS	Prescriptions dispensed in logical order (waiting or calling back prescriptions) PMR used to generate label – check if patient is already registered if not complete the registration process and inform patient they are now included on your system (to satisfy the requirements of the Data Protection Act) Ensure the correct patient is selected if already registered (name address and date of birth) If the prescription is for an item that patient has had before, check that the dose, strength and quantity are the same as used previously before 'repeating' a previously produced label Label in the order the items appear on the prescription form If the PMR displays a drug interaction alert, inform the pharmacist Read the label and ensure it is easy to understand prior to printing Print label Select items to be dispensed from the prescription form, <u>not</u> the accompanying labels Dispense in a clean, clutter free, designated area Label items as they are assembled All items must be dispensed in child-resistant packaging (if patient requests no 'clic-locs' this should be entered on the PMR) Check that a patient information leaflet is included Double check assembled work and initial label in 'dispensed by' box Pass completed prescription form with items dispensed for final accuracy check to designated checking area
RESPONSIBILITY	Dispensing assistants, dispensing technicians, accredited checking technicians and pharmacists
OTHER USEFUL INFORMATION	Any errors spotted at this stage should be noted as this could be due to a process error that could affect others (e.g. adjacent storage of two similarly packaged drugs). Audit performed by the pharmacist
REVIEW	As a result of the audit review, discuss findings and update practices if necessary

Figure 1.6 An example of a standard operating procedure for the label generation and assembly of prescription items within a community pharmacy.

STANDARD OPERATING PROCEDURE – DISPENSING
LABEL GENERATION AND ASSEMBLY OF PRESCRIPTION ITEMS (NHS) – Audit

NAME OF AUDITOR: _____ DATE OF AUDIT: _____

AUDIT QUESTION	SATISFACTORY		AREAS OF NON-COMPLIANCE	RECOMMENDATIONS
	YES	NO		
1. Were the prescriptions labelled in a logical manner?				
2. Were the labels produced in the order they were on the prescription form?				
3. Was the pharmacist alerted to any interactions?				
4. Were the directions on the label easy to follow and accurate?				
5. When assembling the prescription were the items selected from the prescription form?				
6. Is the dispensing bench free from clutter?				
7. Does the dispensed item look presentable and reflect well on the professionalism of the pharmacist or pharmacy technician?				
8. Has a patient information leaflet been included?				
9. Is the item dispensed in a child-resistant container?				

REVIEW DATE: _____ REVIEWED BY: _____

Figure 1.7   An example of an audit form for the audit of a standard operating procedure for the label generation and assembly of prescription items within a community pharmacy.

STANDARD OPERATING PROCEDURE – DISPENSING
ACCURACY CHECK OF PRESCRIPTION ITEMS (NHS)

OBJECTIVES	Prevent the occurrence of dispensing errors Maintain a high level of professional service to patients
SCOPE	Final check of dispensed medication prior to handing out to the patient or their representative
STAGES OF THE PROCESS	The check should preferably be made by someone other than the person who has dispensed the item Check in a designated area Check items in the order they appear on the prescription form Check: 　Product name 　Quantity 　Strength 　Expiry date 　Label – correct patient details, directions, suitable additional warning labels, and legibility 　Professional appearance Initial the appropriate checking box on the label
RESPONSIBILITY	Pharmacists and accredited checking technicians
OTHER USEFUL INFORMATION	Any errors noted at this stage should be recorded on a 'near miss' table [see Figure 1.10] which enables any patterns of error to be observed. Audit performed by pharmacist or accredited checking technician
REVIEW	As a result of the audit review, discuss findings and update practices if necessary

Figure 1.8 An example of a standard operating procedure for the check of prescription items within a community pharmacy.

STANDARD OPERATING PROCEDURE – DISPENSING
ACCURACY CHECK OF PRESCRIPTION ITEMS (NHS) – Audit

NAME OF AUDITOR: _____   DATE OF AUDIT: _____

AUDIT QUESTION	SATISFACTORY		AREAS OF NON-COMPLIANCE	RECOMMENDATIONS
	YES	NO		
1. Is the *near miss* table being used?				
2. Is the checking process taking place in a designated area?				
3. Is the bench free from clutter?				
4. Is the person checking different from the person responsible for dispensing the item?				
5. Are the items checked in the order they appear on the prescription form?				
6. Has the 'checked by' box been initialled by the person checking the item?				

REVIEW DATE: _____   REVIEWED BY: _____

Figure 1.9   An example of an audit form for the audit of a standard operating procedure for the check of prescription items within a community pharmacy.

STANDARD OPERATING PROCEDURE – DISPENSING
DISPENSING 'NEAR MISS' TABLE

WEEK COMMENCING: _____

NAME OF STAFF MEMBER	MONDAY		TUESDAY		WEDNESDAY		THURSDAY		FRIDAY		SATURDAY		TOTAL
	AM	PM	AM	PM	AM	PM	AM	PM	AM	PM	AM	PM	

REVIEW DATE: _____ REVIEWED BY: _____

Key for Entries: Wrong item dispensed: I; Wrong strength selected: S; Wrong form selected: F; Wrong quantity dispensed: Q; Wrong patient name on label: N; Wrong directions on label: D; Labels transposed (switched): T; Item missing from the prescription form: M.

An additional form should be completed by the person making the error detailing the exact time and details of the error.

Figure 1.10   An example of a 'near miss' table.

STANDARD OPERATING PROCEDURE – DISPENSING
HANDING OUT PRESCRIPTION ITEMS (NHS)

OBJECTIVES	To ensure that all legal requirements regarding prescription handling are met To ensure the completed prescription is handed out to the correct person (patient/representative), including items with specific storage requirements (for example, fridge items or items kept in the controlled drugs cupboard) To provide counselling or additional information when necessary or requested To give patients the opportunity to discuss their medication with the pharmacist To inform patients or their representatives if the supply is not complete and items are owing
SCOPE	Handing out of all NHS prescriptions to either the patient or their representative
STAGES OF THE PROCESS	Ask for the name and address of the patient and check it against the prescription form (ask for the details; <u>never</u> give the details to the person collecting) Check whether the pharmacist wishes to communicate with the patient or if an item has specific storage requirements (a 'post-it' sticker system is sometimes employed for this purpose) Counsel discreetly when necessary If the patient requests to speak to pharmacist, ensure this is achieved with the minimum of delay If an item is owing, ensure the person collecting is informed and advised when the supply will be available for collection (the full process would be covered by another SOP) Return the completed prescription form to the dispensary for filing
RESPONSIBILITY	All staff working on the medicines counter: dispensing technicians, accredited checking technicians and pharmacists
OTHER USEFUL INFORMATION	Prescriptions may only be given out in the presence of a pharmacist. Audit carried out by pharmacist (or designated technician/supervisor) using the basic objectives and the stages of the process as a basis of the audit
REVIEW	Following audit make time to review findings with all the staff so that any deficiencies can be rectified and any points of good practice can be implemented within the whole group, not just on an individual basis

Figure 1.11 An example of a standard operating procedure for the handing out of prescription items within a community pharmacy.

STANDARD OPERATING PROCEDURE – DISPENSING
HANDING OUT PRESCRIPTION ITEMS (NHS) – Audit

NAME OF AUDITOR: _____   DATE OF AUDIT: _____

AUDIT QUESTION	SATISFACTORY		AREAS OF NON-COMPLIANCE	RECOMMENDATIONS
	YES	NO		

REVIEW DATE: _____   REVIEWED BY: _____

Figure 1.12 A blank audit form for the audit of a standard operating procedure for the handing out of prescription items within a community pharmacy.

2

NHS supply in the community 1 –
Prescription forms and prescribing

Upon completion of this chapter, you should be able to:

- understand the mechanisms of supply of prescription items via the NHS in the community
- list the different pieces of information that need to be present on NHS prescription forms
- understand the purpose and layout of the different UK *Drug Tariffs*
- define the types of items which may and may not be prescribed on an NHS prescription form
- understand the general restrictions that apply to the supply of items via an NHS prescription form.

2.1 Introduction

This chapter introduces the supply of prescription items via the National Health Service (NHS) in the community. The next chapter (Chapter 3) will cover the different types of NHS prescribers and the dispensing process in the community.

The NHS is the publicly funded healthcare system for England. The devolved administrations of the UK countries are responsible for healthcare in their respective countries. The equivalent organisations in the other countries are called Health and Social Care in Northern Ireland, NHS Scotland and NHS Wales. For the purposes of this book, the term 'NHS' will refer to all four healthcare organisations.

The following topics are covered in this chapter:

- NHS prescription supply
- supplies of prescription items via the NHS within the community
- the different UK *Drug Tariffs*
- items which may be prescribed on an NHS prescription form
- restrictions to supply on an NHS prescription form.

In addition to the supply of prescription items in the community (termed 'primary care'), items may also be supplied to patients within a hospital setting (termed 'secondary care'). The supply of items via the NHS within the hospital setting is covered in Chapter 4. (Items may also be supplied on prescription forms that are not part of the NHS, termed private prescriptions. The supply of prescription items via private prescription forms is covered in Chapter 5.)

2.2 NHS prescription supply

Probably the most common form of prescription supply within community pharmacy is via an NHS prescription form. There are many differing NHS prescription forms in use within the UK, but most follow a similar layout to that shown in Figure 2.1 (front) and Figure 2.2 (back).

The differences between the prescription forms comes from whether the prescription is computer generated (which is more common nowadays) or hand-written, and the identity of the prescriber. In addition, there are differences between the prescription forms used for standard prescribing and those used for instalment prescribing for addicts, which takes place on special larger prescription forms (the extra space is used to record the details of each instalment supplied). Further details on the prescribing for addicts can be found in Section 6.3.5.

In addition to the above, different prescription forms are used in the different countries that make up the UK. Although there are many variants, the different forms can be grouped as follows:

- FP10 – England

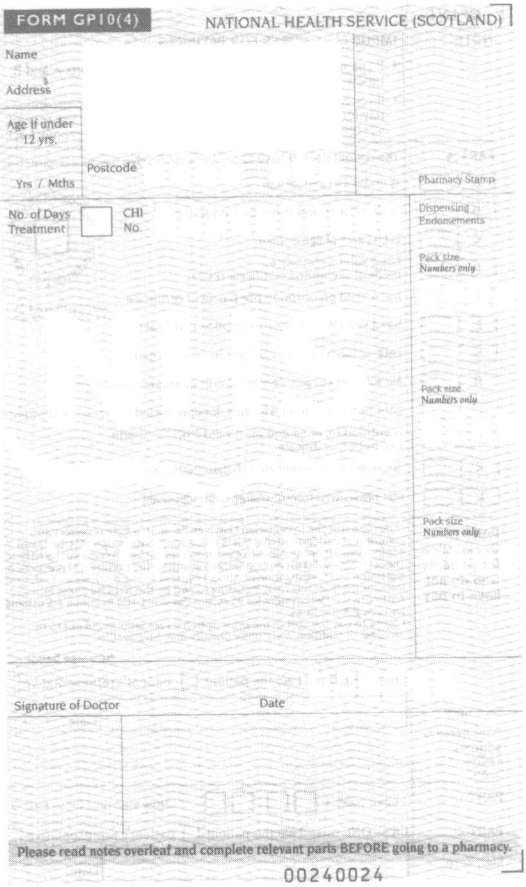

FORM GP10(4) NATIONAL HEALTH SERVICE (SCOTLAND)

Name

Address

Age if under 12 yrs.

Yrs / Mths

Postcode

Pharmacy Stamp

No. of Days Treatment

CHI No.

Dispensing Endorsements

Pack size Numbers only

Pack size Numbers only

Pack size Numbers only

Signature of Doctor

Date

Please read notes overleaf and complete relevant parts BEFORE going to a pharmacy.

00240024

Figure 2.1 The front of a standard NHS prescription form.

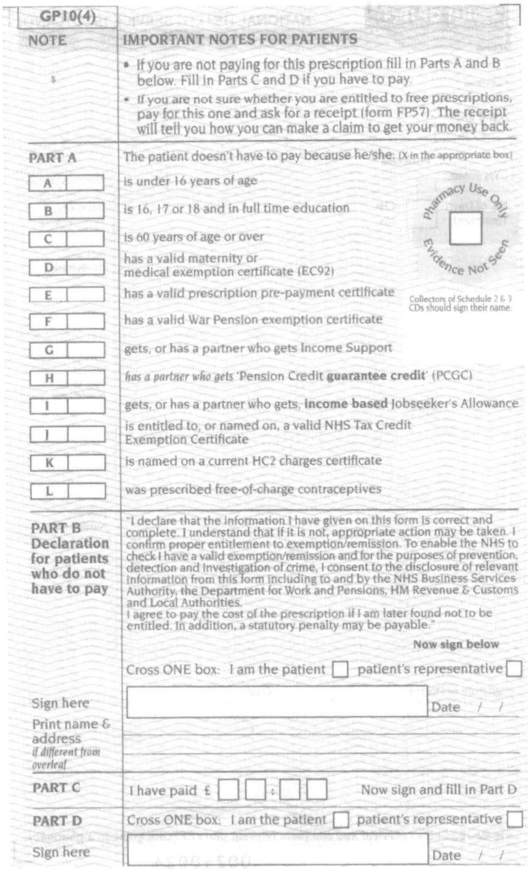

GP10(4)

NOTE

IMPORTANT NOTES FOR PATIENTS

- If you are not paying for this prescription fill in Parts A and B below. Fill in Parts C and D if you have to pay.
- If you are not sure whether you are entitled to free prescriptions, pay for this one and ask for a receipt (form FP57). The receipt will tell you how you can make a claim to get your money back.

PART A

The patient doesn't have to pay because he/she: (X in the appropriate box)

A is under 16 years of age

B is 16, 17 or 18 and in full time education

C is 60 years of age or over

D has a valid maternity or medical exemption certificate (EC92)

E has a valid prescription pre-payment certificate

F has a valid War Pension exemption certificate

G gets, or has a partner who gets Income Support

H *has a partner who gets* 'Pension Credit **guarantee credit**' (PCGC)

I gets, or has a partner who gets, **income based** Jobseeker's Allowance

J is entitled to, or named on, a valid NHS Tax Credit Exemption Certificate

K is named on a current HC2 charges certificate

L was prescribed free-of-charge contraceptives

Pharmacy Use Only

Evidence Not Seen

Collectors of Schedule 2 & 3 CDs should sign their name.

PART B Declaration for patients who do not have to pay

"I declare that the information I have given on this form is correct and complete. I understand that if it is not, appropriate action may be taken. I confirm proper entitlement to exemption/remission. To enable the NHS to check I have a valid exemption/remission and for the purposes of prevention, detection and investigation of crime, I consent to the disclosure of relevant information from this form including to and by the NHS Business Services Authority, the Department for Work and Pensions, HM Revenue & Customs and Local Authorities.

I agree to pay the cost of the prescription if I am later found not to be entitled. In addition, a statutory penalty may be payable."

Now sign below

Cross ONE box: I am the patient ☐ patient's representative ☐

Sign here Date / /

Print name & address *if different from overleaf*

PART C I have paid £ ☐☐.☐☐ Now sign and fill in Part D

PART D Cross ONE box: I am the patient ☐ patient's representative ☐

Sign here Date / /

Figure 2.2 The reverse of a standard NHS prescription form.

Table 2.1 The main different FP10 prescription forms currently in use in England

Standard prescription forms

Computer generated

FP10SS	Green	General practitioners, hospital-based prescribers, nurses, pharmacists and supplementary prescribers

Hand-written

FP10NC	Green	General practitioners
FP10HNC	Green	Hospital-based prescribers
FP10PN	Lilac	Practice nurses
FP10CN	Lilac	Community nurses
FP10SP	Lilac	Supplementary prescribers
FP10D	Yellow	Dentists

Instalment prescription forms

Computer generated

FP10MDA-SS	Blue	General practitioners, hospital-based prescribers, nurses, pharmacists and supplementary prescribers

Hand-written

FP10MDA-S	Blue	General practitioners
FP10HMDA-S	Blue	Hospital-based prescribers
FP10MDA-SP	Blue	Supplementary prescribers

- HS21 – Northern Ireland (and HS21S for stock ordering)
- GP10 or HBP – Scotland (and GP10A for stock ordering)
- WP10 – Wales.

Stock ordering forms in Northern Ireland and Scotland are used by general practitioners to order stock drugs for use in their surgery (for example, vaccinations). There is no equivalent form for ordering stock in England and Wales.

There are also different forms for the Isle of Man (HS10), Jersey (H9) and Guernsey (PS6). There are many forms currently in use, and changes to the forms occur from time to time. The following sections list the more common forms you are likely to encounter in the different administrations within the UK, although it should be remembered that this list must only be used as a guide as changes may have occurred since the list was compiled.

Furthermore, it should be pointed out that some of the codes used in the tables below may be written differently in other publications. For example, 'GP10NSS' (see Table 2.3) may also be seen written as 'GP10N-SS' or 'GP10(N)-SS.'

2.2.1 Prescription supply in England

A summary of the main prescription forms used in England and their respective uses is shown in Table 2.1.

2.2.2 Prescription supply in Northern Ireland

A summary of the main prescription forms used in Northern Ireland and their respective uses is shown in Table 2.2.

Table 2.2 The main different HS21 prescription forms currently in use in Northern Ireland

HS21	Green	General practitioners
HS21S	White	General practitioners (stock orders)
HS21D	Yellow	Dentists
HS21M	Grey	Supplementary prescribers
HS21N	Purple	Independent and supplementary nurse prescribers

Table 2.3 The main different GP10 and associated prescription forms currently in use in Scotland

Standard prescription forms

Computer generated

GP10SS	Orange	General practitioners
GP10NSS	Orange	Supplementary and independent nurse prescriber (community)
HBPSS	Blue	Hospital-based prescribers
HBPNSS	Blue	Supplementary and independent nurse prescribers (hospital)

Hand-written

GP10	Orange	General practitioners
GP10A	Pink	General practitioners (stock orders)
GP10DTS	Pink	Drug Testing Scheme Officer
GP10N	Purple	Supplementary and independent nurse prescribers (community)
CP2	Yellow	Pharmacists (minor ailment patients)
CPUS	Yellow	Pharmacists (urgent supply patients)
GP10P	Blue	Pharmacists supplementary prescribing (community)
HBPP	Blue	Pharmacists supplementary prescribing (hospital)
HBP	Blue	Hospital-based doctors
HBPN	Blue	Supplementary and independent nurse prescribers (hospital)
GP14	Yellow	Dentists

Instalment prescription forms

Computer generated

HBP(A)SS	Pink	Drug addiction/hospital clinics

Hand-written

HBP(A)	Pink	Drug addiction/hospital clinics

2.2.3 Prescription supply in Scotland

A summary of the main prescription forms used in Scotland and their respective uses is shown in Table 2.3.

2.2.4 Prescription supply in Wales

A summary of the main prescription forms used in Wales and their respective uses is shown in Table 2.4.

2.2.5 Other prescription supply

A summary of the main prescription forms used in the Isle of Man, Jersey and Guernsey and their respective uses is shown in Table 2.5.

It is worth noting that prescription forms originating from the Isle of Man, but not Jersey or Guernsey may be dispensed in England, Wales, Scotland and Northern Ireland.

2.2.6 General prescription layout

As can be seen from the previous sections, there are a large number of different prescription forms in use within the UK. However, the prescription forms all follow a basic similar layout as shown in Figure 2.3, which shows a standard NHS prescription form with an indication of where different pieces of information are located.

The front of the prescription form records the patient's details and the details of the medication that is being prescribed. Finally, the prescriber's details are included at the bottom. Prescription forms from independent and

Table 2.4 The main different WP10 prescription forms currently in use in Wales

Standard prescription forms

Computer generated

WP10SS	Green	General practitioners
WP10SPSS	Green	Supplementary prescribers

Hand-written

WP10NC	Green	General practitioners
WP10HP	Green	Hospital-based prescribers
WP10CN	Green	Community nurses
WP10PN	Green	Practice nurses
WP10SP	Green	Supplementary prescribers (community)
WP10HSP	Green	Supplementary prescribers (hospital)
WP10D	Green	Dentists

Instalment prescription forms

WP10MDA	Green	General practitioners
WP10HPAD	Green	Drug treatment centres/ hospitals

Table 2.5 The main different prescription forms currently in use in the Isle of Man, Jersey and Guernsey

Isle of Man

HS10	Pink	General practitioners and dentists
HS10	Green	Hospital-based prescribers

Jersey

H9	White	General practitioners
H9	Yellow	Dentists

Guernsey

PS6	White	General practitioners
PS6	Yellow	Dentists

supplementary prescribers will also indicate on the prescription form the type of prescriber.

Two sections (highlighted in Figure 2.3) deserve particular attention:

Number of days' treatment. N.B. Ensure dose is stated

It is usual for prescribers to write the quantity of each item to be prescribed alongside the item on the prescription form. For example, if a prescription was for amoxicillin 250 mg capsules and the prescriber wanted the patient to take one three times a day for a week, they would usually write '21' (sometimes in a circle) or 'Mitte 21' ('Mitte' meaning 'send' – see Appendix 2).

However, as an alternative, it is possible for the prescriber to indicate the desired number of days' treatment by placing a figure in this box (in the example in the preceding paragraph, this figure would be '7'). As the legend to the box indicates, it is important that the prescriber includes a dose with each prescribed items to enable the pharmacist or pharmacy technician to calculate the number of dosage units to supply.

For dispenser No. of Prescns. on form

This box is completed by the pharmacist or pharmacy technician at the same time as the prescription form is stamped at the top left-hand corner. The figure entered into this box will be the total number of prescription items on the form. This figure will include any items which attract more than one prescription charge (e.g. surgical stockings, some HRT, etc.). For further details on prescription charging, see Section 2.4.1).

It is worth noting at this point that the public will often refer to the form in Figure 2.1 as 'a prescription'. Technically speaking, a prescription is each item that is written on the form. Therefore, each prescription form can contain more than one prescription.

On the reverse of the prescription form, the patient or the patient's representative will complete the form to indicate whether the patient is exempt from prescription charges (and if so, what exemption they are declaring) or an indication of the number of prescription charges paid (see Figure 2.2).

2.2.7 NHS prescription form requirements

All NHS prescription forms will require certain pieces of information to be present. These are as follows (see also Figure 2.3).

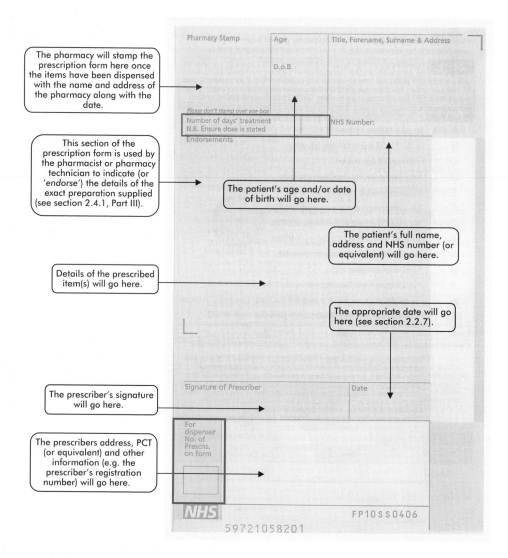

Figure 2.3 The layout of a standard NHS prescription form with an indication of where different pieces of information are located.

The patient's details

The name and address of the patient must be given. It is not essential to give the patient's title (Mr, Mrs, Master, Miss, etc.) but this is sometimes useful if more than one person at the same address has the same name (for example, a father and son).

For patients under 12 years of age, the age *or* date of birth of the patient must be stated but this is not required for older patients. Nowadays,

many computer systems used for generating prescriptions automatically print the patient's age and/or date of birth on the prescription form. This is useful as it helps to identify elderly patients.

Details of the medication to be supplied

Apart from the prescribing of some controlled drugs (see Section 6.3.2) there is no legal requirement to provide particular information about the product prescribed. There will need to be sufficient information provided to enable the accurate and safe supply of medication to the patient and if there is insufficient information on the prescription form, this must be queried with the prescriber before a supply can be made.

It is worth noting that although it would be good practice, the instructions for how to take or use the product do not have to appear on the prescription form. If this information is missing, it will be necessary for the pharmacist to check that the patient understands the prescriber's intentions and advise the patient as to how to take their medication as appropriate.

The signature of the prescriber

The prescriber's signature needs to be present on the prescription form and currently this must be in ink. Electronic signatures or stamps are not currently permitted on paper prescription forms.

To allow the pilots for electronic transmission of prescriptions (ETP) to go ahead in England, the Prescription Only Medicines Order was amended to allow authorised prescribers who were participating in the pilot schemes to sign prescription forms digitally in place of ink signatures.

The address of the prescriber

The prescriber's address, which for most prescribers is usually the practice address, is pre-printed on the prescription form (along with details of the primary care trust (or equivalent) to which the practice belongs). For a nurse employed by a primary care trust, the trust's address is printed on the form and the nurse has to add a code that identifies the patient's GP practice.

An indication of the prescriber type

Particulars to indicate whether the prescriber is a doctor, dentist, nurse, pharmacist or other prescriber need to be included on the prescription form. This does not have to be (and indeed on an NHS prescription form usually is not) the prescriber's qualifications. NHS prescription forms are usually printed with a number to identify the prescriber (see Tables 2.1–2.5).

An appropriate date

A date must appear on the prescription form next to the prescriber's signature. For most prescriptions this is the date the prescriber signed the prescription form but the prescriber is also allowed to put a date before which the prescription should not be dispensed. Prescription forms are valid for six months from the appropriate date (except for some prescriptions for controlled drugs which are only valid for 28 days; see Section 6.3.2).

Post-dated prescription forms are used to prevent patients stockpiling large quantities of medication at home. For example, instead of providing one prescription form for three months' supply, the prescriber could give a patient three appropriately dated prescription forms, each for one month's supply. This will result in the patient having less medication at home (as each supply of medication from the pharmacy would only be for a month) while still saving the patient from visiting the surgery each month.

Key point 2.1

NHS prescription forms will need the following pieces of information to be present:

- the patient's details
- details of the medication to be supplied
- the signature of the prescriber
- the address of the prescriber
- an indication of the prescriber type
- an appropriate date.

The *British National Formulary* also contains advice for prescribers on how to write both hand-written and computer-generated prescriptions clearly.

Any prescriptions that do not contain the necessary information, or are unclear or ambiguous need to be referred back to the prescriber for clarification.

2.3 Supplies of prescription items via the NHS within the community

Community pharmacists and pharmacy technicians are predominantly concerned with the supply of medicines on NHS prescription forms via a registered pharmacy. However, this is not the only method of the supply of medicines against a prescription form within the community and it is important that pharmacists and pharmacy technicians are aware of how patients may obtain medicines or appliances other than through pharmacies.

2.3.1 Dispensing doctors

Although the dispensing of most NHS prescriptions is carried out within a community pharmacy, in some areas of the country it may not be practical for patients to visit a community pharmacy. This will occur in some remote areas of the country where the nearest community pharmacy may be several miles away.

In these situations, dispensing doctors will prescribe and dispense the medication for the patient. In order for the doctor to be reimbursed for the cost of the medicine and to be remunerated for the service, dispensing doctors will submit any prescription forms they have dispensed to the NHS Business Services Authority Prescription Pricing Division (or equivalent) at the end of the month in the same way that pharmacists do (see Section 3.3.8).

2.3.2 Appliance contractors

As well as dispensing doctors, appliance contractors also provide items against NHS prescription forms within the community. In this case, the items supplied are appliances (stoma equipment, etc.) and not drugs.

There is a very large range of appliances that may be prescribed on the NHS and it is not practical for community pharmacies to stock all available products. Appliance contractors are set up to provide these items to patients, often direct to their homes. In addition, they provide advice and guidance on how to use the various items. Appliance contractors will also submit any prescription forms they have dispensed to the NHS Business Services Authority Prescription Pricing Division (or equivalent) at the end of the month in the same way that pharmacists do (see Section 3.3.8).

Key point 2.2

NHS prescriptions may be dispensed by:

- pharmacists via registered pharmacies
- dispensing doctors (geographical restrictions apply)
- appliance contractors (appliances only).

2.4 The Drug Tariffs

One of the most important non-clinical reference sources for the supply of items on an NHS prescription form is the *Drug Tariff*. Produced monthly, the *Drug Tariff* is the guide as to what can and cannot be prescribed on an NHS prescription form. In addition, it also provides information on the amount pharmacies will be reimbursed and remunerated for dispensing items on NHS prescription forms and performing other NHS services.

It should be noted that three separate *Drug Tariffs* exist (one for England and Wales, one for Northern Ireland and one for Scotland) and although similar in nature, the contents and the layout of the different sections does differ between the three.

The *Drug Tariff* is probably not the easiest book to use and navigate your way around; however, it is vital that pharmacists and pharmacy technicians involved in the dispensing process are familiar with its layout. As discussed in Section 2.3, there are different classes of individuals who supply items against NHS prescriptions (pharmacists, dispensing doctors and appliance contractors) and so the *Drug Tariff* contains information for all three types of supplier (i.e. it is not solely a reference source for pharmacists and pharmacy technicians).

It is suggested that student pharmacists and pharmacy technicians either obtain a paper copy of the *Drug Tariff* or (for England and Wales) access the contents on-line via the Prescription Pricing Division website (part of the NHS Business Services Authority). Unlike the on-line versions of many pharmaceutical texts, the on-line version of the *Drug Tariff for England and Wales* mirrors the paper version in both content and layout and so the on-line version can be used to learn how to navigate around the various parts of the paper version. On-line versions of the *Scottish Drug Tariff* and the *Northern Ireland Drug Tariff* also exist.

It is beyond the scope of this text to provide detailed information on all parts of the three *Drug Tariffs*, however, below is a summary of what can be found in them at the time of publication. Details of the contents of the *Drug Tariff for England and Wales* have been provided, along with a summary of the contents of the other two (the *Northern Ireland Drug Tariff* and the *Scottish Drug Tariff*) and how the contents of these two map to the content of the *Drug Tariff for England and Wales*.

2.4.1 *Drug Tariff for England and Wales*

Part I – Requirements for the supply of drugs, appliances and chemical reagents

The first part provides some background information on what may and may not be supplied via an NHS prescription form and some background information on claims for payments.

Part II – Requirements enabling payments to be made for the supply of drugs, appliances and chemical reagents

This part provides details on how calculations for payments to suppliers are made and details of prescription form endorsing. It also provides advice on the quantity to be supplied in special circumstances (for example, see Part II, Clause 10).

It also contains the list of drugs for which discount is not deducted (see also Part V).

Part IIIA – Professional fees (pharmacy contractors)

This lists the professional fees pharmacies will be paid for supplying various items via NHS prescription forms. Almost all items dispensed on an NHS prescription form will attract a flat fee, which will be supplemented by an additional fee for certain items.

In many cases, the amount reimbursed for supplying an item on a prescription is fixed (see also Part VIII). However, in some cases, it will be necessary for the pharmacist or pharmacy technician to 'endorse' the prescription form with the details of what was actually supplied against the prescription so that the correct reimbursement can be made. This part also gives details of these endorsements

Additional endorsements may also be required to ensure that the correct payments are paid to pharmacies (for example, endorsing 'MF' if the pharmacy measured and fitted a patient for elastic hosiery).

Nowadays, the computer system in many community pharmacies is set up to automatically endorse the side of the prescription form with the correct information by feeding the prescription form into a printer after the items have been dispensed.

Part IIIB – Scale of fees (appliance contractors)

This lists the professional fees appliance contractors will be paid for supplying differing appliances against NHS prescriptions.

Part IV – Containers

This part includes information on providing a suitable container for items supplied via an NHS prescription form. To cover the cost of containers and other items which may need to be supplied to patients (for example, a 5-mL plastic measuring spoon) every prescription (except an oxygen prescription) will attract a flat fee for supplying a container, whether or not one was supplied.

Part V – Deduction scale (pharmacy contractors)

In general, community pharmacies will purchase most of the items they dispense via one or two local wholesalers. In return for this business, wholesalers will provide a discount on the cost of the items to the pharmacy. As pharmacies will be reimbursed the cost of the medication via the Prescription Pricing Division or Health Solutions Wales, a deduction percentage is applied to the items being reimbursed. This aims to prevent the NHS having to pay more for any prescription items than the pharmacy contractor paid the wholesaler. This deduction is based on a scale, set against the monthly total of the price of the items dispensed. Details of this scale can be found in Part V.

It should be noted that some items will not attract a discount from the wholesaler when purchased by the pharmacy contractor. These items were known as 'zero discount' or 'ZD' items. The list of drugs for which discount is not deducted can be found in Part II of the *Drug Tariff.*

Part VIA – Payment for essential services (pharmacy contractors)

This part contains details of and information on the payment of essential services provided by pharmacy contractors.

Part VIB – Scale of on-cost allowances (appliance contractors)

This part contains information on the percentage on-cost allowance for appliance contractors, based on the number of prescriptions dispensed during that month.

Part VIC – Advanced services (pharmacy contractors)

This part contains information on the payment of advanced services to pharmacy contractors.

Part VID – Enhanced services (pharmacy contractors)

This part contains information on the payment of enhanced services to pharmacy contractors.

Part VII – Drugs with common pack sizes

This part contains a list of those drugs with common pack sizes. If a drug specified in this list is supplied but the relative prescription form is not endorsed payment will be calculated on the basis of the price for the pack size listed.

Part VIII – Basic prices of drugs

This part contains a list of drugs where the price that will be reimbursed has been set (as detailed in Part II, Clause 8). Therefore, irrespective of what item was supplied against a prescription, the price that will be used to calculate the reimbursement cost is fixed and detailed within this part. There are five categories of items within this part, the difference being how the price of the item listed in the *Drug Tariff* is calculated. These categories are:

- *Category A* – Drugs which are readily available. Endorsement of pack size is required if more than one pack size is listed. Broken bulk (see below) may be claimed if necessary.
- *Category B* – Drugs whose usage has declined over time. No endorsement is required other than a claim for broken bulk if necessary.
- *Category C* – Priced on the basis of a particular brand or particular manufacturer. Endorsement of pack size is required if more than one pack is listed. Broken bulk may be claimed if necessary.
- *Category E* – Extemporaneously prepared items for which the fee listed for extemporaneous dispensing in Part IIIA will be claimed. No endorsement is required. Broken bulk is not allowed, but may be paid on the ingredients.
- *Category M* – Drugs which are readily available, where the Department of Health calculate the reimbursement price based on information submitted by manufacturers. Endorsement of pack size is required if more than one pack size is listed. Broken bulk may be claimed if necessary.

'Broken bulk' is where a pharmacy contractor may claim for the remainder of a container if only part was supplied and if they are unlikely to use the remainder before it expires (see Part

II, Clause 11). For example, if a contractor had to supply 50 tablets of a drug that came in a pack size of 100, they would have to purchase 100 in order to be able to supply the 50. However, if it was a drug that was rarely used, the pharmacy contractor will be financially disadvantaged if they did not supply the remainder against a prescription before the end of the item's shelf-life. Therefore, for certain items the Prescription Pricing Division will pay for the entire container (not just the proportion supplied). If a further prescription is received for the same item within six-months of a broken bulk request, the Prescription Pricing Division will assume that the supply has been made from the remainder and the only payments which will be made are professional fees and container allowances until the remainder has been used up.

Key point 2.3

If an item is listed in Part VIII of the *Drug Tariff for England and Wales*, that is the price that the pharmacy will be reimbursed for supplying the item, irrespective of the brand supplied.

Part VIII of the *Drug Tariff* is important for pharmacy contractors. If an item is listed within this part, supplying a more expensive alternative will render the pharmacy financially disadvantaged.

If a drug is prescribed in the community using a proprietary name, the proprietary product must be supplied (different rules apply in hospitals – see Section 4.3.4). However, if a drug is prescribed by its generic name, in most cases, any generic or proprietary equivalent may be supplied. If a proprietary version is supplied against a generic prescription and the generic drug is listed in Part VIII, as the proprietary version is likely to be more expensive, it is likely that the cost (even when a discount is applied) will be more than the reimbursement price listed. Therefore, pharmacies are financially-better off if they supply the cheaper generic drug

against a generic prescription. By forcing the supply of the cheaper presentations of drugs, this part of the *Drug Tariff* assists in keeping down the cost of prescribed medication via the NHS.

The exception to this is the case of some sustained-release preparations where the release properties of different brands may vary (for example modified-release diltiazem or theophylline preparations). In these cases, it is usual for patients to be maintained on one particular brand to prevent fluctuations in plasma concentration. See the *British National Formulary* for further details.

Key point 2.4

If a drug is prescribed in the community using a proprietary name, the proprietary product must be supplied. However, if a drug is prescribed by its generic name, in most cases (except, for example, in the case of some sustained-release preparations), any generic or proprietary equivalent may be supplied.

NCSO – No cheaper stock obtainable

The only exception to the fixed reimbursement price listed in Part VIII of the *Drug Tariff* is where in the opinion of the Secretary of State for Health and the National Assembly for Wales there is no product available to pharmacies at the appropriate price (for example if there were manufacturing shortages of a generic item and only a proprietary equivalent was available). In these cases, endorsements of brand name or of manufacturer or wholesaler of the product and pack size so used may be accepted.

The *Drug Tariff* states that

contractors shall not so endorse unless they have made all reasonable efforts to obtain the product at the appropriate price but have not succeeded. The endorsement shall be initialled and dated by or on behalf of the contractor, and shall be further endorsed 'no cheaper stock obtainable' or 'NCSO' to indicate that the contractor has taken all such responsible steps.

Part IXA – Appliances

This part lists those appliances which may be prescribed on an NHS prescription form. Further details on this part can be found in Section 2.5.2.

Part IXB – Incontinence appliances

This part lists those incontinence appliances which may be prescribed on an NHS prescription form. Further details can be found in Section 2.5.2.

Part IXC – Stoma appliances

This part lists those stoma appliances which may be prescribed on an NHS prescription form. Further details can be found in Section 2.5.2.

Part IXR – Chemical reagents

This part lists those chemical reagents which may be prescribed on an NHS prescription form. Further details can be found in Section 2.5.3.

Part X – Home oxygen therapy service

This part provides detailed information for those pharmacy contractors providing a home oxygen therapy service. Traditionally, patients who required oxygen to be supplied at home would obtain their supplies via a community pharmacy (often delivered to the patient's home by a member of staff from the community pharmacy).

Recently, home oxygen supply services have been contracted out to specialist suppliers (similar in nature to the supply of appliances by appliance contractors – see Section 2.3.2) so oxygen supplies from community pharmacies have declined.

Part XI – Exit payments (pharmacy contractors)

This part provides information for pharmacy contractors on exit payments to be paid to contractors who decide no longer to provide pharmaceutical services from the pharmacy.

Part XII – Essential Small Pharmacies Scheme (ESPS)

Under the Essential Small Pharmacies Scheme (ESPS) pharmacies with a low monthly prescription volume, located in an area not served by another pharmacy, may apply for additional payment to compensate for the low prescription volume.

Part XIII – Payments in respect of pre-registration trainees

This part provides details of the payments to be made to pharmacy contractors who provide the pre-registration training experience needed by pharmacy graduates and certain undergraduates for admission to the Royal Pharmaceutical Society of Great Britain's Register of Pharmaceutical Chemists.

Part XIV – Reward scheme – fraudulent prescription forms

This part provides details on the reward scheme that allows pharmacists (pharmacies) to claim a financial reward where they have identified a fraudulent prescription form and thereby either prevented fraud or contributed with valuable information to the investigation of fraud.

Part XV – Borderline substances

This part provides information on those products classified as borderline substances. Further details can be found in Section 2.6.1.

Part XVI – Notes on charges

In principle, in England, one prescription charge is payable for each prescription item. This charge is fixed and is irrespective of the cost of the item or the number of dosage units. Patients who are not exempt from paying prescription charges will be charged one prescription charge per item (this is not the case in Wales where all prescription items are free if prescribed via an NHS prescription form).

Although initially this would appear straightforward, there are a number of more complex

Key point 2.5

In England, one prescription charge is payable for each prescription item. This charge is fixed and is irrespective of the cost of the item or the number of dosage units.

charging scenarios which may occur. This part of the *Drug Tariff* summarises these potential situations and provides suitable examples to enable pharmacists and pharmacy technicians to ensure they charge patients the correct amount.

This is important as the pharmacy is acting on behalf of the NHS in collecting the prescription charges. As the pharmacy will keep these charges, the Prescription Pricing Division will deduct the amount collected from the monies it will pay to the pharmacy at the end of the month. This deduction will be based on what the pharmacy *should* have collected, irrespective of what they *did* collect. Therefore, if a pharmacy does not take the correct number of prescription charges, they will be financially disadvantaged. This is especially important for preparations containing more than one medicinal product (for example tablets for hormone replacement therapy where there may be 21 tablets containing one drug and seven containing a different drug in the same packet). These preparations will attract more than one prescription charge as although there is only one 'box', there is more than one preparation within.

The charging rules are summarised in Table 2.6.

Key point 2.6

There are a number of situations where a single prescription item will attract more than one prescription charge. Student pharmacists and pharmacy technicians should study this part of the *Drug Tariff* and become familiar with the different charging models.

Table 2.6 Summary of charging rules	
Single prescription charge payable	The same drug or preparation is supplied in more than one container
	Different strengths of the same drug in the same formulation are ordered as separate prescriptions on the same prescription form
	More than one appliance of the same type (other than hosiery[a]) is supplied
	A set of parts making up a complete appliance is supplied
	Drugs are supplied in powder form with the solvent separate for subsequent admixing
	A drug is supplied with a dropper, throat brush or vaginal applicator
	Several flavours of the same preparation are supplied
Multiple prescription charges payable	Different drugs, types of dressing or appliances are supplied
	Different formulations or presentations of the same drug or preparation are prescribed and supplied
	Additional parts are supplied together with a complete set of apparatus or additional dressing(s) together with a dressing pack
	More than one piece of elastic hosiery[a] is supplied

[a]Anklet, legging, knee-cap, below-knee, above knee or thigh stocking.

Exercise 2.1

You receive an NHS prescription form at your pharmacy in England for the following two items:

- prednisolone tablets 1 mg
- prednisolone tablets 2.5 mg enteric coated.

The patient is not exempt from paying prescription charges. How many prescription charges should you take?

Exercise 2.2

You receive an NHS prescription form at your pharmacy in England for the following item:

- 1 pair thigh stockings – class II.

The patient is not exempt from paying prescription charges. How many prescription charges should you take?

Part XVIIA – Dental prescribing

Dentists may only prescribe items listed in Part XVIIA of the *Drug Tariff* on an NHS prescription form in England and Wales. Further details can be found in Section 3.2.2.

Key point 2.7

Dentists may only prescribe, on an NHS prescription form, those items listed in the Dental Practitioners' Formulary (DPF) in the *Drug Tariff*.

Part XVIIB(i) – Nurse prescribers' formulary for community practitioners (in Wales district nurses and health visitors)

In a similar way to dental prescribing on an NHS prescription form, certain nurses (termed community practitioner nurse prescribers) may prescribe certain items for patients within their care in England and Wales on an NHS prescription form. These items are listed within this part of the *Drug Tariff*. Further details can be found in Section 3.2.3.

Part XVIIB(ii) – Nurse and pharmacist independent prescribing

This part provides information on nurse and pharmacist independent prescribing. Further details on independent non-medical prescribing can be found in Section 3.2.5.

Part XVIIC – National out-of-hours formulary

This part contains the minimum list of drugs that patients should be able to access. Exact mechanisms for the provision of these drugs should be decided locally, taking into account existing treatment protocols. At the time of going to press this information applied only to England, as the National Assembly for Wales had not adopted the formulary.

Part XVIIIA – Drugs and other substances not to be prescribed under the NHS pharmaceutical services

There are restrictions on the prescribing of some drugs and other substances on an NHS prescription form. This part of the *Drug Tariff* lists those drugs and other substances not to be prescribed on an NHS prescription form. Further details can be found in Section 2.6.2.

Part XVIIIB – Drugs to be prescribed in certain circumstances under the NHS pharmaceutical services

In a similar fashion to the restrictions placed on the prescribing of certain drugs and other substances on an NHS prescription form in Part XVIIIA, Part XVIIIB lists those drugs and other substances which may only be prescribed on an NHS prescription form in certain circumstances. Further details can be found in section 2.6.3

Part XVIIIC – Criteria notified under the transparency directive

This part details the six criteria that the UK

Government has applied to certain products to exclude them from NHS prescription supply.

Part XIX – Payments to chemists suspended by a primary care trust or by direction of the FHSAA

This part details how payments will be calculated to those pharmacies who have had their contract with their local Primary Care Trust in England or Local Health Board in Wales suspended or who are suspended by direction of the FHSAA (Family Health Services Appeal Authority). Suspension of a contract would be imposed, for example, to protect patients if there is evidence of substandard clinical practice or personal behaviour.

Part XX – Private prescriptions for controlled drugs

Although not NHS prescribing, this part of the *Drug Tariff* provides details on the private prescribing of controlled drugs. From 1 April 2006 all private prescriptions issued for controlled drugs in Schedule 2 or 3 of the Misuse of Drugs Regulations 2001 for dispensing in the community (for human use) must be ordered using the prescription form designed specially for this purpose (FP10PCD) (see Section 6.3.3).

Following dispensing, FP10PCD prescription forms must be submitted to the NHS Business Services Authority (NHSBSA) Prescription Pricing Division or Health Solutions Wales for audit purposes and the arrangements for this submission are detailed in this part of the *Drug Tariff*. Further details on the prescribing of controlled drugs (including private prescribing) can be found in Chapter 6 (see Section 6.3.3).

2.4.2 Northern Ireland Drug Tariff

The *Northern Ireland Drug Tariff* contains similar information to the *Drug Tariff for England and Wales*. It is divided into 13 parts (including the general notes) as detailed below.

General notes

The General Notes section contains background information on what may and may not be supplied on an NHS prescription form and some background information on claims for payments. This part is similar in composition to Parts II and III of the *Drug Tariff for England and Wales* (see Section 2.4.1).

Part I – List of drugs and preparations with tariff prices

This lists those drugs and preparations with *Drug Tariff* prices and is similar in composition to Part VIII of the *Drug Tariff for England and Wales* (see Section 2.4.1).

Part II – Approved list of chemical reagents

This part lists those chemical reagents which may be prescribed on an NHS prescription form and is similar in composition to Part IXR of the *Drug Tariff for England and Wales* (see Section 2.4.1).

Part III – List of appliances

This lists those appliances that may be prescribed on an NHS prescription form and is similar in composition to Part IXA of the *Drug Tariff for England and Wales* (see Section 2.4.1).

Part IV – Domiciliary oxygen therapy service

This part provides detailed information for those contractors providing a home oxygen therapy service and is similar in composition to Part X of the *Drug Tariff for England and Wales* (see Section 2.4.1).

Part V – Containers

This part gives further information (to that in the General Notes) regarding the supply of containers to patients and is similar in composition to Part IV of the *Drug Tariff for England and Wales* (see Section 2.4.1).

Part VI – Net ingredient cost scale for chemist contractors

This part contains information on the net ingredient cost scale for chemist (pharmacist) contractors and is similar in composition to Part V of the *Drug Tariff for England and Wales* (see Section 2.4.1).

Part VII – List of drugs and threshold above which an additional fee will be paid

This part contains the list of drugs and threshold above which an additional fee will be paid.

Part VIII – Prescription charges

This part contains information on the NHS prescription charging system and is similar in composition to Part XVI of the *Drug Tariff for England and Wales* (see Section 2.4.1). As in Scotland (see Section 2.4.3), there has been talk in Northern Ireland of abolishing prescription charges altogether.

Part IXA – List of preparations approved by the Department which may be prescribed by dentists on form HS21D

Part IXA contains the dental prescribing formulary and is similar in composition to Part XVIIA of the *Drug Tariff for England and Wales* (see Section 2.4.1).

Part IXB – List of preparations approved by the Department which may be prescribed by nurses on form HS21N

Part IXB contains the nurse prescribing formulary (for community nurses and health visitors) and is similar in composition to Part XVIIB(i) of the *Drug Tariff for England and Wales* (see Section 2.4.1).

Part IXC

This part provides information on nurse independent prescribing, including the prescribing of controlled drugs by nurse independent prescribers. It is similar in composition to Part XVIIB(ii) of the *Drug Tariff for England and Wales* (see Section 2.4.1). Further details on independent non-medical prescribing can be found in Section 3.2.5.

Part X – Borderline substances

This part provides information on those products classified as borderline substances and is similar in composition to Part XV of the *Drug Tariff for England and Wales* (see Section 2.4.1). Further details on this can be found in Section 2.6.1.

Part XIA – Drugs and other substances not to be prescribed under Health Service pharmaceutical services

This part lists those drugs and other substances not to be prescribed on an NHS prescription form. It is similar in composition to Part XVIIIA of the *Drug Tariff for England and Wales* (see Section 2.4.1). Further details can be found in Section 2.6.2.

Part XIB – Drugs to be prescribed in certain circumstances under Health Service pharmaceutical services

This part contains information on drugs to be prescribed in certain circumstances on an NHS prescription form and is similar in composition to Part XVIIIB of the *Drug Tariff for England and Wales* (see Section 2.4.1). Further details can be found in Section 2.6.3.

Part XIC – Criteria notified under the Transparency Directive

This part details the six criteria that the UK Government has applied to certain products to exclude them from NHS prescription supply and is similar in composition to Part XVIIIC of the *Drug Tariff for England and Wales* (see Section 2.4.1).

Part XII – List of technical specifications

This part provides information on how pharmacists may obtain information on technical specifications for certain items which may be prescribed on an NHS prescription form (hypodermic syringes, catheters, etc.).

2.4.3 Scottish Drug Tariff

As with the *Northern Ireland Drug Tariff* (see Section 2.4.2) the *Scottish Drug Tariff* contains similar information to the *Drug Tariff for England and Wales* (see Section 2.4.1). It is divided into 14 parts as detailed below.

Part 1 – General information

This part is subdivided into a number of sections and provides general background information. The sections contained within this part are as follows:

- Scope and application of the *Scottish Drug Tariff*
- Frequency of publication
- Details of amendments since last published edition
- Standards of quality for drugs
- Items which may not be prescribed by statute
- Appliances
- Chemical reagents
- Domiciliary oxygen therapy service
- Reimbursement in respect of drugs which may be prescribed by dental practitioners
- Reimbursement in respect of drugs which may be prescribed by nurse prescribers
- Pharmaceutical services remuneration
- Reimbursement arrangements for medicinal products
- Reimbursement of medical devices, reagents and other items
- Weights and packaging
- Calculation of net ingredient costs
- Broken bulk
- Out of pocket expenses
- Payments in exceptional cases where drugs ordered are subject to market shortages
- Timing and amounts of payment arrangements
- Prescription charges
- Arrangements for updating this tariff
- Information enquiries.

In addition, there are three Annexes to Part 1. These are:

- *Annex A – Zero Discount List*: This contains information on the Zero Discount List and is similar in composition to Part II of the *Drug Tariff for England and Wales* (see Section 2.4.1).
- *Annex B – Prescription Charges*: This contains

information on the NHS prescription charging system and is similar in composition to Part XVI of the *Drug Tariff for England and Wales* (see Section 2.4.1). However, it is worth noting that there are plans to abolish prescription charges in Scotland, which may start with the abolition of charges to the chronically ill as early as 2008, with total abolition by 2011.

- *Annex C – Community Pharmacy Contractor Remuneration Arrangements*: This contains information on the remuneration arrangements for community pharmacy contractors providing pharmaceutical services.

Part 2 – Dressings

This part lists those dressings which may be prescribed on an NHS prescription form and is similar in composition to Part IXA of the *Drug Tariff for England and Wales* (see Section 2.4.1).

Part 3 – Appliances

This part lists those appliances which may be prescribed on an NHS prescription form and is similar in composition to Part IXA of the *Drug Tariff for England and Wales* (see Section 2.4.1).

Part 4 – Elastic hosiery

This part lists those elastic hosiery items which may be prescribed on an NHS prescription form and is similar in composition to Part IXA of the *Drug Tariff for England and Wales* (see Section 2.4.1).

Part 5 – Incontinence appliances

This part lists those incontinence appliances which may be prescribed on an NHS prescription form and is similar in composition to Part IXB of the *Drug Tariff for England and Wales* (see Section 2.4.1).

Part 6 – Stoma appliances

This part lists those stoma appliances which may be prescribed on an NHS prescription form and is similar in composition to Part IXC of the

Drug Tariff for England and Wales (see Section 2.4.1).

Part 7 – Drugs and preparations with tariff prices

This part lists those drugs and preparations with *Drug Tariff* prices and is similar in composition to Part VIII of the *Drug Tariff for England and Wales* (see Section 2.4.1).

Part 8 – Dental and nurse prescribing formularies

Part 8A – Dental practitioner formulary

Part 8A contains the dental prescribing formulary and is similar in composition to Part XVIIA of the *Drug Tariff for England and Wales* (see Section 2.4.1).

Part 8B – Nurse prescriber formulary

Part 8B contains the nurse prescribing formulary (for community nurses and health visitors) and is similar in composition to Part XVIIB(i) of the *Drug Tariff for England and Wales* (see Section 2.4.1).

Part 9 – Chemical reagents

This part lists those chemical reagents which may be prescribed on an NHS prescription form and is similar in composition to Part IXR of the *Drug Tariff for England and Wales* (see Section 2.4.1).

Part 10 – Domiciliary oxygen service

This part provides detailed information for those contractors providing a home oxygen therapy service and is similar in composition to Part X of the *Drug Tariff for England and Wales* (see Section 2.4.1).

Part 11 – Net ingredient cost scale for pharmacist contractors

This part contains information on the net ingredient cost scale for pharmacist contractors and is similar in composition to Part V of the *Drug Tariff for England and Wales* (see Section 2.4.1).

Part 12 – Drugs to be prescribed in certain circumstances under the NHS pharmaceutical services

This part contains information on drugs to be prescribed in certain circumstances on an NHS prescription form and is similar in composition to Part XVIIIB of the *Drug Tariff for England and Wales* (see Section 2.4.1). Further details can be found in Section 2.6.3.

Criteria notified under the Transparency Directive

This part of the *Drug Tariff* details the six criteria that the UK Government has applied to certain products to exclude them from prescription NHS supply and is similar in composition to Part XVIIIC of the *Drug Tariff for England and Wales* (see Section 2.4.1).

Part 13 – Items on short supply

This part contains details of the items in respect of which endorsements on the grounds of short supply are permitted for the stated month. This is similar to the NCSO rules in the *Drug Tariff for England and Wales* (see Section 2.4.1, Part VIII).

Part 14 – Business rules of NHS National Services Scotland Practitioner Services Division

This part contains the rules which set out the basic requirement for reimbursement of items presented on NHS primary care prescription forms in Scotland.

2.5 Items which may be prescribed on an NHS prescription form

For ease of understanding, it is best to separate prescribing of items on NHS prescription forms into three categories:

- medicinal products (i.e. drugs)
- appliances (for example, stoma equipment)
- chemical reagents (for example, diabetic test strips).

2.5.1 Medicinal products

All medicinal products may be prescribed on an NHS prescription form (providing that the prescriber is authorised to prescribe that item – see Section 3.2) and that the item is not subject to any specific restrictions. For details of the different restrictions, see Section 2.6.

Key point 2.8

All medicinal products may be prescribed on an NHS prescription form, providing that the prescriber is authorised to prescribe that item and the item is not subject to any specific restrictions.

2.5.2 Appliances

Only those appliances listed within the respective *Drug Tariff* may be prescribed on an NHS prescription form. If an appliance is not listed, then it may not be prescribed on an NHS prescription form and if a pharmacist dispenses an appliance not listed within the *Drug Tariff*, then they would not be reimbursed the cost of the item.

Key point 2.9

Only those appliances listed within the respective *Drug Tariff* may be prescribed on an NHS prescription form.

All approved appliances for England and Wales can be found in Part IX of the *Drug Tariff*.

* Part IXA contains an alphabetical list of appliances (e.g. atomizers, peak flow meters) and dressings that are allowed to be prescribed on an NHS prescription form. All items included in Part IXA will be listed in the index at the back of the *Drug Tariff*.
* Part IXB contains a list of incontinence appliances that are allowed to be prescribed on an NHS prescription form. At the front of Part IXB there is an index of component headings, and each section thereafter is listed alphabetically by manufacturer name.
* Part IXC contains a list of stoma appliances that are allowed to be prescribed on an NHS prescription form. The format of this section follows the same pattern as Part IXB.

The *Northern Ireland Drug Tariff* lists approved appliances in Part III and similar lists can be found in the *Scottish Drug Tariff*. Each Part of the *Scottish Drug Tariff* starts with an alphabetical list of product types and within each type, individual products are listed in alphabetical order.

* Part 2 – Dressings
* Part 3 – Appliances
* Part 4 – Elastic hosiery
* Part 5 – Incontinence appliances
* Part 6 – Stoma appliances.

2.5.3 Chemical reagents

As with the prescribing of appliances, the only chemical reagents that may be prescribed on an NHS prescription form are those listed within the respective *Drug Tariff*. If a reagent is not listed, then it may not be prescribed on an NHS prescription and if a pharmacist dispenses a reagent not listed within the *Drug Tariff*, then they would not be reimbursed the cost of the item.

Key point 2.10

Only those chemical reagents listed within the respective *Drug Tariff* may be prescribed on an NHS prescription form.

In England and Wales, all approved reagents can be found in Part IXR of the *Drug Tariff*. A sentence at the beginning of this section explains the order in which the products are listed. They are also listed by brand name in the index at the back of the *Drug Tariff*. For Northern Ireland all approved reagents can be found in Part II of the *Northern Ireland Drug Tariff* (see Section 2.4.2) and for Scotland, all approved reagents can be found in Part 9 of the *Scottish Drug Tariff* (see Section 2.4.3).

2.6 Restrictions to supply on an NHS prescription form

In addition to any clinical and patient-specific considerations that need to be taken into consideration when supplying an item against a prescription, there are a number of additional restrictions that are placed upon certain items being prescribed (and therefore dispensed) on an NHS prescription form. It should be remembered that these restrictions are based upon the nature of the item and are specific to NHS prescription forms (i.e. the item may be prescribed on a private prescription form – see Chapter 5).

Appropriate prescribers may prescribe any medicinal product on an NHS prescription form, within their approved areas unless it is prohibited by the *Drug Tariff*. These restrictions can be divided into three groups:

- borderline substances (ACBS restrictions) (see Section 2.6.1)
- drugs and other substances not to be prescribed under the NHS pharmaceutical services (see Section 2.6.2)
- drugs to be prescribed in certain circumstances under the NHS pharmaceutical services (SLS restrictions) (see Section 2.6.3).

2.6.1 Borderline substances

Details of borderline substances can be found in Part XV of the *Drug Tariff for England and Wales* (see Section 2.4.1) and Part X of the *Northern Ireland Drug Tariff* (see Section 2.4.2). Information can also be found in Appendix 7 of the *British National Formulary*.

Borderline substances are described by the *Drug Tariff for England and Wales* as follows:

> In certain conditions some foods and toilet preparations have characteristics of drugs and the Advisory Committee on Borderline Substances advises as to the circumstances in which such substances may be regarded as drugs.

Therefore, these items are not drugs as such; they are foods or toiletries that may in certain circumstances be prescribed on an NHS prescription form.

The relevant part of the *Drug Tariffs* is divided into two lists: List A and List B. List A gives an alphabetical index of products which the Advisory Committee on Borderline Substances (ACBS) has recommended for the management of the conditions shown under each product. List B is an index cross-linking clinical conditions and the products which the ACBS has approved for the management of those conditions. It is normal to consult List A first.

So, for an item in List A of Part XV of the *Drug Tariff* to be prescribed on an NHS prescription form, the patient should be being treated for a listed condition. To indicate that this criterion has been met, the prescriber should endorse the prescription 'ACBS'.

Pharmacists may dispense any item listed in Part XV of the *Drug Tariff* even if it has not been endorsed 'ACBS' by the prescriber. However, items listed in Part XV of the *Drug Tariff* that are not endorsed 'ACBS' by the prescriber may result in him or her being asked by their PCT (or equivalent) to justify why the product has been supplied at NHS expense.

It is important that pharmacists are aware of the contents of the relevant part of the *Drug Tariffs*. Each *Drug Tariff* is updated on a monthly basis and so is the primary reference source for information on borderline substances. However, the *British National Formulary* does also indicate whether an item would need to be endorsed 'ACBS' before being supplied by listing the various product in Appendix 7.

Pharmacists and pharmacy technicians should always remember that the *British National Formulary* is only updated once every six months and so is usually less up-to-date than the *Drug Tariff*. Therefore, wherever possible

---

Key point 2.11

Borderline substances are foods or toiletries that may in certain circumstances be prescribed on an NHS prescription form. For items on the borderline substances list, the prescriber should endorse the prescription 'ACBS' to indicate that the patient is being treated for a listed condition.

pharmacists and pharmacy technicians should use their respective *Drug Tariff* for information on borderline substances.

2.6.2 Drugs and other substances not to be prescribed under the NHS pharmaceutical services

Part XVIIIA of the *Drug Tariff for England and Wales* and Part XIA of the *Northern Ireland Drug Tariff* lists those drugs and other substances not to be prescribed on an NHS prescription form. These sections were colloquially referred to as the 'black list', although this is a term that is not used much nowadays. Similar information for Scotland is contained in Schedule 10 to the NHS (General Medical Services) Regulations 1992.

If a medicinal product appears on this list, then it cannot be prescribed on an NHS prescription form (and therefore should not be dispensed). Many of the items on this list are proprietary items, for example, Calpol Infant Suspension. However, so long as the generic name for the items does not also appear on the list, the item may be prescribed generically. Therefore, in this example, Calpol Infant Suspension could be supplied against a prescription for paracetamol suspension 120 mg/5 mL, although the reimbursement to the pharmacy would not take into account that a more expensive proprietary brand had been supplied.

It is important that pharmacists are aware of the contents of their respective parts of the *Drug Tariff*. The *Drug Tariff* is updated on a monthly basis and so is the primary reference source for information on drugs and other substances not to be prescribed on an NHS prescription form. However, the *British National Formulary* does also indicate if an item is not to be prescribed on the NHS by annotating the monograph in the text with a crossed-out 'NHS' (see Figure 2.4).

Figure 2.4 This entry next to an item's monograph in the British National Formulary indicates that it is not to be prescribed on an NHS prescription form.

Key point 2.12

Each *Drug Tariff* lists those items that must not be prescribed on an NHS prescription form. These lists used to be colloquially referred to as the 'black list'.

However, pharmacists and pharmacy technicians should always remember that the *British National Formulary* is only updated once every six months and so is usually less up-to-date than the respective *Drug Tariff*.

2.6.3 Drugs to be prescribed in certain circumstances under the NHS pharmaceutical services (SLS restrictions)

Part XVIIIA of the *Drug Tariff for England and Wales,* Part XIB of the *Northern Ireland Drug Tariff* and Part 12 of the *Scottish Drug Tariff* lists those drugs which may only be prescribed on an NHS prescription form for certain conditions or for certain patients, along with a list of those conditions and/or patients. This section is similar to borderline substances (see above) except in that case we were dealing with items that may or may not have been prescribed for medical reasons (i.e. foods and toiletries). In this case, the items are all drugs, but they may only be prescribed in certain conditions or for certain patients.

To indicate that the criteria within this part of the *Drug Tariff* have been met, the prescriber must endorse the prescription 'SLS' (Selective List Scheme) (or 'S. 11' in Northern Ireland). Pharmacists should not dispense any item listed in these respective Parts of the *Drug Tariff* unless it has been endorsed 'SLS' (or 'S. 11') by the prescriber. It is not the role of the pharmacist to verify that the patient is indeed being treated for a listed condition; this is the responsibility of the prescriber.

It is important that pharmacists are aware of the contents of their respective parts of the *Drug Tariff*. The *Drug Tariff* is updated on a monthly basis and so is the primary reference source for information on SLS restrictions. However, the

British National Formulary does also indicate whether an item would need to be endorsed 'SLS' before being supplied by annotating the monograph in the text 'SLS'. However, pharmacists and pharmacy technicians should always remember that the *British National Formulary* is only updated once every six months and so is usually less up-to-date than the respective *Drug Tariff*.

Key point 2.13

In addition to borderline substances, each *Drug Tariff* lists those drugs that must only be prescribed on an NHS prescription form in certain circumstances. The drugs and the circumstances in which they may be prescribed can be found in the respective *Drug Tariffs*.

2.7 Chapter summary

This chapter has covered the key basics behind the supply of medication via an NHS prescription form in the community. It is important that these concepts are understood before the student pharmacist or pharmacy technician tackles the actual mechanics of medicines supply via the NHS in the community. Chapter 3 will take the concepts covered in this chapter and show their detailed use in the supply of medicinal products via NHS prescription forms in the community. This will then be followed by a collection of worked examples.

3

NHS supply in the community 2 – Prescribers and the dispensing process

Upon completion of this chapter, you should be able to:

- list which types of prescriber may prescribe items via an NHS prescription form and what restrictions are placed on each type of prescriber
- comprehend the general dispensing procedure for NHS prescriptions in the community
- understand the role and function of Patient Group Directions (PGDs)
- complete a number of worked examples of NHS prescriptions and the dispensing process.

> **Key point 3.1**
>
> NHS prescriptions can be written by:
>
> - doctors
> - dentists
> - nurses
> - supplementary prescribers
> - independent non-medical prescribers.
>
> Different restrictions on what may be prescribed on an NHS prescription form will apply to different prescribers.

3.1 Introduction

The material in this chapter will follow on from Chapter 2 by covering the supply of prescription items via the National Health Service (NHS) in the community. The following topics are covered:

- NHS prescribers
- the dispensing procedure for NHS prescriptions
- Patient Group Directions (PGDs)

- a collection of worked examples
- a chapter summary.

3.2 NHS prescribers

NHS prescriptions are written by the following groups of prescribers:

- doctors (see Section 3.2.1)
- dentists (see Section 3.2.2)
- nurse prescribers (see Section 3.2.3)

- supplementary prescribers (see Section 3.2.4)
- independent non-medical prescribers (see Section 3.2.5).

Each of these differing prescribers will have different restrictions as to what they may prescribe on an NHS prescription form.

3.2.1 NHS prescriptions written by doctors

Doctors may prescribe any licensed (i.e. products with a UK marketing authorisation) or unlicensed medicinal product on an NHS prescription form (unless the item is specifically prohibited by the relevant *Drug Tariff* – see Section 2.6). In addition they may prescribe any licensed or unlicensed product on a private prescription form (see Section 5.1). NHS prescriptions written by doctors for dispensing in the community will usually either be written by general practitioners (GPs) or (less commonly) by hospital doctors. Prescriptions for patients written by hospital doctors that are to be dispensed within the hospital are written on hospital-specific forms (see Section 4.2).

3.2.2 NHS prescriptions written by dentists

Dentists are regarded as practitioners and can legally prescribe any licensed or unlicensed medicinal product on a private prescription form (see Section 5.1), although they are ethically expected to limit their prescribing to within their individual area(s) of competence.

However, dentists may also prescribe medicinal products on an NHS prescription form. For England and Wales, this prescribing must be limited to those items listed in Part XVIIA of the *Drug Tariff for England and Wales* (see Section 2.4.1), for Northern Ireland, those items listed in Part IXA of the *Northern Ireland Drug Tariff* (see Section 2.4.2) and for Scotland those items listed on Part 8A of the *Scottish Drug Tariff* (see Section 2.4.3). Only those items listed within these parts of the respective *Drug Tariffs* may be prescribed by a dentist on an NHS dental prescription form.

It is worth noting that some of the entries within these parts of the *Drug Tariffs* are for particular strengths or presentations of a particular drug. Where only one strength or presentation of a medicinal product is listed, only this strength or presentation may be prescribed and therefore supplied via an NHS dental prescription form. For example, dentists may prescribe erythromycin tablets, but not capsules.

It is important that pharmacists are aware of the contents of the respective parts of the *Drug Tariff(s)* dealing with dental prescribing on the NHS. The *Drug Tariffs* are updated on a monthly basis and so are the primary reference source for information on dental prescribing. The *British National Formulary* also indicates whether an item would be allowed to be prescribed on an NHS dental prescription form by listing the Dental Practitioners' Formulary (DPF). However, pharmacists and pharmacy technicians should always remember that the *British National Formulary* is only updated once every six months and so is usually less up-to-date than the respective *Drug Tariffs*.

3.2.3 NHS prescriptions written by nurses

There are three types of nurse prescribers: community practitioner nurse prescribers (sometimes called district nurses or health visitors) who may prescribe from a restricted list of items, nurses who are supplementary prescribers (see Section 3.2.4) and nurses who are independent prescribers (see Section 3.2.5).

For nurses who are prescribing from a restricted list of items, this prescribing must be limited to those items listed in Part XVIIB(i) of the *Drug Tariff for England and Wales* (see Section 2.4.1), Part IXB of the *Northern Ireland Drug Tariff* (see Section 2.4.2) or Part 8B of the *Scottish Drug Tariff* (see Section 2.4.3). Only those items listed within these parts of the respective *Drug Tariffs* may be prescribed by a community practitioner nurse prescriber on an NHS prescription form.

As in the case of dentists (see Section 3.2.2), these lists may specify the strength, form and/or presentation of items which may be prescribed on a community nurse NHS prescription form. Where only one strength or presentation of a medicinal product is listed, only this strength or presentation may be prescribed and therefore supplied via an NHS prescription.

In a similar way to dental prescribing in the NHS (see Section 3.2.2) it is important that pharmacists are aware of the contents of the respective parts of the *Drug Tariff(s)* dealing with nurse prescribing on the NHS. The *British National Formulary* also indicates whether an item would be able to be prescribed on an NHS prescription by a nurse by listing the *Nurse Prescribers' Formulary for Community Practitioners*. However, the *British National Formulary* is not usually as up to date as the *Drug Tariff* as indicated above.

3.2.4 NHS prescriptions written by supplementary prescribers

Recently, the Department of Health has introduced supplementary prescribing, which is described as:

> A voluntary prescribing partnership between an independent prescriber and a supplementary prescriber, to implement an agreed patient-specific clinical management plan with the patient's agreement.

A number of different health professional groups may qualify as supplementary prescribers and are able to prescribe medicinal products on the NHS. Different supplementary prescribers are able to prescribe different medicinal products depending on their area(s) of expertise.

Supplementary prescribers are able to prescribe from a range of medicines for a broad range of medical conditions under the terms of a clinical management plan (CMP). The plan will be drawn up, with the patient's agreement, in consultation with an independent prescriber (the independent prescriber is a doctor or (less commonly) a dentist).

Health professionals who may qualify as supplementary prescribers currently include individuals from the following groups (although other health professional groups may be added to this list in due time):

- chiropodists/podiatrists
- midwives
- nurses
- optometrists
- pharmacists
- physiotherapists
- radiographers (diagnostic or therapeutic).

3.2.5 NHS prescriptions written by independent non-medical prescribers

In addition to supplementary prescribing by non-medical practitioners (see Section 3.2.4), independent non-medical prescribing has also recently been introduced. Currently this is limited to suitably qualified nurses and pharmacists, although as with supplementary prescribing, independent prescribing may be extended to other health professional groups in due time.

Nurse independent prescribers are able to prescribe any licensed medicinal product including some controlled drugs. Pharmacist independent prescribers have similar prescribing rights; however, currently they may not prescribe any controlled drugs (although this may change in the future).

Further information on independent nurse and pharmacist prescribing can be found in Part XVIIB(ii) of the *Drug Tariff for England and Wales* (see Section 2.4.1). This states that nurse independent prescribers and pharmacist independent prescribers:

- can prescribe licensed medicines independently for uses outside their licensed indications (so-called 'off-licence' or 'off-label'). They must accept clinical/legal responsibility for that prescribing, and should only prescribe off-licence/off-label where it is accepted clinical practice
- may prescribe any appliances/dressings that are listed in Part IX of the *Drug Tariff*; must not prescribe drugs and other substances listed in Part XVIIIA of the *Drug Tariff* at NHS expense
- may prescribe drugs listed in Part XVIIIB of the *Drug Tariff* at NHS expense, but only in the specified circumstances, and/or for the specified patient groups listed in the *Drug Tariff*
- must not prescribe unlicensed medicines
- may prescribe borderline substances, which have been approved by the Advisory

Committee on Borderline Substances (ACBS). A list of ACBS approved products and the circumstances under which they can be prescribed, can be found in part XV of the Drug Tariff. Although this is a non-mandatory list, Nurse Independent Prescribers should normally restrict their prescribing of borderline substances to items on the ACBS approved list.

The controlled drugs that independent nurse prescribers are able to prescribe are listed in Part XVIIB(ii) of the *Drug Tariff for England and Wales* (see Section 2.4.1), along with the indication and route of administration. Independent nurse prescribers may only prescribe those controlled drugs listed in Part XVIIB(ii) and only for the indications listed and for administration via the route(s) listed.

3.3 The dispensing procedure for NHS prescriptions

This section details the procedure to be followed when dispensing an NHS prescription. Upon receipt of an NHS prescription form, the following procedure should be followed:

1. Check the legality of the NHS prescription form (see Section 3.3.1).
2. Identify the prescriber (see Section 3.3.2).
3. Check that the prescriber is allowed to prescribe the item(s) on an NHS prescription form (see Section 3.3.3).
4. Perform a clinical check on the prescription (see Section 3.3.4).
5. Dispense and label the item(s) (see Section 3.3.5).
6. Check the item(s) dispensed is/are correct and labelled appropriately. Ideally this check would be performed by a colleague (i.e. an independent check) but when working alone, the pharmacist will need to check the item(s) themselves (see Section 3.3.6).
7. Pass the item(s) to the patient and counsel the patient in the use of the medication (see Section 3.3.7)
8. Process the prescription form (see Section 3.3.8).

> ## Key point 3.2
>
> The dispensing procedure for NHS prescriptions:
>
> 1. Check the legality of the NHS prescription form.
> 2. Identify the prescriber.
> 3. Check that the prescriber is allowed to prescribe the item(s) on an NHS prescription form.
> 4. Perform a clinical check on the prescription.
> 5. Dispense and label the item(s).
> 6. Check the item(s) dispensed is/are correct and labelled appropriately.
> 7. Pass the item(s) to the patient and counsel the patient in the use of the medication.
> 8. Process the prescription form.

3.3.1 Checking the legality of the NHS prescription form

All prescription forms received by pharmacists or pharmacy technicians need to be checked to ensure that they are legally correct. Only prescriptions on forms that meet the requirements should be dispensed. If a prescription form is not legally correct, it should be referred to the prescriber for amendment before dispensing.

Details of what needs to be present on an NHS prescription form can be found in Section 2.2.7. In summary, this is:

1. The patient's details. This must include the age or date of birth of the patient if they are under 12 years of age.
2. Sufficient details of the medication to be supplied. Except in the prescribing of controlled drugs (see Section 6.3.2), there is no legal requirement to provide particular information about the product. However, there will need to be sufficient information provided to enable the accurate and safe supply of medication to the patient and if there is insufficient information on the

prescription form, this must be queried with the prescriber before a supply can be made.

3. The signature of the prescriber.
4. The address of the prescriber.
5. An indication as to the prescriber type.
6. An appropriate date.

Key point 3.3

NHS prescription forms will need the following pieces of information to be present before the prescription can be dispensed:

- the patient's details
- details of the medication to be supplied
- the signature of the prescriber
- the address of the prescriber
- an indication of the prescriber type
- an appropriate date.

3.3.2 Identifying the prescriber

It is important to identify who the prescriber is so that you can ensure that they are able to prescribe the item(s) on an NHS prescription. Different prescribers have different restrictions on the items they may prescribe and may use differing prescription forms (see Section 2.2). Information on who may prescribe items on an NHS prescription is detailed in Section 3.2 and can be divided into:

- doctors (see Section 3.2.1)
- dentists (see Section 3.2.2)
- community practitioner nurse prescribers (see Section 3.2.3)
- supplementary prescribers (see Section 3.2.4)
- independent non-medical prescribers (see Section 3.2.5).

3.3.3 Checking that the prescriber is allowed to prescribe the item(s) on an NHS prescription

Once the identity of the prescriber has been confirmed, a check can then be made to confirm that the item(s) is/are allowed to be prescribed

on NHS prescription forms. This will involve two stages:

1. Verification that the item(s) may be prescribed on an NHS prescription form.
2. If the item(s) may be prescribed on an NHS prescription form, verification that the prescriber is able to prescribe the item(s) (as different NHS prescribers have differing restrictions as to what they may prescribe on an NHS prescription form).

The first part of this process involves verifying that the item(s) prescribed may be prescribed on an NHS prescription form (i.e. that prescribing the item by any prescriber on an NHS prescription is not prohibited). As discussed earlier in this chapter, certain restrictions have been placed on the prescribing of certain items (e.g. borderline substances – see Section 2.6.1). Further details on these restrictions can be found in Section 2.6.

Once it has been established that the item(s) may be prescribed on an NHS prescription, the pharmacist or pharmacy technician needs to establish whether the prescriber who has prescribed the item(s) is able to do so. For doctors, this is simple as long as the item is able to be prescribed on an NHS prescription form (i.e. the first part of this process has been completed and the item is not restricted), they will be able to prescribe the item.

For other NHS prescribers, differing restrictions have been placed on their prescribing. These prescribers can be divided into dentists (see Section 3.2.2), community practitioner nurse prescribers (see Section 3.2.3), supplementary prescribers (see Section 3.2.4) and independent non-medical prescribers (see Section 3.2.5).

3.3.4 Performing a clinical check on the prescription

It is beyond the scope of this text to go into detail on the clinical use of different medicinal agents. However, it is a fundamental role of the supplying pharmacist that they have checked the suitability of all medication that they supply. For all prescription items the following points need to be considered:

- the patient
- the dose of the medication
- the patient's condition
- other medication the patient may be taking.

Key point 3.4

When dispensing medication against a prescription, pharmacists and pharmacy technicians should always consider the following points for every prescription:

- the patient
- the dose of the medication
- the patient's condition
- other medication the patient may be taking.

The patient

First and foremost, who is the patient? Is it a child, an adult or an elderly person? This needs to be established first as many of the other decisions you may make about the patient's therapy will utilise this information. However, it is not always easy to identify the age of the patient.

For children under the age of 12 years, the age or date of birth will be present on the prescription as this is a legal requirement. Nowadays, it is common for all NHS prescription forms to detail the patient's date of birth (or age, or sometimes both). However, it is not a legal requirement for the age (or date of birth) of patients over 12 to be stated on a prescription and so it may not always be present.

If the prescription is for a female of childbearing age, consideration will need to be given to whether she may be pregnant or breast-feeding.

The dose of the medication

Is the dose of the prescribed item suitable for the patient? Doses of medication will differ for different patients. For example, for many drugs,

a child's dose will be less than that for an adult. However, this is not always the case. In addition, there are a number of patient-specific factors that will alter the dose.

If you are unfamiliar with the dose of the medication, this will need to be checked. The best reference source for this is the *British National Formulary* or the *British National Formulary for Children*, or the Summary of Product Characteristics (SPC), which each pharmaceutical company is obliged to produce for each individual medicinal product.

The patient's condition

What is the condition of the patient? Is their renal (kidney) or hepatic (liver) system compromised? Are they pregnant or breast-feeding? Is their condition one that would dictate the form of the medication to be supplied (for example, an elderly infirm patient who cannot swallow solids may require their medication in liquid form)?

As patients age, they are more likely to suffer from liver impairment or reduced renal function. However, this is a generalisation and many young patients suffer from conditions that affect their liver and/or kidneys. If a drug is metabolised by the liver or excreted by the kidneys, patients who have liver disease or reduced renal function may require alteration of the drug's dosage or substitution of a different drug. The *British National Formulary* provides a summary of drugs to be avoided or used with caution in liver disease (Appendix 2) or renal impairment (Appendix 3).

Certain drugs may not be prescribed or only used with caution in patients who are pregnant or breast-feeding. Pregnancy is divided into three (roughly three-month) periods known as 'trimesters'. It is important, when checking the prescription for a pregnant patient, that you are aware of the stage of the pregnancy. Some drugs are not suitable for administration in particular trimesters, while being considered safe in other trimesters. Appendix 4 of the *British National Formulary* provides a summary of drugs to be avoided or used with caution in pregnancy.

In addition, certain drugs will be excreted in breast milk and as such, should be avoided in patients who are breast-feeding. Appendix 5 of the *British National Formulary* provides a list of drugs present in breast milk.

Further to general considerations, some drugs may not be used in specific patient groups. These restrictions (termed contraindications) are detailed in the individual drug entry within the *British National Formulary* or *British National Formulary for Children*, or the manufacturer's SPC.

Other medication the patient may be taking

In addition to the patient's condition, consideration needs to be given to any other medication the patient may be taking. Some medication may not be suitable for particular patients based on the patient's condition. In addition, some medication may not be suitable for a patient, or the dose of the medication may need to be altered because of other medication the patient may be taking.

For example, imagine a patient who has been taking a maintenance dose of 250 micrograms of digoxin every morning for heart failure for a number of years, and has just been prescribed a loading dose of amiodarone for cardiac arrhythmias (200 mg three times a day for one week, followed by 200 mg twice a day for one week, followed by 200 mg once a day). The addition of the amiodarone will increase the plasma concentration of the digoxin. This increase in the amount of digoxin in the plasma will effectively increase the patient's dose (even though they are not taking any more of the drug by mouth). In this case, the dose of digoxin that the patient is taking will need to be halved.

This above situation is called a drug interaction. Summary information on drug interactions can be found in Appendix 1 of the *British National Formulary*. In some cases, it is necessary to find out further details on how a drug interaction occurs and the possible effects on the patient. In these cases, suitable information can be found in *Stockley's Drug Interactions*.

Drug interactions can vary widely in complexity and it is important that pharmacists and pharmacy technicians are aware of how they can occur. Drug interactions can be categorised into two groups: pharmacodynamic interactions and pharmacokinetic interactions.

Pharmacodynamic drug interactions

Pharmacodynamic drug interactions are interactions between drugs that have either similar or antagonistic actions. Although drug interactions will affect different patients differently, pharmacodynamic drug interactions are easy to predict and occur in a majority of patients who take the drugs affected. These interactions will, for example, include drugs that compete at the same receptor site or affect the same body systems. A pharmacist or pharmacy technician, using their knowledge of body systems, can make a decision as to the importance of the interaction.

 Example 3.1
A pharmacodynamic drug interaction

A prescription is received by the pharmacy for captopril (an ACE inhibitor) 12.5 mg bd and bendroflumethiazide (a diuretic) 2.5 mg om. The pharmacist notices that Appendix 1 of the *British National Formulary* states that there is an enhanced hypotensive effect when ACE inhibitors are administered with diuretics. What should the pharmacist do?

This is a good example of where a theoretical interaction is being used to treat the patient. In this case, the patient's hypertension (high blood pressure) cannot be controlled with one drug. The prescriber has added a second antihypertensive agent to further lower the patient's blood pressure. Therefore, in this case it is appropriate that the patient takes both drugs.

Pharmacokinetic drug interactions

Compared with pharmacodynamic interactions, pharmacokinetic drug interactions are harder to predict and will have an increased variability between patients. In pharmacokinetic interactions, one of the drugs alters the absorption, distribution, metabolism or excretion of the other. This results in an increase or decrease in the amount of drug available to have a pharmacological effect.

Example 3.2
A pharmacokinetic drug interaction

A prescription is received by the pharmacy for cimetidine (an H_2 receptor antagonist) 400 mg bd and theophylline (a bronchodilator) (as Slo-Phyllin), 250 mg bd. The pharmacist notices that Appendix 1 of the *British National Formulary* states that cimetidine inhibits the metabolism of theophylline (therefore increasing the plasma concentration of the theophylline). What should the pharmacist do?

In this example, it is necessary to obtain a little more of the patient's drug history. Upon further questioning, the pharmacist ascertains that the patient has been taking theophylline for a number of years and has just been prescribed the cimetidine for the first time. As the cimetidine inhibits the metabolism of the theophylline, raising the plasma levels, it would alter the effective dose of the theophylline.

In this case, there are two options. First, the dose of the theophylline could be reduced while the patient is taking the cimetidine. Although this is a possibility, in reality this would not be the option of choice as it would not be easy to suggest a suitable alternative dose that would reduce the amount taken while still remaining therapeutic. The second option would be to change the cimetidine for an alternative drug that did not have the same interaction. In this case, any of the other H_2 receptor antagonists would be suitable (as they do not cause the same effect).

The pharmacist should contact the prescriber, outlining the potential drug interaction and suggest an alternative H_2 receptor antagonist.

Key point 3.5

Drug interactions can be categorised into two groups:

- Pharmacodynamic drug interactions occur between drugs that have either similar or antagonistic actions. Although drug interactions will affect different patients differently, pharmacodynamic drug interactions are easy to predict and occur in a majority of patients who take the drugs affected.
- Pharmacokinetic drug interactions occur where one drug affects the absorption, distribution, metabolism or excretion of the other. Pharmacokinetic drug interactions are harder to predict than pharmacodynamic drug interactions and in many cases, affect different patients differently.

3.3.5 Dispensing and labelling the item(s)

Once it has been established that the item(s) on the prescription form are safe and suitable for the patient, the label(s) can be generated and the item(s) dispensed.

Generate the label(s)

It is good practice to generate the labels for every item for each patient before dispensing that patient's items. This allows the labels to be applied to the items as soon as they have been dispensed. If the items were dispensed before the labels were generated, it would allow more opportunity for the item(s) to be incorrectly labelled (as the items could not be labelled as soon as they are dispensed).

Almost all modern pharmacies use a computer to generate the labels for dispensed prescriptions. In addition to generating labels, the pharmacy computer can be used to collate individual patient medication records (PMRs) and highlight any potential drug interactions, both with medication that is currently being supplied and with previous medication that the patient may still be taking (using the PMR system). However, it is still the responsibility of the pharmacist or pharmacy technician dispensing the item to ensure that the label is correct. The accuracy of the label is of paramount importance as it conveys essential information to the patient on the use of the preparation.

Although the pharmacist or pharmacy technician may counsel the patient on the use of the medication when it is handed over, it is unlikely that the patient will be able to remember all the information that they are given verbally. The label therefore acts as a permanent reminder of the key points that the patient needs to know.

Key point 3.6

The label of a pharmaceutical product has many functions:

- to indicate clearly the contents of the container
- to indicate clearly to the patient how and when the medicinal product should be taken or used
- to indicate clearly to the patient how the product should be stored and for how long
- to indicate clearly to the patient any warnings or cautions of which they need to be made aware.

Label appearance

The label must be clean, secure and affixed in the correct position:

- Clean – Ensure the container is clean before packing the product, and then clean the outside before affixing the label. Never pour any liquids into a pre-labelled container as this risks spoiling the label with drips of the medicament.
- Secure – Ensure that the label is secure before dispensing the product to the patient. The main reason for labels not sticking to product containers is because of a dirty or greasy container.

- Correct position – Ensure that the patient can open the container without destroying the label (e.g. when labelling cartons). Ensure the label is positioned with care and is straight, not crooked. Use a position appropriate to the type of container:
  - *Medicine bottles* – The label should be on the front, about a third of the way down the bottle. The front of an internal bottle is the curved side and the front of a fluted (external) bottle is the plain side.
  - *Cartons* – The label should be placed on the larger side of the carton. If there is not enough room on a single side of the carton for the entire label, it should be placed around the carton, ensuring that all the information is visible.
  - *Ointment jars* – The label should be placed on the side of the jar, ensuring that the words on the label are visible when the top is placed on the jar.

Information

The information on the label must be legible, concise, adequate, intelligible and accurate:

- Legible – Always check label print size and quality to ensure that it can be read clearly. If there is too much information to place on one label, consider placing the additional information on a secondary label, rather than reducing the size of the print or trying to include too much information on a single label.
- Concise – Although it is important that sufficient information is placed on the label, it must be remembered that it is essential not to confuse the patient by placing too much information on the label. If the label contains too much information the patient may feel overwhelmed and unwilling to read any of the information.
- Adequate – Ensure that sufficient information is given, for example the term 'when required' leaves the questions: How much? How often? When required for what?
- Intelligible – The wording of the information on the label must be in plain English, be easily understandable and use unambiguous terms. It must always be remembered that

patients may feel embarrassed to ask for further clarification of the meaning of complicated words used on the label.

- Accurate – It is important that the title is accurate, the instructions are accurate and the patient's name is complete and accurate.

Key point 3.7

Remember, the label of a pharmaceutical product must be in the right place and contain the right information. The following need to be taken into consideration:

- *Appearance*
  - correct position
  - clean
  - secure
- *Information*
  - legible
  - concise
  - adequate
  - intelligible
  - accurate.

In the UK, detailed requirements for labelling of medicinal products are contained in the Medicines Act 1968 and in amendments to that Act made by Statutory Instrument. The legislation distinguishes between labelling of a medicinal product for sale and the labelling for a dispensed product when lesser requirements apply. The following is a list of both legal and good practice requirements for the labelling of a dispensed medicinal product.

1. All labels for dispensed medicines must have the name of the patient, preferably the full name, not just initials and if possible the title of the patient (Mr, Mrs, Miss, Master, Ms, etc.) as this helps to distinguish between family members. The date and the name and address of the pharmacy are also legally required. This will normally automatically appear on most computer labelling systems with the date being reset automatically. The words 'Keep out of the reach of children' are also legally required, but most labels used for dispensing purposes are already pre-printed with these words. (The Royal Pharmaceutical Society of Great Britain has advised that it would be better to use the phrase 'Keep out of the reach and sight of children' on pharmacy labels, although this is a good practice suggestion, rather than a legal requirement.)

2. All labels must state the name of the product dispensed, the strength where appropriate and the quantity dispensed.
   (a) All directions on labels should use active rather than passive verbs. For example 'Take TWO' (not 'TWO to be taken'), 'Use ONE' (not 'ONE to be used'), 'Insert ONE' (not 'ONE to be inserted'), etc.
   (b) Where possible, adjacent numbers should be separated by the formulation name. For example 'Take TWO THREE times a day' could allow for easy misinterpretation by the patient; ideally the wording on this label would include the formulation, e.g. 'Take TWO tablets THREE times a day'. The frequency and quantity of individual doses is always expressed as a word rather than a numeral (i.e. 'TWO' not '2').
   (c) Liquid preparations for internal use usually have their dose expressed as a certain number of 5 mL doses. This is because a 5 mL spoon is the normal unit provided to the patient to measure their dose from the dispensed bottle. Therefore if a prescription called for the dosage instruction 10 mL tds this would be expressed as 'Take TWO 5 mL spoonfuls THREE times a day'. Paediatric prescriptions may ask for a 2.5 mL dose; in this case the label would read 'Give a 2.5 mL dose using the oral syringe provided'. Note here the use of the word 'Give' as the preparation is for a child and would be given to the patient by the parent or guardian.
   (d) Remember that the label on a medicine is included so that the item can be identified and the patient instructed as to the directions for use. Therefore, simple language should always be used.
      - Never use the word 'Take' on a preparation that is not intended for the oral route of administration.
      - Use 'Give' as a dosage instruction on

products for children as a responsible adult should administer them.

- Only use numerals when quoting the number of millilitres to be given or taken. All other dosage instructions should use words in preference to numerals.
- Always be prepared to give the patient a verbal explanation of the label.

(e) Where multiple containers of the same medication are supplied, it is good practice for this to be indicated on the label in the form of, for example, '1 of 2 containers', etc. This additional information is designed to prevent patients mistakenly thinking that they have to administer a dose from each container.

3. Warning labels may also be required. These may be pharmaceutical or pharmacological warnings (see Appendix 9 in the *British National Formulary*). Generally if there is a choice between two warning labels with equivalent meaning, the positive one should be chosen (e.g. 'For rectal use only' is preferable to 'Do not swallow' for suppositories).

Within the UK, the term 'For external use only' is used on any preparation intended for external use. The Medicines Act 1968 defines products for external use as embrocations, liniments, lotions, liquid antiseptics, other liquids or gels for external use.

However, traditionally, for the following dosage forms, alternative labels have been employed instead of 'For external use only' to more closely reflect the intended purpose of the product. These alternative labels are:

- enemas – 'For rectal use only'
- gargles and mouthwashes – 'Not to be taken'
- inhalations – 'Not to be taken'
- nasal drops – 'Not to be taken'
- pessaries – 'For vaginal use only'
- suppositories – 'For rectal use only'.

Pharmacists should use their professional judgement when deciding which auxiliary labels should be applied to different pharmaceutical dosage forms.

Extemporaneously dispensed items can require additional information on the label. For further details, consult *Pharmaceutical Compounding and Dispensing*.

Dispense the item(s)

Once the label(s) has/have been generated, the item(s) may be dispensed. There are many items which may be prescribed via an NHS prescription form and it is important that pharmacists and pharmacy technicians ensure that the correct item(s) are being supplied. Remember, within community pharmacy, if a drug is prescribed using a proprietary name, the proprietary product must be supplied. However, if a drug is prescribed by its generic name, in most cases, any generic or proprietary equivalent may be supplied. (The exception to this is for some sustained-release preparations where the release properties of different brands may vary.)

Key point 3.8

In the community, if a drug is prescribed using a proprietary name, the proprietary product must be supplied. However, if a drug is prescribed by its generic name, in most cases (except, for example, in the case of some sustained-release preparations), any generic or proprietary equivalent may be supplied.

In addition, the pharmacist or pharmacy technician should be sure that the correct presentation of a particular drug is being supplied. Some drugs may be presented in a variety of different forms, for example, modified-release and non-modified-release, tablets and capsules, etc. Furthermore, as these different presentations may be produced by the same pharmaceutical manufacturing company, the packaging may appear very similar.

Key point 3.9

Pharmacists and pharmacy technicians should ensure that they are supplying the correct drug and the correct presentation of the drug (e.g. not supplying a modified-release preparation when a standard (non-modified-release) was requested).

3.3.6 Checking the item(s) dispensed is/are correct and labelled appropriately

Once all the above points have been followed, it is important that the label(s) and dispensed item(s) are checked against the prescription form to ensure they are correct.

Ideally, this check will be performed by a second competent colleague. However, there may be some situations where the pharmacist is working alone. In these cases, a second check still needs to take place and the pharmacist will need to perform this second check him- or herself.

3.3.7 Passing the item(s) to the patient and counselling the patient in the use of the medication

Once dispensed and checked, the item(s) will be passed to the patient or their representative. At this point, three things need to occur:

1. The pharmacist or pharmacy technician passing the medication to the patient or their representative needs to confirm that the item(s) is/are going to the right patient.
2. The pharmacist or pharmacy technician needs to pass certain key information to the patient or their representative verbally.
3. The pharmacist or pharmacy technician needs to verify that the patient or their representative understood what they have been told and check to see if they have any questions.

Confirming the patient's identity

It is usual for the pharmacist or pharmacy technician to ask the patient or their representative for the patient's address. The prescription may be for Mrs Smith and there may be three Mrs Smiths in that community pharmacy at that time. If the pharmacist or pharmacy technician called out 'Prescription for Mrs Smith' and handed it out to the first person who said 'Yes,' there would be a 67% chance the medication had been given to the wrong patient!

By asking for the patient's address, the pharmacist or pharmacy technician can confirm that it is indeed the correct patient. Please note that we ask the patient or patient's representative for the address, rather than saying, for example, '1 Station Road, is that correct?' By asking for the patient or their representative to give you the address, you are ensuring that the address is correct as they have to actively give you the information. In the second method, the patient or their representative could easily mishear and just answer 'Yes', or be in such a rush to catch the next bus, for example, they assume the medication is for them and just collect it from the pharmacist or pharmacy technician. Although it appears that you have checked properly, the medication could still go to the wrong patient.

Passing on key information

In addition to the information contained on the label and in the patient information leaflet supplied with the product, it is usual for the pharmacist or pharmacy technician to pass on key information verbally. It is important that the patient or their representative is not overwhelmed with too much information. Therefore, it is usual for only the key information to be given verbally, for example, a reinforcement of the dose of the medication and a reminder of any specific warnings.

However, there may be certain situations where it is necessary to pass on additional information to ensure that the patient uses the medication correctly, for example in the case of eye drops, inhalers or suppositories. Further general information on patient counselling can be found in Chapter 8, with information on specific dosage forms in Chapter 9.

Verification and checking

Finally, it is usual for the pharmacist or pharmacy technician to verify that the patient or their representative has understood what they have been told and whether they have any questions. It is important to ask if the patient or their representative has any questions as they are much more likely to ask a question if the opportunity to do so is offered to them. As useful phrase for this part of the dispensing process is:

'Are you happy with those instructions? Do you have any questions? Feel free to call back any time'.

Key point 3.10

Once dispensed and checked, the item(s) will be passed to the patient or their representative. At this point, three things need to occur. The pharmacist or pharmacy technician passing the medication to the patient or their representative needs:

- to confirm that the item(s) is/are going to the right patient;
- to pass certain key information to the patient or their representative verbally, and;
- to verify that the patient or their representative understood what they have been told and check to see if they have any questions.

3.3.8 Processing the prescription form

Finally, once the prescription item(s) have been passed to the patient or the patient's representative, the pharmacist or pharmacy technician should confirm that the prescription form has been endorsed properly (to ensure that the pharmacy will be correctly reimbursed and remunerated for the supply – see Section 2.4.1, Part IIIA) and the prescription form can then be filed ready for submission at the end of the month. In England, this will be to the Prescription Pricing Division (PPD) of the NHS Business Services Authority; in Northern Ireland, the Central Services Agency; in Scotland, Practitioner Services Division (PSD) of NHS National Services Scotland; and in Wales, Health Solutions Wales (HSW).

At the end of the month, all NHS prescription forms are sorted into two main groups (exempt from prescription charge and prescription charge paid) and then by prescriber type (doctor, dentist, etc.) and finally by individual prescriber,

and then submitted to the relevant organisation for processing and payment.

If the receiving organisation receive any forms that require further annotation, either by the prescriber (e.g. the omission of 'SLS' – see Section 2.6.3) or the pharmacist (e.g. missing endorsements – see Section 2.4.1, Part IIIA), they will return them to the community pharmacy for the missing information to be added. Analysis of these returns can be used to audit the dispensing process (see Section 1.4.3 and Figure A1).

3.4 Patient Group Directions (PGDs)

3.4.1 Background to Patient Group Directions

The preferred way for patients to receive their medicines is for a trained healthcare professional to examine them and then prescribe on an individual patient basis. However in some circumstances it may be advantageous for patients to receive medications from other specially trained healthcare professionals, for example, paramedics.

In order to achieve this legally, in August 2000 Patient Group Directions (PGDs) were introduced, enabling certain healthcare professionals to administer or supply medicines to specified groups of patients without the need for a prescription. An example of this would be the supply of emergency hormonal contraception from a community pharmacy. Patient Group Directions are authorised by NHS Trusts and are designed to help patients' access to healthcare while not compromising patient safety.

The definition of a Patient Group Direction is:

A written instruction for the sale, supply and/or administration of named medicines in an identified clinical situation. It applies to groups of patients who may not be individually identified before presenting for treatment.

From *Practical Group Directions – A practical guide and framework of competencies for all professionals using patient group directions*. Liverpool: National Prescribing Centre, 2004. www.npc.co.uk

Patient Group Directions have been specifically developed to allow first contact services to supply or administer medicines without the patient first needing to see a doctor or a dentist. A first contact service is a service that a patient would make contact with when seeking unscheduled care under the umbrella of the NHS and include:

- accident and emergency services
- ambulance services
- community pharmacies
- minor injury clinics
- NHS walk-in centres
- out-of-hours services.

Patient Group Directions are intended to help healthcare professionals to work in a more flexible manner and develop a more patient centred approach to medicines that is safe and effective. They are an extra layer of exemptions in addition to the long standing exemptions already in medicines legislation (e.g. the supply of medication to patients by chiropodists, optometrists, etc.).

The use of Patient Group Directions means that designated healthcare professionals may supply (for example, an inhaler or tablets) or administer (for example, an injection) directly to a patient without the need for that patient to first obtain a prescription from a prescriber. Patient Group Directions are intended for short-term, usually urgent, care; it is not intended that they would be used to manage a patient's condition in the long term.

Patient Group Directions are particularly suited to minor injuries as they often can be easily treated with medicines that could be provided by the first contact care team without the need to refer to a GP or hospital doctor for a prescription.

Healthcare professionals who work under Patient Group Directions do not need an additional formal qualification, unlike supplementary (see Section 3.2.4) or independent (see Section 3.2.5) prescribers.

Scotland has introduced a system whereby Patient Group Directions can be used by pharmacists in the urgent supply of medicines or appliances. For specific details on the use of Patient Group Directions in the urgent supply of medicines or appliances to patients in Scotland, see Section 7.3.

3.4.2 The format of Patient Group Directions

Patient Group Directions are drawn up by a group of professionals from different disciplines, including a senior doctor (or dentist), a senior pharmacist and a senior member of the profession working under the direction.

Legislation states that Patient Group Directions must contain the following information:

- the name of the business to which the direction applies
- the date the direction comes into force and the date it expires
- a description of the medicine(s) to which the direction applies
- the class of health professional who may supply or administer the medicine
- a signature of a doctor or dentist, as appropriate, and a pharmacist
- a signature from an appropriate health organisation
- the clinical condition or situation to which the direction applies
- a description of those patients excluded from treatment under the direction
- a description of the circumstances in which further advice should be sought from a doctor (or a dentist, as appropriate) and arrangements for referral
- details of appropriate dosage and maximum total dosage, quantity, pharmaceutical form and strength, route and frequency of administration, and minimum or maximum

period over which the medicine should be administered

- relevant warnings, including potential adverse reactions
- details of any necessary follow-up action and the circumstances
- a statement of the records to be kept for audit purposes.

The regulations state that the following health professionals may supply or administer medicines under a Patient Group Direction. It should be noted that these professionals may only work under the Patient Group Direction on an individually named basis:

- registered dieticians
- registered health visitors
- registered midwives
- registered nurses
- registered occupational therapists
- registered ophthalmic opticians
- registered orthotists and prosthetists
- registered pharmacists
- registered speech and language therapists
- state registered chiropodists
- state registered orthoptists
- state registered paramedics or individuals who hold a certificate of proficiency in ambulance paramedic skills issued by the Secretary of State, or issued with his or her approval
- state registered physiotherapists
- state registered radiographers.

Patient Group Directions are used in both the NHS and private sector. Organisations that may sell or supply/administer medicines under a Patient Group Direction are:

- a doctor or dentist's practice in the provision of NHS services
- a non-NHS organisation providing treatment under an arrangement made with an NHS Trust or Primary Care Organisation (PCO) (e.g. a 'walk-in centre', family planning clinic or community pharmacy)
- healthcare services provided by the medical service for the armed forces
- healthcare services provided by the police force
- healthcare services provided by the prison service

- independent hospitals, agencies and clinics registered under the Care Standards Act 2000
- NHS Trusts and Primary Care Organisations
- services funded by the NHS but provided by the private, voluntary or charitable sector
- special health authorities.

If a medicine is supplied using a Patient Group Direction under NHS guidelines, a prescription charge will be levied and if outside the NHS, a charge will be made but this will not be subject to VAT.

3.4.3 Examples of Patient Group Directions

Figure 3.1 contains a sample template for a Patient Group Direction, Figure 3.2 contains an example of a Patient Group Direction for the administration of fusidic acid cream/ointment 2% by a community pharmacist and Figure 3.3 contains an example of a Patient Group Direction for the administration of trimethoprim 200 mg tablets by community nurses for the management of patients with cystitis.

Reference is made, in the following examples, to whether the drug is a 'black triangle' drug. The black triangle symbol (▼) is used within the *British National Formulary* to indicate drugs or certain preparations of drugs that are under closer monitoring by the Medicines and Healthcare products Regulatory Agency (MHRA). These may be, for example, a newly licensed medicine or an established medicine being used for a new condition or administered via a new route.

Key point 3.12

The black triangle symbol (▼) is used within the *British National Formulary* to indicate drugs or certain preparations of drugs that are under closer monitoring by the Medicines and Healthcare products Regulatory Agency (MHRA). These may be, for example, a newly licensed medicine or an established medicine being used for a new condition or administered via a new route.

TEMPLATE PATIENT GROUP DIRECTION

Patient Group Direction for [Name of Drug]:

Name of body authorising the PGD:

PGD comes into effect	[Appropriate date]
PGD to be reviewed	[Appropriate date]
Supply/administration of	[Name of drug including form and strength]
Legal classification	[POM, P, GSL]
Black triangle?	[If yes, state the reason for inclusion]
Outside terms of SPC?	[If yes, state the reason for inclusion]
Clinical situations for which medicine is to be used	[Clinical conditions for which the medicine can be supplied or administered]
Clinical criteria for inclusion	[Clinical criteria under which a person shall be eligible for treatment]
Criteria for exclusion	[Clinical criteria under which a person shall not be eligible for treatment]
Reasons for seeking further advice from doctor/dentist	[What circumstances should further advice be sought, if any]
Dosage	[Applicable dose/maximum dosage]
Route of administration	[As appropriate]
Frequency of administration	[As appropriate]
Period of administration	[Maximum/minimum period of administration as appropriate]
Warnings	[Applicable warnings to note]
Follow-up	[What follow-up is appropriate, if any]
Arrangements for referral	[As appropriate]
Details of records to be kept	[As appropriate]
Names of individuals permitted to supply/administer under the PGD	[Names of all individuals who are permitted to supply/administer under the PGD. All must belong to one of the designated classes of healthcare professional]
Signed by:	[Relevant authorising body*]
Signed by:	[Doctor/dentist as appropriate]
Signed by:	[Pharmacist]
Signed by:	[Doctor/dentist whom the supply is to assist, where the PGD is to assist doctors/dentists in providing primary care NHS facilities]

*e.g. Relevant NHS body, registered service provider in the private sector, signed by or on behalf of the prison governor in prison service or the Chief Constable in police a police force. In case of Her Majesty's forces, signed by or on behalf of the Surgeon General, a medical director general or a chief executive of an executive agency of the Ministry of Defence.

Figure 3.1   A template for a Patient Group Direction.

PATIENT GROUP DIRECTION FOR USE BY:

COMMUNITY PHARMACISTS

Patient Group Direction for *Fusidic acid Cream/Ointment 2%*

Authorised by: *Anytown Primary Care Trust*

PGD comes into effect	*July 2008*
PGD to be reviewed	*July 2010*
Supply/administration of	*Fusidic acid cream/ointment 2%*
Legal classification	*POM*
Black triangle?	*No*
Outside terms of SPC?	*No*
Clinical situations for which medicine is to be used	*To treat acute impetigo caused by staphylococcal skin infection*
Clinical criteria for inclusion	*Any patient showing primary infection, small localised area*
Criteria for exclusion	• *Large non-localised areas of infection* • *Previous occurrence of impetigo within the last three months* • *Pregnant or breast-feeding* • *Hypersensitivity to fusidic acid or any excipients of the cream/ointment* • *Secondary infection of wound already being treated/dressed with another topical preparation* • *Patients registered with a doctor's surgery outside Anytown PCT* • *If patient refuses to give consent* • *Any patient that is excluded from treatment as above*
Reasons for seeking further advice from doctor	• *If fails to respond to treatment after 3 days* • *If condition worsens* • *Adverse reaction to cream/ointment*
Dosage	• *Apply three to four times a day* • *Soften and remove crusting lesions with warm soapy water prior to application of cream*
Route of administration	*Topical*
Frequency of administration	*As above*
Period of administration	*Apply for 7 days*
Warnings	• *For external use only* • *Wash hands before and after application* • *Do not share towels/flannels/pillows* • *Avoid touching spots* • *Avoid close contact with others and children should not attend nursery until crusting of lesions has stopped and there is no leakage of fluid* • *Keep nails cut short*
Follow-up	*Referral to GP if treatment fails*

Figure 3.2   An example of a Patient Group Direction for the administration of fusidic acid cream/ointment 2% by community pharmacists. (Continued overleaf.)

Arrangements for referral	*Refer direct to GP along with documented evidence of any advice given*
Details of records to be kept	• *Name of supplying pharmacist* • *Name and address of patient, date of birth if under 16 years* • *Product supplied, manufacturer, batch number and expiry date* • *Any adverse effects experienced by the patient*
Names of individuals permitted to supply/ administer under the PGD	*See attached list*
Signed by:	*Clinical governance lead*
Signed by:	*Doctor/dentist as appropriate*
Signed by:	*Pharmacist*
Signed by:	*N/A*

Name	Address	Qualification	Signature
Mr T. K. Pill	Scratby Pharmacy	MRPharmS	
Miss R. U. Well	Long Itchington Pharmacy	MRPharmS	
Mrs N. E. Simtoms	Itchingfield Pharmacy	MRPharmS	
Mr Ivor Cure	Bishop Itchington Pharmacy	MRPharmS	

Figure 3.2   continued

PATIENT GROUP DIRECTION FOR USE BY:

NURSES IN MINOR TREATMENT CENTRES OF OUT OF HOURS SERVICE

Patient Group Direction for *Trimethoprim*

Authorised by: *Anytown Primary Care Trust*

PGD comes into effect	*July 2008*
PGD to be reviewed	*July 2009*
Supply/administration of	*Trimethoprim tablets 200 mg*
Legal classification	*POM*
Black triangle?	*No*
Outside terms of SPC?	*No*
Clinical situations for which medicine is to be used	*Management of patients with cystitis*
Clinical criteria for inclusion	*Women presenting with cystisis who are:* • *Sexually active* • *Not pregnant* • *Had previous infection but not in past 2 weeks*
Criteria for exclusion	• *Previous occurrence of cystitis in past 2 weeks that was treated with antibiotics*

Figure 3.3   An example of a Patient Group Direction for the administration of trimethoprim 200 mg tablets by community nurses for the management of patients with cystitis. (Continued opposite.)

	• Previous occurrence of cystitis more than twice in last 12 months • High temperature (may be pyelonephritis) • Pregnant or breast-feeding • Hypersensitivity to trimethoprim or any excipients of the tablets • Known renal impairment • Known blood dyscrasias • Children • Men • Non-sexually active women • Interaction with current medication • If patient refuses to give consent
Reasons for seeking further advice from doctor	• If fails to respond to treatment after 3 days • If condition worsens • Adverse reaction to trimethoprim
Dosage	200 mg
Route of administration	Oral
Frequency of administration	Every 12 hours
Period of administration	3 days
Warnings	• May reduce effectiveness of combined oral contraceptives; advise regarding use of alternative contraception • Take regularly and complete the course even if the condition appears to have cleared up • Warn of risk of gastro-intestinal upset and skin rash
Follow-up	• Referral to GP if treatment fails • If patient is excluded as above
Arrangements for referral	Refer direct to GP along with documented evidence of any advice given
Details of records to be kept	• Supply recorded on patient's medical records • Date, quantity and dose supplied • Name of health professional providing treatment
Names of individuals permitted to supply/administer under the PGD	See attached list
Signed by:	Clinical governance lead
Signed by:	Doctor/dentist as appropriate
Signed by:	Pharmacist
Signed by:	Dr R. U. Better

Name	Title	Qualification	Signature
Peggy Legge	Miss	RGN	
Lynne C. Doyle	Mrs	RGN	
N. E. Hash	Mrs	RGN	
U. B. Bettasoon	Mr	RGN	

Figure 3.3   continued

Certain medications are given special consideration before being used as part of a Patient Group Directive. In October 2003 the Misuse of Drugs Regulations 2001 were amended to allow some controlled drugs (see Chapter 6) to be supplied. Under Patient Group Directions, the following controlled drugs may be supplied or administered:

- diamorphine – only for treatment of cardiac pain by nurses working in coronary care units and accident and emergency units
- all Schedule 4 controlled drugs (e.g. benzodiazepines) except anabolic steroids
- all Schedule 5 controlled drugs
- from January 2008, midazolam became a Schedule 3 controlled drug and will be the only Schedule 3 controlled drug that can be included in a PGD.

Patient Group Directions for antimicrobials are drawn up with caution because of the issue of antimicrobial resistance. Any Patient Group Direction for antimicrobials must be consistent with local policies and should be regularly reviewed.

Medicines used outside their Summary of Product Characteristics and black triangle drugs (i.e. those recently licensed and subject to special reporting arrangements for adverse drug reactions) are also only included in Patient Group Directions in exceptional circumstances. Dressings and unlicensed drugs cannot be supplied using Patient Group Directions.

GSL medicines do not require a Patient Group Direction nor do P medicines if supplied by a pharmacist, but in all other instances a Patient Group Direction would be required.

3.4.4 Patient Group Directions – a summary

In summary, Patient Group Directions contain two separate but linked sets of information. Primarily the information concerns the medicine but linked with this is the review and monitoring process. We could therefore split the Patient Group Direction as shown below.

Name of medication:

- clinical condition/indications included

- inclusion criteria
- exclusion criteria
- supply and administration details
- adverse reactions
- action to be taken in the case of adverse reactions
- audit arrangements.

Review and monitoring processes:

- minimum qualification requirements
- additional training requirements
- names of the authors of Patient Group Direction
- names and signatures of professionals taking clinical responsibility
- implementation date
- review date
- audit arrangements.

3.5 Worked examples

This section contains examples of NHS prescription forms for dispensing within a community pharmacy. Although a number of different examples are used in this section, from a variety of different prescribers, all prescription forms can be addressed by using a standard systematic approach (see Section 3.3 for NHS prescription forms, and Section 5.4 for non-NHS (private) prescription forms).

3.5.1 Framework for systematic dispensing/ supply in the community

This approach is summarised in Figure 3.4 (this framework does not cover the supply of items from a pharmacy to non-practitioners; see Section 5.2.8).

3.5.2 Examples of NHS prescriptions and the dispensing process

The following section contains examples of NHS prescriptions that may be encountered in a community pharmacy. In each case, the following sections are completed to guide you through the dispensing process:

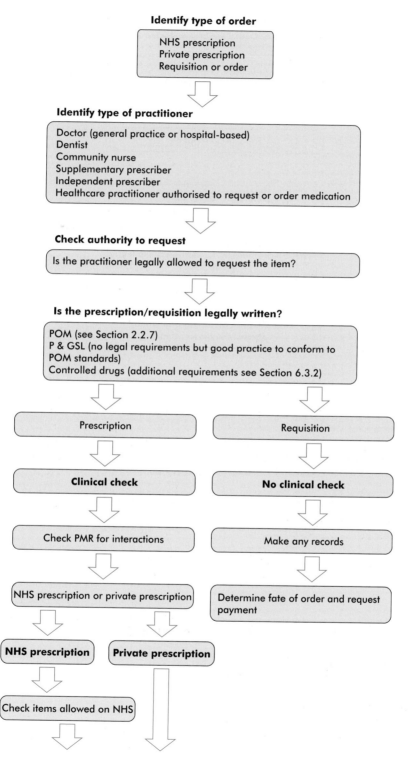

Figure 3.4   Framework for systematic dispensing/supply in the community. (Continued overleaf.)

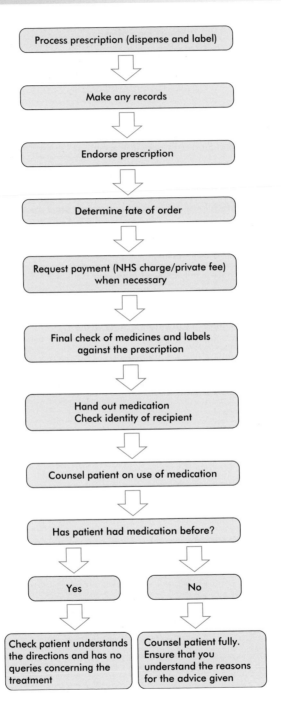

Figure 3.4   continued

1. Identity of order
2. Prescriber
3. Legally written?
4. Clinical check (complete the following table):

DRUG	INDICATIONS	DOSE CHECK	REFERENCE

5. Interactions

6. Suitability for patient
7. Item(s) allowable on the NHS
8. Records to be made (including copies of the record(s))
9. Process prescription (including example of label(s))
10. Endorse prescription
11. Destination of paperwork
12. Identity check/counselling.

Example 3.3

You receive the prescription shown below in your pharmacy:

Pharmacy Stamp

Age

Title, Forename, Surname & Address

D.o.B

27/07/50

Barbara Ache
3 Pain Close
Anytown
AT3 6PC

Please don't stamp over age box

Number of days' treatment
N.B. Ensure dose is stated

NHS Number: 1234567890

Endorsements

Lederfen Capsules
300mg

1 om and 2 on

Mitte 168

FP10SS0403

Signature of Prescriber

Date
Today's

For dispenser
No. of
Prescns.
on form

DR. R. U. BETTER Anytown PCT
Anytown Health Centre 123456
ANYTOWN
AT1 1RB
01674 343536

NHS   PATIENTS – please read the notes overleaf

20742603476

Example 3.3 Continued

1. *Identity of order*: NHS prescription (FP10SS).
2. *Prescriber*: Doctor (general practitioner).
3. *Legally written?* No. The doctor failed to sign the prescription. The prescription will need to be returned to the prescriber for addition of signature prior to dispensing.
4. *Clinical check (complete the following table)*:

DRUG	INDICATIONS	DOSE CHECK	REFERENCE
Fenbufen.	Pain and inflammation	300 mg in the morning and 600 mg at night	*British National Formulary* 54th edition, section 10.1.1

5. *Interactions*: There is only one drug on the prescription. However, it would also be advisable for the pharmacist or pharmacy technician to check the patient medication record (PMR) for any concurrent medication that could cause an interaction.
6. *Suitability for patient*: Item prescribed is safe and suitable for a patient of this age and the dose ordered on the prescription is within the recommended dose limits.
7. *Item(s) allowable on the NHS*: Yes (see *Drug Tariff*)
8. *Records to be made (including copies of the record(s))*: Make a note of the intervention on a clinical intervention form (see Figure 1.5).
9. *Process prescription (including example of label(s))*:
   - 168 capsules have been ordered. The product comes in packs of 84, so it would be sensible to prepare two labels, one for each pack of 84.
   - Check Appendix 9 of the *British National Formulary* for supplementary labelling requirements. Fenbufen: *British National Formulary* label number 21.
   - Select two packs (also called two 'OPs' or two original packs), remembering to check the expiry date and taking care that both packs are 300 mg capsules (the packaging of other strengths/forms is very similar).
   - Perform final check of item, label and prescription.
   - Pack in a suitable bag ready to give to the patient or patient's representative.

   Labels (we have assumed that the name and address of the pharmacy and the words 'Keep out of the reach and sight of children' are pre-printed on the label):

Lederfen 300 mg capsules   **84**
Take ONE capsule in the morning and TWO at night.
Take with or after food.
1 of 2 containers.
Ms Barbara Ache   Date of dispensing

Lederfen 300 mg capsules   **84**
Take ONE capsule in the morning and TWO at night.
Take with or after food.
2 of 2 containers.
Ms Barbara Ache   Date of dispensing

Example 3.3 Continued

10. *Endorse prescription*: Stamp with pharmacy stamp to indicate completion.
11. *Destination of paperwork*: Send to the PPD at the end of the month.
12. *Identity check/counselling*:
    - Check patient's name and address.
    - Reinforce the dosage instructions; advise that the capsules are best taken with or after food to help prevent stomach irritation. Taking with milk will also 'protect' the stomach
    - Occasionally fenbufen causes skin to become more sensitive to sunlight. Use a sunscreen if affected and avoid sun beds.
    - Initially some patients may experience dizziness. Do not drive or operate machinery if affected.
    - Draw patient's attention to the patient information leaflet (PIL) and ask if she has any questions.

Example 3.4

You receive the following prescription in your pharmacy.

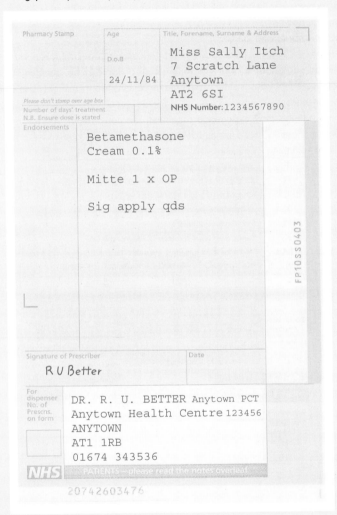

1. *Identity of order*: NHS prescription (FP10SS).
2. *Prescriber*: Doctor (general practitioner).
3. *Legally written?* No. The doctor failed to date the prescription. The prescription will need to be returned to the prescriber for addition of the date prior to dispensing.
4. *Clinical check (complete the following table)*:

DRUG	INDICATIONS	DOSE CHECK	REFERENCE
Betamethasone valerate	Severe inflammatory skin disorders	Apply thinly once or twice a day	*British National Formulary* 54th edition, section 13.4

Example 3.4 Continued

5. *Interactions*: There is only one item on the prescription form. However, it would also be advisable for the pharmacist or pharmacy technician to check the patient medication record (PMR) for any concurrent medication that could cause an interaction. In this case, the patient's PMR indicated that she also used E45 cream (an emollient).

6. *Suitability for patient*: Item prescribed is safe and suitable for a patient of this age but the instructions for use on the prescription (i.e. to apply four times a day) are not within the recommended limits. Contact prescriber to check his or her intentions and arrange for the prescription to be changed to a more acceptable frequency (for example, twice a day).

7. *Item(s) allowable on the NHS*: Yes (see Drug Tariff).

8. *Records to be made (including copies of the record(s))*: Make a note of the intervention on a clinical intervention form (see Figure 1.5).

9. *Process prescription (including example of label(s))*:
   - Prepare label for product.
   - Check Appendix 9 of the *British National Formulary* for supplementary labelling requirements. Betamethasone valerate: *British National Formulary* label number 28.
   - Remember to add pharmaceutical cautions to the label (For external use only).
   - Select tube of cream, remembering to check the expiry date and taking care that the cream and not the ointment has been selected (packaging of different forms may be very similar). As '1 × op' has been requested, the smallest pack size (30 g) should be supplied.
   - Label the primary container (i.e. the tube not the box).
   - Perform final check of item, label and prescription.
   - Pack in a suitable bag ready to give to patient/patient's representative.

   Labels (we have assumed that the name and address of the pharmacy and the words 'Keep out of the reach and sight of children' are pre-printed on the label):

Betamethasone Valerate Cream 0.1%	**30 g**
Apply TWICE a day.	
Spread thinly.	
For External Use Only.	
Miss Sally Itch	Date of dispensing

10. *Endorse prescription*: Stamp with pharmacy stamp to indicate completion.

11. *Destination of paperwork*: Send to the PPD at the end of the month.

12. *Identity check/counselling*.
    - Check patient's name and address.
    - Advise patient of change in directions of use without alarming the patient.
    - Reinforce new dosage instructions and advise to apply the cream thinly and that it is for external use only.
    - Draw patient's attention to the patient information leaflet (PIL) and ask if she has any questions.
    - She asks whether she should apply the cream before or after application of her E45 cream. What would be your answer be? You should advise the patient to apply her steroid cream (the betamethasone valerate cream) first. Allow an hour before applying the emollient (the E45 cream) to prevent the emollient from diluting the steroid cream.

Example 3.5

You receive the following prescription in your pharmacy:

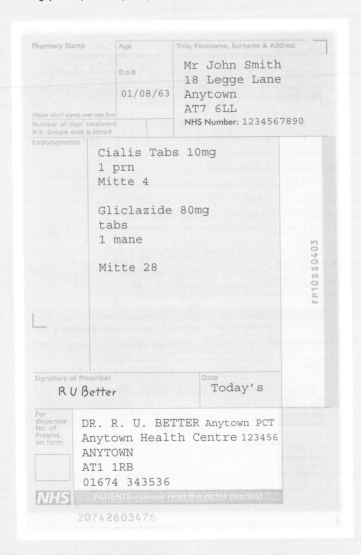

Pharmacy Stamp	Age	Title, Forename, Surname & Address
	D.o.B 01/08/63	Mr John Smith 18 Legge Lane Anytown AT7 6LL NHS Number: 1234567890

Please don't stamp over age box
Number of days' treatment
N.B. Ensure dose is stated
Endorsements

Cialis Tabs 10mg
1 prn
Mitte 4

Gliclazide 80mg
tabs
1 mane

Mitte 28

FP10SS0403

Signature of Prescriber
R U Better

Date
Today's

For dispenser
No. of
Prescns.
on form

DR. R. U. BETTER Anytown PCT
Anytown Health Centre 123456
ANYTOWN
AT1 1RB
01674 343536

NHS   PATIENTS – please read the notes overleaf

20742603476

1. *Identity of order*: NHS prescription (FP10SS).
2. *Prescriber*: Doctor (general practitioner).
3. *Legally written?* Yes.

Example 3.5 Continued

4. *Clinical check (complete the following table)*:

DRUG	INDICATIONS	DOSE CHECK	REFERENCE
Tadalafil	Erectile dysfunction	Initially 10 mg adjusted up to 20 mg as a single dose at least 30 minutes before sexual activity	*British National Formulary* 54th edition, section 7.4.5
Gliclazide	Diabetes mellitus	Initially 40–80 mg daily adjusted according to response max 160 mg as a single dose	*British National Formulary* 54th edition, section 6.1.2.1

5. *Interactions*: There is no interaction between tadalafil and gliclazide. However, it would also be advisable for the pharmacist or pharmacy technician to check the patient medication record (PMR) for any concurrent medication that could cause an interaction. In this case, the patient's PMR indicated that he has taken gliclazide for some time.

6. *Suitability for patient*: Items prescribed are safe and suitable for a patient of this age and the doses ordered on the prescription are within the recommended dose limits.

7. *Item(s) allowable on the NHS*: Yes, see *Drug Tariff*. The medication ordered indicates that the patient is diabetic therefore tadalafil may be prescribed under the selected list scheme. Return the prescription to the prescriber to ask him to add 'SLS' to the body of the prescription next to the order for Cialis so that it will be passed for payment by the PPD.

8. *Records to be made (including copies of the record(s))*: Make a note of the intervention on a clinical intervention form (see Figure 1.5).

9. *Process prescription (including example of label(s))*:
   - Prepare a label for each product.
   - Check Appendix 9 of the *British National Formulary* for supplementary labelling requirements (there are none).
   - Perform final check of items, labels and prescription.
   - Pack in a suitable bag ready to give to patient/patient's representative.
     Labels (we have assumed that the name and address of the pharmacy and the words 'Keep out of the reach and sight of children' are pre-printed on the label):

Cialis 10 mg Tablets   **4**
　　　Take ONE tablet when required.

Mr John Smith   Date of dispensing

Gliclazide 80 mg Tablets   **28**
　　　Take ONE tablet in the morning.

Mr John Smith   Date of dispensing

Example 3.5 Continued

10. *Endorse prescription*: Stamp with pharmacy stamp to indicate completion.
11. *Destination of paperwork*: Send to the PPD at the end of the month.
12. *Identity check/counselling*:
    - Check patient's name and address.
    - Reinforce the doses of the medication; remind him that gliclazide is best taken with breakfast.
    - Advise him that tadalafil should only be taken once per day as it may still be effective up to 36 hours after taking the tablet. Reassure him that tadalafil has few side-effects but should he have any problems with the medication you will be happy to discuss them with him.
    - Draw patient's attention to the patient information leaflets (PILs) and ask if he has any questions.

Example 3.6

You receive the following prescription in your pharmacy:

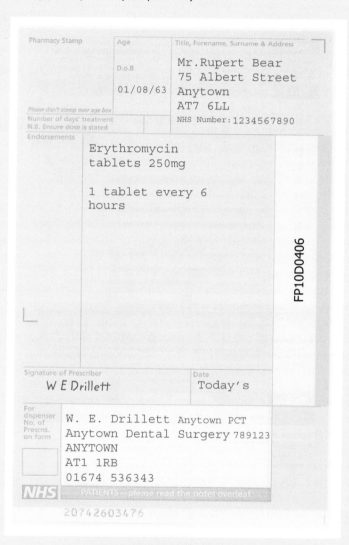

1. *Identity of order*: NHS prescription (FP10D).
2. *Prescriber*: Dentist.
3. *Legally written?* Yes.

Example 3.6 Continued

4. *Clinical check (complete the following table)*:

DRUG	INDICATIONS	DOSE CHECK	REFERENCE
Erythromycin	Oral infections	250–500 mg every 6 hours	*British National Formulary* 54th edition, section 5.1.5
Metronidazole	Oral infections	200 mg three times a day for 3 days	*British National Formulary* 54th edition, section 5.1.11

5. *Interactions*: There is only one drug on the prescription. However, it would also be advisable for the pharmacist or pharmacy technician to check the patient medication record (PMR) for any concurrent medication that could cause an interaction. In this case, the patient's PMR indicated that he has epilepsy stabilised on carbamazepine. There is an interaction between carbamazepine and erythromycin (the plasma concentration of carbamazepine is increased by erythromycin). You also note the patient is penicillin sensitive.

6. *Suitability for patient*: The item prescribed (erythromycin) is unsuitable for this patient as it will interact with his carbamazepine. You need to advise the dentist of the potentially serious interaction between erythromycin and carbamazepine and suggest an alternative. A usual alternative antibiotic would be a penicillin; however, you are also aware that the patient is penicillin sensitive. Therefore, another choice would be metronidazole 200 mg tds for 3 days (see 4 above) which will not interact with the carbamazepine, is suitable for a penicillin-sensitive patient and is allowable on NHS dental prescriptions. Ask the dentist to provide a new prescription.

7. *Item(s) allowable on the NHS*: Yes, see *Drug Tariff*.

8. *Records to be made (including copies of the record(s))*: Make a note of the intervention on a clinical intervention form (see Figure 1.5).

9. *Process prescription (including example of label(s))*:
   - Prepare label for product.
   - Check Appendix 9 of the *British National Formulary* for supplementary labelling requirements. Metronidazole: *British National Formulary* labels number 4, 9, 21, 25 and 27.
   - Perform final check of item, label and prescription.
   - Pack in a suitable bag ready to give to patient/patient's representative.
   Labels (we have assumed that the name and address of the pharmacy and the words 'Keep out of the reach and sight of children' are pre-printed on the label):

Metronidazole 200 mg Tablets   **9**

Take ONE tablet THREE times a day with or after food
with plenty of water.
Warning. Avoid alcoholic drink.
Take at regular intervals. Complete the prescribed course
unless otherwise directed.
Swallowed whole, not chewed.

Mr Rupert Bear   Date of dispensing

Example 3.6 Continued

10. *Endorse prescription*: Stamp with pharmacy stamp to indicate completion.
11. *Destination of paperwork*: Send to the PPD at the end of the month.
12. *Identity check/counselling*:
    • Check patient's name and address.
    • Explain change in medication without alarming the patient.
    • Reinforce the dose of the medication; explain need to avoid alcohol, take the medication at regular intervals (8 hourly) and complete the prescribed course, swallow the tablets whole and take with or after food with plenty of water.
    • Draw patient's attention to the patient information leaflet (PIL) and ask if he has any questions. The patient asks how long it will be before he can have a drink after completing the course of metronidazole as he will be going to a wedding next week. What answer would you give him? You should advise the patient that they should not drink alcohol during the antibiotic course and for 48 hours after taking the last tablet as the combination of the medication and alcohol causes unpleasant side-effects. This, along with additional information, can be found in the patient information leaflet (PIL).

Example 3.7

You receive the following prescription in your pharmacy:

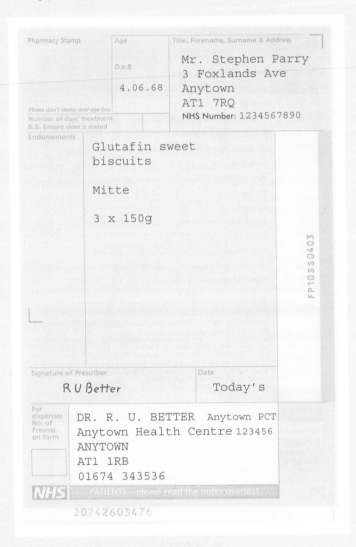

1. *Identity of order*: NHS prescription (FP10SS).
2. *Prescriber*: Doctor (general practitioner).
3. *Legally written?* Yes.

Example 3.7 Continued

4. *Clinical check (complete the following table):*

DRUG	INDICATIONS	DOSE CHECK	REFERENCE
Glutafin sweet biscuits	Gluten-sensitive enteropathies, coeliac disease	N/A	*British National Formulary* 54th edition, Appendix 7

5. *Interactions*: There is only one item on the prescription form. However, it would also be advisable for the pharmacist or pharmacy technician to check the patient medication record (PMR) for any concurrent medication that could cause an interaction. In this case, the patient's PMR indicated that there no interactions with any previous or concurrent medication.

6. *Suitability for patient*: Item prescribed is safe and suitable for a patient of this age.

7. *Item(s) allowable on the NHS*: Yes, provided it is prescribed as recommended by the Advisory Committee on Borderline Substances. Although the prescriber does not legally have to add 'ACBS' to the prescription it is good practice and indicates he is prescribing in accordance with the committee's advice. Return the prescription to the doctor to add 'ACBS' in the body of the prescription which will ensure the prescription will be passed for payment without further investigation.

8. *Records to be made (including copies of the record(s))*: Make a note of the intervention on a clinical intervention form (see Figure 1.5).

9. *Process prescription (including example of label(s))*:
   • Prepare 3 labels for the product.
   • Check Appendix 9 of the *British National Formulary* for supplementary labelling requirements (there are none).
   • Perform final check of item, label and prescription.
   • Pack in a suitable bag ready to give to patient/patient's representative.

Labels (we have assumed that the name and address of the pharmacy and the words 'Keep out of the reach and sight of children' are pre-printed on the label):

Glutafin Sweet Biscuits	**150 g**
Take as directed. 1 of 3 containers.	
Mr Stephen Parry	Date of dispensing

Glutafin Sweet Biscuits	**150 g**
Take as directed. 2 of 3 containers.	
Mr Stephen Parry	Date of dispensing

Glutafin Sweet Biscuits	**150 g**
Take as directed. 3 of 3 containers.	
Mr Stephen Parry	Date of dispensing

Example 3.7 Continued

10. *Endorse prescription*: Stamp with pharmacy stamp to indicate completion.
11. *Destination of paperwork*: Send to the PPD at the end of the month.
12. *Identity check/counselling*:
    • Check patient's name and address.
    • Give the patient the opportunity to ask any questions.
    You may wish to advise the patient of other items that are available on NHS prescription forms for patients with gluten sensitive enteropathies. Where would you find the necessary information? Information as to which products can be prescribed on an NHS prescription can be found by consulting the *Drug Tariff* (see Section 2.4). Specific foods (i.e. borderline substances) can be found in the respective parts of the *Drug Tariff for England and Wales* (see Section 2.4.1, Part XV) or the *Northern Ireland Drug Tariff* (see Section 2.4.2, Part X) or in Appendix 7 of the *British National Formulary* (see Section 2.6.1).

Example 3.8

You receive the following prescription in your pharmacy:

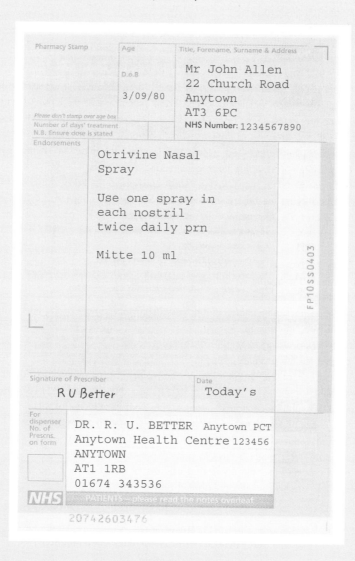

Pharmacy Stamp	Age	Title, Forename, Surname & Address
	D.o.B 3/09/80	Mr John Allen 22 Church Road Anytown AT3 6PC

Please don't stamp over age box

Number of days' treatment
N.B. Ensure dose is stated

NHS Number: 1234567890

Endorsements

Otrivine Nasal
Spray

Use one spray in
each nostril
twice daily prn

Mitte 10 ml

FP10SS0403

Signature of Prescriber

R U Better

Date

Today's

For
dispenser
No. of
Prescns.
on form

DR. R. U. BETTER Anytown PCT
Anytown Health Centre 123456
ANYTOWN
AT1 1RB
01674 343536

NHS PATIENTS – please read the notes overleaf

20742603476

1. *Identity of order*: NHS prescription (FP10SS).
2. *Prescriber*: Doctor (general practitioner).
3. *Legally written?* Yes.

Example 3.8 Continued

4. *Clinical check (complete the following table)*:

DRUG	INDICATIONS	DOSE CHECK	REFERENCE
Xylometazoline 0.1%	Symptomatic relief of nasal congestion	One spray in each nostril two–three times daily as necessary	*British National Formulary* 54th edition, section 12.2.2

5. *Interactions*: There is only one item on the prescription form. However, it would also be advisable for the pharmacist or pharmacy technician to check the patient medication record (PMR) for any concurrent medication that could cause an interaction. In this case, the patient's PMR indicated that there no interactions with any previous or concurrent medication.

6. *Suitability for patient*: Item prescribed is safe and suitable for a patient of this age and the dose ordered on the prescription is within the recommended dose limits.

7. *Item(s) allowable on the NHS*: No. Otrivine Nasal Spray is in the list of drugs and other substances not to be prescribed under the NHS Pharmaceutical Services (see Section 2.6.2). Contact prescriber and suggest he orders the item generically as xylometazoline 0.1% nasal spray (as xylometazoline is not in the list of drugs and other substances not to be prescribed under the NHS Pharmaceutical Services).

   Ask prescriber to provide a new prescription or (if the patient is not exempt from prescription charges) as this item is available for purchase from pharmacies (a 'P' medicine – see Section 1.3.2), offer to sell the item to the patient.

8. *Records to be made (including copies of the record(s))*: Make a note of the intervention on a clinical intervention form (see Figure 1.5).

9. *Process prescription (including example of label(s))*:
   - Prepare a label for the product.
   - Check Appendix 9 of the *British National Formulary* for supplementary labelling requirements (there are none).
   - Remember to add pharmaceutical cautions to the label (Not to be taken).
   - Perform final check of item, label and prescription (take care that the nasal spray has been selected and not similarly packed nasal drops).
   - Pack in a suitable bag ready to give to patient/patient's representative.

   Labels (we have assumed that the name and address of the pharmacy and the words 'Keep out of the reach and sight of children' are pre-printed on the label):

Xylometazoline 0.1% Nasal Spray	**10 ml**
Use ONE spray in each nostril TWICE daily when required.	
Not to be taken	
Mr John Allen	Date of dispensing

10. *Endorse prescription*: Stamp with pharmacy stamp to indicate completion.

Example 3.8 Continued

11. *Destination of paperwork*: Send to the PPD at the end of the month.
12. *Identity check/counselling*:
    - Check patient's name and address.
    - Reinforce the dosage instructions (see Section 9.7).
        - Blow your nose gently so that your nostrils are clear.
        - Wash your hands.
        - Shake the bottle.
        - Take the cap off the bottle.
        - Tilt your head slightly forward.
        - Close one nostril by gently pressing against the side of your nose with your finger.
        - Insert the tip of the nasal spray into the other nostril and start to breathe in slowly through your nose.
        - While you are still breathing in squirt one spray into the nostril, keeping the bottle upright.
        - Remove the spray from the nostril and breathe out through your mouth.
        - Tilt your head backwards to allow the spray to drain into the back of the nose. Repeat in other nostril.
        - Replace the cap on the bottle.
    - Some nasal sprays give an unpleasant taste as they drain into the back of the throat. A drink of water or other liquid will help to take this taste away.
    - Draw patient's attention to the patient information leaflet (PIL) and ask if he has any questions.

Example 3.9

You receive the following prescription in your pharmacy:

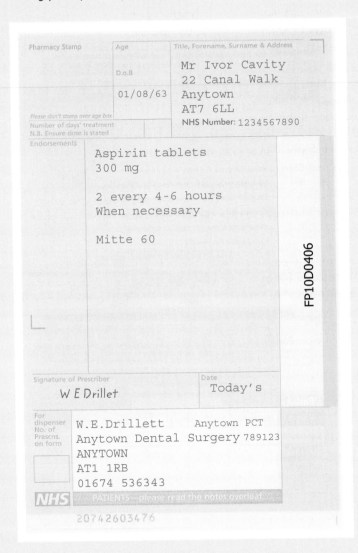

Pharmacy Stamp	Age	Title, Forename, Surname & Address
	D.o.B 01/08/63	Mr Ivor Cavity 22 Canal Walk Anytown AT7 6LL NHS Number: 1234567890

Please don't stamp over age box

Number of days' treatment
N.B. Ensure dose is stated

Endorsements

Aspirin tablets
300 mg

2 every 4-6 hours
When necessary

Mitte 60

FP10D0406

Signature of Prescriber   Date

W E Drillet   Today's

For dispenser
No. of
Prescns.
on form

W.E.Drillett   Anytown PCT
Anytown Dental Surgery 789123
ANYTOWN
AT1 1RB
01674 536343

NHS PATIENTS – please read the notes overleaf

20742603476

1. *Identity of order*: NHS prescription (FP10D).
2. *Prescriber*: Dentist.
3. *Legally written?* Yes.

Example 3.9 Continued

4. *Clinical check (complete the following table)*:

DRUG	INDICATIONS	DOSE CHECK	REFERENCE
Aspirin	Dental and orofacial pain	300–900 mg every 4–6 hours when necessary. Max 4 g daily	*British National Formulary* 54th edition, section 4.7.1

5. *Interactions*: There is only one item on the prescription form. However, it would also be advisable for the pharmacist or pharmacy technician to check the patient medication record (PMR) for any concurrent medication that could cause an interaction. In this case, the patient's PMR indicated that there no interactions with any previous or concurrent medication.
6. *Suitability for patient*: Item prescribed is safe and suitable for a patient of this age and the dose ordered on the prescription is within the recommended dose limits.
7. *Item(s) allowable on the NHS*: No. The *Dental Practitioner's Formulary* indicates that dentists are only allowed to prescribe aspirin dispersible tabs 300 mg on an NHS prescription form. Return prescription to the dentist for the addition of 'dispersible' or (if the patient is not exempt from prescription charges) as this item is available for purchase from pharmacies (a 'P' medicine – see Section 1.3.2), offer to sell the item to the patient.
8. *Records to be made (including copies of the record(s))*: Make a note of the intervention on a clinical intervention form (see Figure 1.5).
9. *Process prescription (including example of label(s))*:
   • Prepare a label for the product.
   • Check Appendix 9 of the *British National Formulary* for supplementary labelling requirements. Aspirin: *British National Formulary* labels number 13 and 21.
   • Perform final check of item, label and prescription.
   • Pack in a suitable bag ready to give to patient/patient's representative.
   Labels (we have assumed that the name and address of the pharmacy and the words 'Keep out of the reach and sight of children' are pre-printed on the label):

> **Aspirin 300 mg Dispersible Tablets**   **60**
> Dissolve TWO tablets in water and take every FOUR to
> SIX hours when necessary.
> Take with or after food.
> Dissolve or mix with water before taking.
>
> Mr Ivor Cavity   Date of dispensing

10. *Endorse prescription*: Stamp with pharmacy stamp to indicate completion.
11. *Destination of paperwork*: Send to the PPD at the end of the month.
12. *Identity check/counselling*:
    • Check patient's name and address.
    • Explain change in medication without alarming the patient.
    • Reinforce the dose of the medication, explain need to dissolve the tablets in water prior to taking and that best to take after food.
    • Draw patient's attention to the patient information leaflet (PIL) and ask if he has any questions.

Example 3.10

You receive the following prescription in your pharmacy.

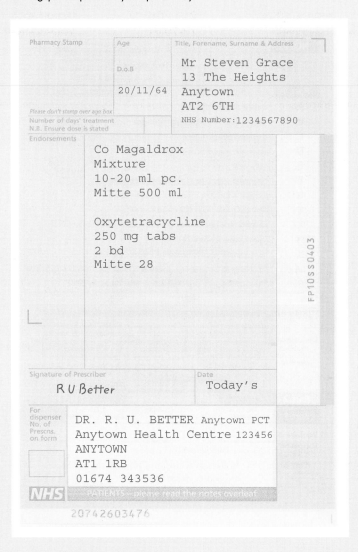

1. *Identity of order*: NHS prescription (FP10SS).
2. *Prescriber*: Doctor (general practitioner).
3. *Legally written?* Yes.

Example 3.10 Continued

4. *Clinical check (complete the following table):*

DRUG	INDICATIONS	DOSE CHECK	REFERENCE
Co-magaldrox	Dyspepsia	10–20 mL 20–60 minutes after food and at bedtime or when required	*British National Formulary* 54th edition, section 1.1.1
Oxytetracycline	Rosacea	500 mg twice daily	*British National Formulary* 54th edition, section 13.6.2

5. *Interactions*: There is an interaction between the antacid (co-magaldrox) and the tetracycline anti-bacterial (oxytetracycline). The tetracycline chelates with the aluminium and magnesium ions in the co-magaldrox, reducing the absorption of the tetracycline. However, the two medications can be taken concurrently providing there is a suitable dosing interval. Therefore, in this situation there is no need to contact the prescriber as simply advising the patient of how to take medications in order to get optimum benefit will suffice.

   However, it would also be advisable for the pharmacist or pharmacy technician to check the patient medication record (PMR) for any additional concurrent medication that could cause an interaction. In this case, the patient's PMR indicated that they are not taking any additional medication.

6. *Suitability for patient*: The items prescribed are safe and suitable for a patient of this age.
7. *Item(s) allowable on the NHS*: Yes.
8. *Records to be made (including copies of the record(s))*: None.
9. *Process prescription (including example of label(s))*:
   - Prepare a label for each product.
   - Check Appendix 9 of the *British National Formulary* for supplementary labelling requirements. Co-magaldrox: no additional *British National Formulary* labels but the pharmaceutical caution to 'Shake the bottle' should be added for the suspension. Oxytetracycline: *British National Formulary* labels number 7, 9 and 23.
   - Perform final check of items, labels and prescription.
   - Pack in a suitable bag ready to give to patient/patient's representative.

Labels (we have assumed that the name and address of the pharmacy and the words 'Keep out of the reach and sight of children' are pre-printed on the label):

e.g.   **Example 3.10** Continued

Co-magaldrox Mixture   **500 ml**

Take TWO to FOUR 5 ml spoonfuls after food.
Shake the bottle.

Mr Steven Grace   Date of dispensing

Oxytetracycline 250mg Tablets   **28**

Take TWO tablets TWICE a day an hour before food
or on an empty stomach.
Do not take milk, indigestion remedies, or medicines
containing iron or zinc at the same time of day
as this medicine.
Take at regular intervals. Complete the prescribed course
unless otherwise directed.

Mr Steven Grace   Date of dispensing

---

10. *Endorse prescription*: Stamp with pharmacy stamp to indicate completion.
11. *Destination of paperwork*: Send to the PPD at the end of the month.
12. *Identity check/counselling*:
    - Check patient's name and address.
    - Advise patient to take the oxytetracycline two tablets twice a day, at regular intervals and to take an hour before food or on an empty stomach. Do not take milk, indigestion remedies or medicines containing iron or zinc at the same time as they will react with the oxytetracycline and prevent its absorption.
    - Advise patient to take the co-magaldrox two to four 5 mL spoonfuls after food. This preparation is an antacid and therefore could interact with the oxytetracycline. However if you separate the dose of antibiotic and antacid by 2–3 hours there should be no significant interaction. If after taking oxytetracycline you remain in an upright position rather than lying down this should also help to speed up the passage of the drug through the digestive system and speed up its absorption.
    - Draw patient's attention to the patient information leaflets (PILs) and ask if he has any questions. He asks if he can drink alcohol while taking the antibiotics. What would be your response? You should advise the patient that it is alright to drink alcohol (in moderation) while taking oxytetracycline tablets.

Example 3.11

You receive the following prescription in your pharmacy:

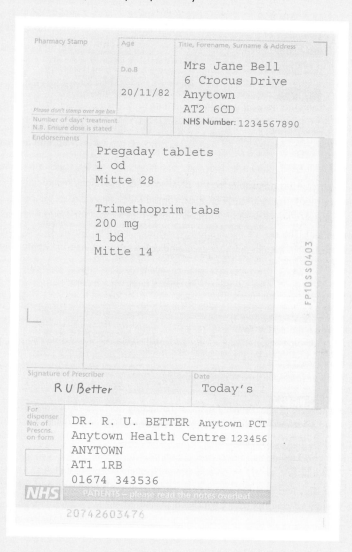

Pharmacy Stamp	Age	Title, Forename, Surname & Address
	D.o.B 20/11/82	Mrs Jane Bell 6 Crocus Drive Anytown AT2 6CD NHS Number: 1234567890

Please don't stamp over age box
Number of days' treatment
N.B. Ensure dose is stated
Endorsements

Pregaday tablets
1 od
Mitte 28

Trimethoprim tabs
200 mg
1 bd
Mitte 14

FP10SS0403

Signature of Prescriber   *R U Better*

Date   Today's

For dispenser
No. of
Prescns.
on form

DR. R. U. BETTER Anytown PCT
Anytown Health Centre 123456
ANYTOWN
AT1 1RB
01674 343536

NHS   PATIENTS – please read the notes overleaf

20742603476

1. *Identity of order*: NHS prescription (FP10SS).
2. *Prescriber*: Doctor (general practitioner).
3. *Legally written?* Yes.

Example 3.11 Continued

4. *Clinical check (complete the following table)*:

DRUG	INDICATIONS	DOSE CHECK	REFERENCE
Iron and folic acid	Prevention of iron and folate deficiency in pregnancy	1 tablet daily	*British National Formulary* 54th edition, section 9.1.1.1
Trimethoprim	Lower urinary tract infections	200 mg every 12 hours	*British National Formulary* 54th edition, section 5.1.13
Amoxicillin	Lower urinary tract infections	3 g repeated after 10–12 hours	*British National Formulary* 54th edition, section 5.1.13

5. *Interactions*: There is no interaction between the Pregaday tablets and the trimethoprim tablets. However, it would also be advisable for the pharmacist or pharmacy technician to check the patient medication record (PMR) for any additional concurrent medication that could cause an interaction. In this case, the patient's PMR indicated that they are not taking any additional medication.
6. *Suitability for patient*: The use of the Pregaday suggests that the patient is pregnant and so the use of folate antagonists, like trimethoprim, is contraindicated. You will need to contact the prescriber with a suggested alternative.
    Amoxicillin is safe to use in pregnancy and therefore would be the drug of choice assuming patient is not penicillin sensitive. Ask prescriber to change to amoxicillin sachets 3 g, 1 every 12 hours, mitte 2 (see 4 above).
7. *Item(s) allowable on the NHS*: Yes.
8. *Records to be made (including copies of the record(s))*: Make a note of the intervention on a clinical intervention form (see Figure 1.5).
9. *Process prescription (including example of label(s))*:
    • Prepare a label for each product.
    • Check Appendix 9 of the *British National Formulary* for supplementary labelling requirements. Pregaday: no additional *British National Formulary* labels. Amoxicillin sachets: *British National Formulary* labels number 9 and 13.
    • Perform final check of items, labels and prescription.
    • Pack in a suitable bag ready to give to patient/patient's representative.
Labels (we have assumed that the name and address of the pharmacy and the words 'Keep out of the reach and sight of children' are pre-printed on the label):

Example 3.11 Continued

Pregaday Tablets   **28**
                     Take ONE daily.

Mrs Jane Bell   Date of dispensing

Amoxicillin 3 g Sachets   **2**
Take the contents of ONE sachet every TWELVE hours.
        Dissolve or mix with water before taking.
    Take at regular intervals. Complete the prescribed
            course unless otherwise directed.

Mrs Jane Bell   Date of dispensing

---

10. *Endorse prescription*: Stamp with pharmacy stamp to indicate completion.
11. *Destination of paperwork*: Send to the PPD at the end of the month.
12. *Identity check/counselling*:
    - Check patient's name and address.
    - Advise patient to take one Pregaday tablet daily.
    - Advise of the change in antibiotic without alarming the patient and explain treatment consists of two sachets to be taken 12 hours apart.
    - Explain how to dissolve the contents of each sachet in water prior to taking it.
    - Reassure the patient that the treatment is safe during pregnancy.
    - Draw patient's attention to the patient information leaflets (PILs) and ask if she has any questions. She asks if she can drink alcohol while taking the antibiotics. What would be your response? You should advise the patient that it is alright to drink alcohol while taking amoxicillin tablets. However, if the patient is pregnant, it would be advisable to avoid alcohol during her pregnancy to prevent any harm to the fetus.

Example 3.12

You receive the following prescription in your pharmacy:

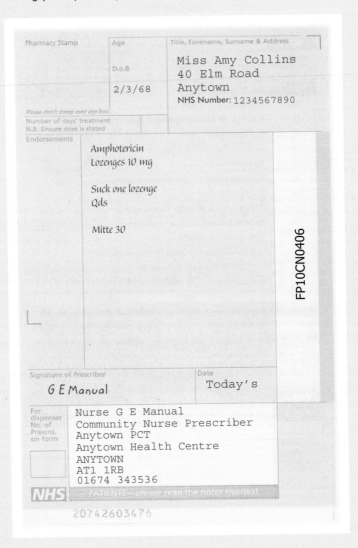

1. *Identity of order*: NHS prescription (FP10CN).
2. *Prescriber*: Community nurse.
3. *Legally written?* Yes.

Example 3.12 Continued

4. *Clinical check (complete the following table):*

DRUG	INDICATIONS	DOSE CHECK	REFERENCE
Amphotericin	Oral and perioral fungal infections	One lozenge four times a day for 10–15 days	*British National Formulary* 54th edition, section 12.3.2
Nystatin	Oral and perioral fungal infections	100 000 Units four times a day after food usually for seven days Continue for 48 hours after lesions have resolved	*British National Formulary* 54th edition, section 12.3.3

5. *Interactions*: There is only one item on the prescription form. However, it would also be advisable for the pharmacist or pharmacy technician to check the patient medication record (PMR) for any concurrent medication that could cause an interaction. In this case, the patient's PMR indicated that there no interactions with any previous or concurrent medication.

6. *Suitability for patient*: Item prescribed is safe and suitable for a patient of this age and the dose ordered on the prescription is within the recommended dose limits.

7. *Item(s) allowable on the NHS*: No, see *Drug Tariff*. The amphotericin are not listed in the *Nurse Prescribers' Formulary* for community practitioners and so cannot be prescribed by a community nurse on an NHS prescription form (see Section 3.2.3).

    Contact the nurse and suggest nystatin oral suspension 1 mL (100 000 units) four times a day as an alternative that she is allowed to prescribe (see 4 above). Ask her to provide a new prescription. She explains that the patient had previously been prescribed amphotericin by the doctor but as she now realises it is outside the list from which she may prescribe she will provide a new prescription for nystatin oral suspension.

8. *Records to be made (including copies of the record(s))*: Make a note of the intervention on a clinical intervention form (see Figure 1.5).

9. *Process prescription (including example of label(s))*:
   - Prepare a label for the product.
   - Check Appendix 9 of the *British National Formulary* for supplementary labelling requirements. Nystatin oral suspension: *British National Formulary* labels number 9 (and counselling – use of pipette, hold in mouth after food).
   - Remember to add pharmaceutical cautions to the label (Shake the bottle).
   - Perform final check of item, label and prescription.
   - Pack in a suitable bag ready to give to patient/patient's representative.

Labels (we have assumed that the name and address of the pharmacy and the words 'Keep out of the reach and sight of children' are pre-printed on the label):

Example 3.12 Continued

> **Nystatin Oral suspension (100,000 Units/ml) 30 ml**
> Apply the contents of ONE dropper (1 mL) to the
> mouth and gums.
> FOUR times a day after food.
> Take at regular intervals. Complete the prescribed course
> unless otherwise directed.
> Shake the bottle.
>
> Miss Amy Collins   Date of dispensing

10. *Endorse prescription*: Stamp with pharmacy stamp to indicate completion.
11. *Destination of paperwork*: Send to the PPD at the end of the month.
12. *Identity check/counselling*:
    - Check patient's name and address.
    - Explain change in medication without alarming the patient.
    - Reinforce the dosage instructions:
      – Fill the dropper to the '1 mL' mark.
      – Squirt the contents of the dropper around the mouth and gums.
      – Keep the suspension in the mouth as long as possible.
      – Do not eat or drink anything for one hour after using the suspension.
      – If you wear dentures remove them before applying the suspension.
    - Draw patient's attention to the patient information leaflet (PIL) and ask if she has any questions.

3.6 Chapter summary

This chapter has taken the concepts covered in Chapter 2 and has used them to discuss the points it is necessary to become familiar with in order to supply medication via an NHS prescription form in the community. This includes details on the different prescribers who prescribe on NHS prescription forms, a discussion of the general dispensing procedure for NHS prescriptions in the community and information on the role and function of Patient Group Directions (PGDs).

A collection of worked examples has been provided and it is suggested that the student pharmacist or pharmacy technician works though these examples and ensures that they are familiar with the key learning points.

The next chapter (Chapter 4) will cover NHS medication supply within hospitals and some other residential healthcare establishments.

4

NHS supply within hospitals

Upon completion of this chapter, you should be able to:

- understand the supply of medication to hospital in-patients including:
  - in-patient drug charts
  - discharge medication (TTOs/TTAs)
  - patients' own drugs (POD) schemes
  - dispensing for discharge schemes
  - self-medication schemes
- understand the supply of medication to hospital out-patients
- complete a number of worked examples of NHS hospital prescriptions and the dispensing process.

4.1 Introduction

This chapter will cover the supply of medicines via the National Health Service (NHS) within hospitals. Throughout this chapter, the term 'hospital' is used, but the types of supply described may also apply to other residential style care establishments, for example, some care homes and hospices. It should be noted that the procedures discussed in this chapter for NHS hospitals will be equally applicable to the supply of medication within a private sector establishment. The only difference being that the medication and care is entirely funded by the patient (or their healthcare insurance company).

The dispensing process within hospitals is similar in a number of ways to the supply of items on NHS prescriptions within community pharmacy (see Chapters 2 and 3). The main difference is that the supply is not usually on an NHS prescription form (except in some cases where the prescription originates from a prescriber within a hospital but it is intended to be dispensed within the community).

4.1.1 In-patient drug charts

All hospital in-patients will have a personal drug chart. This chart details all the medication that is supplied to a patient during their stay. Each hospital has its own style of drug chart, but they are similar in layout.

Commonly, in-patient drug charts are approximately A4 in size and consist of four sides (i.e. when opened out are approximately A3 in size). The front page contains the patient's details at the top of the page, along with any known sensitivities (both medication sensitivities and sensitivities to other items, such as latex). This is often followed by a section detailing 'one-off' drugs. These are drugs that were or are to be given to patients at a particular time, but will not necessarily require repeated administration. A good example would be drugs administered in theatre during a surgical procedure. The front page is often completed by a section detailing any 'when required' or 'PRN' drugs. This section details medication that can be administered if required, for example some analgesics or medication for intermittent constipation. Figure 4.1 shows an example of the front page of an in-patient drug chart.

Pages 2 and 3 of the in-patient drug chart usually detail the regular medication to be administered. Each different drug is detailed in a separate section of the chart, giving the drug name, strength, frequency and any other administration details. An example is shown in Figure 4.2.

The final page of an in-patient drug chart usually details the administration of any intravenous fluids. In addition, some hospitals have a section detailing the patient's discharge medication. In other hospitals, the discharge medication is listed on a separate discharge prescription (see Section 4.2.2). An example of the final page of an in-patient drug chart is shown in Figure 4.3.

4.1.2 The role of the ward pharmacist

The ward pharmacist is an important member of any hospital healthcare team with a number of key responsibilities. They will review each patient's drug chart on a daily basis and annotate the chart as appropriate:

- If the drug name is unclear or written on the drug chart as a proprietary product, the ward pharmacist will annotate the entry with the correct generic name (hospital prescribing is not constrained by the same rules regarding the supply of proprietary items as those NHS prescription forms originating in the community (see Section 2.4.1, Part VIII)). If the

drug's bioavailability varies with different proprietary presentations, the brand of the drug is usually added in brackets after the generic name.
- The ward pharmacist will annotate the 'Pharmacy' box on the chart with information to help the nursing staff to locate the medication. This will include annotating whether the item is a ward stock item (see Section 4.2.1), an item that the patient has brought into the hospital (which is suitable for use during their stay) (see Section 4.2.2) or an item that has been specifically ordered by the ward pharmacist for administration to the patient during their stay (see Section 4.2.1) according to the directions of the prescriber.

4.2 Supply of medication within a hospital setting

The supply of medication by the pharmacy department within a hospital can be divided into three main categories:

- in-patient supply (see Section 4.2.1)
- discharge medication (see Section 4.2.2)
- out-patient supply (see Section 4.2.3).

> ### Key point 4.1
>
> The supply of medication by the pharmacy department within a hospital can be divided into three main categories:
>
> - in-patient supply
> - discharge medication
> - out-patient supply.

4.2.1 In-patient supply

Many patients admitted to hospital will require some form of medication to be administered at some point during their stay. The type of medication supplied may depend on the reason for admission but patients may be on other

AH NHS Trust	Anywhere Hospital Anywhere

Surname:		Ward:	
First Name:		Consultant:	
Patient Number:		Date of Birth:	
Known Sensitivities:			

Once only medication

Date	Time	Drug	Dose	Route	Signature
Pharmacy		Administered		Time	
Date	Time	Drug	Dose	Route	Signature
Pharmacy		Administered		Time	
Date	Time	Drug	Dose	Route	Signature
Pharmacy		Administered		Time	
Date	Time	Drug	Dose	Route	Signature
Pharmacy		Administered		Time	

As required medication

Drug name:	Dose	Route	Date	Time	Dose	Admin
Frequency:	Date	Pharmacy				
Signature:						
Drug name:	Dose	Route	Date	Time	Dose	Admin
Frequency:	Date	Pharmacy				
Signature:						
Drug name:	Dose	Route	Date	Time	Dose	Admin
Frequency:	Date	Pharmacy				
Signature:						
Drug name:	Dose	Route	Date	Time	Dose	Admin
Frequency:	Date	Pharmacy				
Signature:						

Figure 4.1 An example of the front page of an in-patient drug chart.

Surname:				Ward:					
First Name:				Consultant:					
Patient Number:				Date of Birth:					
Regular medication		Date:							
Drug name:	Frequency	08.00							
		10.00							
Signature:	Route	12.00							
		14.00							
Pharmacy	Date	18.00							
		22.00							
Drug name:	Frequency	08.00							
		10.00							
Signature:	Route	12.00							
		14.00							
Pharmacy	Date	18.00							
		22.00							
Drug name:	Frequency	08.00							
		10.00							
Signature:	Route	12.00							
		14.00							
Pharmacy	Date	18.00							
		22.00							
Drug name:	Frequency	08.00							
		10.00							
Signature:	Route	12.00							
		14.00							
Pharmacy	Date	18.00							
		22.00							
Drug name:	Frequency	08.00							
		10.00							
Signature:	Route	12.00							
		14.00							
Pharmacy	Date	18.00							
		22.00							
Drug name:	Frequency	08.00							
		10.00							
Signature:	Route	12.00							
		14.00							
Pharmacy	Date	18.00							
		22.00							
Drug name:	Frequency	08.00							
		10.00							
Signature:	Route	12.00							
		14.00							
Pharmacy	Date	18.00							
		22.00							

Figure 4.2   An example of the second and third page of an in-patient drug chart.

Anywhere Hospital NHS Trust					
Surname:				Ward:	
First Name:				Consultant:	
Patient Number:				Date of Birth:	
Intravenous medication					
Date	Time	Drug and dose	Duration	Route	Signature
Pharmacy		Administered		Time	
Date	Time	Drug and dose	Duration	Route	Signature
Pharmacy		Administered		Time	
Date	Time	Drug and dose	Duration	Route	Signature
Pharmacy		Administered		Time	
Date	Time	Drug and dose	Duration	Route	Signature
Pharmacy		Administered		Time	
Date	Time	Drug and dose	Duration	Route	Signature
Pharmacy		Administered		Time	
Date	Time	Drug and dose	Duration	Route	Signature
Pharmacy		Administered		Time	
Discharge medication					
Drug		Dosage and Instructions			Pharmacy
Prescriber's name:					
Prescriber's bleep:					
Prescriber's signature:					
Date:					

Figure 4.3   An example of the final page of an in-patient drug chart.

medication which is not related to the reason for admission (for example, a hypertensive patient admitted to hospital for the removal of their appendix will need to continue their antihypertensive medication along with any additional medication that may be prescribed for their appendectomy).

More often than not, patients admitted for medical conditions will require a greater range of drugs than those admitted for surgical procedures, who may only require analgesics and antibiotics to be administered. In view of these differences, different wards within a hospital will have a different range of 'stock' drugs. If a patient is prescribed medication which is available from the ward stock, this can simply be administered from the stock each time. Maintaining a supply of these drugs is then a simple matter of maintaining the relevant stock levels, a task usually undertaken by pharmacy assistants, under the supervision of a pharmacy technician.

However, it is likely that many patients will require drugs which are not stock items on the particular ward on which they are staying. In these cases, a patient-specific in-patient order is completed (commonly by the ward pharmacist) to order this specific item for the patient. Although the item is normally labelled, it is usually with a reduced set of information (for example, usually just the title of the item, the batch number and expiry date). There are two reasons for this: (a) the item will not be given to the patient to take, it will be administered by the nurses from the drugs trolley, and (b) the dose of the item may alter during the patient's stay and as any changes will be noted on the patient's drug chart, the dosage instructions on the chart may differ from those on the label, leading to potential dosing errors.

Key point 4.2

In-patient medication is an item ordered for a specific patient for use during their stay on the ward. In-patient orders will be for medication not usually kept as 'stock' on the patient's ward.

An example of an in-patient order form is shown in Figure 4.4. The order will usually specify the name of the patient, the patient's ward and the name and strength of the drug required. Note that the dosage of the drug is not usually specified on the order as this will be detailed on the patient's drug chart. The dosage would only be specified on the order (and therefore the label) if the medication was being supplied as part of a dispensing for discharge scheme (see Section 4.2.2).

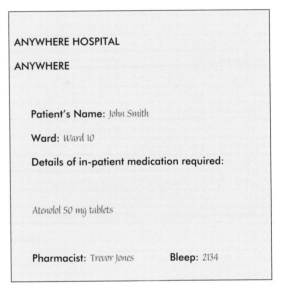

ANYWHERE HOSPITAL

ANYWHERE

Patient's Name: John Smith

Ward: Ward 10

Details of in-patient medication required:

Atenolol 50 mg tablets

Pharmacist: Trevor Jones   Bleep: 2134

Figure 4.4 An example of an in-patient order.

4.2.2 Discharge medication

Discharge medication, also termed TTO (to take out) or TTA (to take away) medication, is a supply of medication given to a patient on discharge. Enough medication is supplied to allow for the discharge letter to be sent to the patient's general practitioner (GP) and for them to take over the regular prescribing of the patient's medication (usually 14 days' supply). TTOs are either written on a specific section of the patient's drug chart (see Figure 4.3) or on hospital-specific forms (Figure 4.5). TTOs require the same information as any other prescription (including directions for administration for the patient to follow), the difference being that they may only be dispensed within the hospital.

ANYWHERE HOSPITAL

ANYWHERE

DISCHARGE MEDICATION

Patient's Name: *John Smith*

Patient's address: *10 Canal Street, Anywhere*

Ward: *Ward 10*

Details of in-patient medication required:

Drug	Dosage and Instructions	Pharmacy
Atenolol	*50 mg om*	

Prescriber: *William Henry*   Bleep: *5432*

Figure 4.5   An example of a TTO (discharge medication).

Key point 4.3

Discharge medication is also termed TTO (to take out) or TTA (to take away) medication. It is a hospital-based prescription for a specific patient used to provide the patient with a supply (usually 14 days) of medication upon discharge.

Patients' own drugs (PODs)

Recent changes in hospital procedures have allowed the use of drugs brought into hospital by patients. This prevents unnecessary wastage and reduces the hospital's drugs bill.

Before these schemes were introduced, patients were asked to bring any medication they were taking into hospital so that doctors could gather an accurate patient medication history upon admission. This information was transferred to the patient's in-patient chart and subsequent administration of the medication in the hospital took place either via ward stock or patient-specific in-patient orders (see Section 4.2.1). Upon discharge, patients were given a standard 14-day supply of medication via a TTO. In many cases, the patient's original medication was not returned to them and was just discarded.

With a patients' own drugs scheme, patients still bring in their medication from home and this is then assessed by the ward pharmacist during the admission process. If there is sufficient medication left, in a suitable condition and labelled appropriately, this is added to the drugs trolley and used for that patient during drug rounds. Upon discharge, if there is still sufficient medication remaining and there has been no change to the dosage, etc., the patient is given their own medication back, rather than receiving newly dispensed medication from the hospital pharmacy. In addition to the obvious cost savings, if all the medication the patient is to be discharged on is their own, this will also speed up the discharge process.

Key point 4.4

Patients' own drugs (POD) schemes allow the use of medication brought into the hospital by patients. Medication is checked by the ward pharmacists for suitability and the patient's drug chart annotated appropriately.

Dispensing for discharge

In addition to POD schemes, another system recently introduced into hospital medication supply practice is the dispensing for discharge scheme. This is a combination of an in-patient order and a TTO. Any medication required as an in-patient order is labelled as for a TTO. When the patient is then discharged, the medication and labelling is re-checked by the ward pharmacist and if suitable, the medication is then used as TTO medication.

In order for this system to work effectively, more than 14 days' supply is usually supplied in the first place to allow for both the in-patient and TTO supply. This reduces the instances of items being dispensed twice for a patient (i.e. once as an in-patient order and once as a TTO) and therefore reduces both dispensing time and cost.

Key point 4.5

Dispensing for discharge schemes allow in-patient medication to be labelled for use upon discharge. Usually, in excess of 14 days' supply is provided to allow for use both during the patient's stay and upon discharge. Before discharge, the ward pharmacist will verify that the medication is still suitable for use (for example, checking that the dose has not altered since original dispensing).

Self-medication schemes

Under some circumstances the use of self-medication schemes is appropriate. Here, instead of the medication being placed on the ward drugs trolley for administration by the nursing staff, the patient is given the medicine for self-administration. The medication may be kept in a locked cupboard by the patient's bed, for example, and a key given to the patient.

Patients operating within this scheme are first assessed for suitability (usually by the ward pharmacist). Although this scheme would not be suitable for many patients, there are a significant number of patients who are perfectly capable of self-administration of medication. This not only enables a patient to be in control of their own medication, but also helps to reduce staff workload.

4.2.3 Out-patient supply

Patients also visit hospitals for out-patient appointments. This is where the patient comes to the hospital to see a specialist, usually in a specific clinic. Depending on the individual circumstances, an out-patient may require a supply of prescribed drugs. This prescribing will usually be the role of the patient's GP, however, as with the prescribing of TTO medication (see Section 4.2.2) it may take time for the details of the medication to be prescribed to reach the patient's GP by letter.

In these circumstances, it may be necessary for the hospital doctor to provide a supply of the medication. This is usually achieved via an internal out-patient supply form, which can only be dispensed within the hospital pharmacy. Out-patients supply forms are specific to each hospital and contain the same type of information as an NHS prescription form.

Although it is usual for any prescriptions issued by hospital prescribers to out-patients to be dispensed within the hospital (and therefore via an out-patient supply form), there may be situations where it is necessary for the item to be supplied within the community. In these situations, it is necessary for the prescriber to prescribe the item(s) via an NHS prescription form (see Section 2.2).

4.3 The dispensing procedure for hospital supply

As with the supply of medication against an NHS prescription form (see Chapter 3), the supply of medication within a hospital setting can be divided into a number of distinct sections.

Upon receipt of an order for medication within a hospital, the following procedure should be followed:

1. Identify the order type (see Section 4.3.1 below).
2. Check all necessary information is present on the order (see Section 4.3.2).
3. If appropriate, perform a clinical check on the prescription (see Section 4.3.3).

4. Dispense and label the item(s) as necessary (see Section 4.3.4).
5. Check the item(s) dispensed is/are correct and labelled appropriately. Ideally this check would be performed by a colleague (i.e. an independent check) but when working alone, the pharmacist will need to check the item(s) themselves (see Section 4.3.5).
6. If appropriate, pass the item(s) to the patient and counsel the patient in the use of the medication (see Section 4.3.6).

Key point 4.6

The dispensing procedure for hospital orders:

1. Identify the order type.
2. Check all necessary information is present on the order.
3. If appropriate, perform a clinical check on the prescription.
4. Dispense and label the item(s) as necessary.
5. Check the item(s) dispensed is/are correct and labelled appropriately.
6. If appropriate, pass the item(s) to the patient and counsel the patient in the use of the medication.

4.3.1 Identify the order type

As discussed above, medication orders within the hospital setting will fall into one of three types:

- in-patient orders (see Section 4.2.1) (Remember that some in-patient orders may be labelled for use upon discharge – dispensing for discharge (see Section 4.2.2).)
- TTOs (see Section 4.2.2)
- out-patient prescriptions (see Section 4.2.3).

It is important to establish which type of medication order has been presented as different orders will have different requirements (for example, labelling).

4.3.2 Check all necessary information is present on the order

Different hospital orders will require differing pieces of information to be present.

- In-patient orders (see Figure 4.4) will usually specify the name of the patient, the ward they are on and the name and strength of the drug required. Note that the dosage of the drug is not usually specified on the order as this will be detailed on the patient's drug chart. The dosage would usually only be specified on the order (and therefore the label) if the medication was being supplied as part of a dispensing for discharge scheme (see Section 4.2.2).
- TTOs are either written on a specific section of the patient's drug chart (see Figure 4.3) or on hospital-specific forms (see Figure 4.5). TTOs require the same information as an NHS prescription form (see list below), the difference being that these may only be dispensed within the hospital.
- Out-patient prescription forms are specific to each hospital and contain the same type of information as an NHS prescription form.

TTOs and out-patient prescription forms will include the following (see Section 2.2.7):

- the patient's details
- details of the medication to be supplied
- the signature of the prescriber
- the address of the prescriber
- an indication of the prescriber type
- an appropriate date.

Key point 4.7

- In-patient orders will usually specify the name of the patient, the ward the patient is on and the name and strength of the drug required.
- TTOs and out-patient prescription forms will specify the patient's details, details of the medication to be supplied, the signature of the prescriber, the address of the prescriber, an indication of the prescriber type and an appropriate date.

4.3.3 If appropriate, perform a clinical check on the prescription

In addition to the patient's name and details of the ward they are staying on, *in-patient orders* will usually only contain the name and strength of the drug required. Therefore, it is the responsibility of the ward pharmacist to perform the clinical check on the medication on the ward. This will involve checking the dose and frequency of administration (as details of the dose and frequency of administration will be detailed in the in-patient drug chart).

For *out-patient prescriptions*, it is the responsibility of the pharmacist to perform a clinical check on the prescription. This will follow the same stages that are followed when performing a clinical check on an NHS prescription (see Section 3.3.4). The main key difference is that the hospital pharmacy staff will not have access to the patient's patient medical record (PMR) as this is usually held on the computer of the patient's usual community pharmacy. Therefore, it will not usually be possible to check for interactions with previously prescribed medication. In summary, the following points need to be considered:

- the patient
- the dose of the medication
- the patient's condition
- other medication the patient may be taking.

For *TTOs*, the clinical check (as outlined above) will happen in one of two ways. The first is for the clinical check to be performed by a pharmacist in the hospital pharmacy when the TTO arrives for dispensing (usually accompanied by the patient's in-patient drug chart to enable a full clinical check to be performed).

Alternatively, the ward pharmacist will perform the clinical check on the ward and 'sign off' the TTO for dispensing before sending it down to the hospital pharmacy. In this case, it would be possible for the items on the TTO to be dispensed by a pharmacy technician and then the dispensing check could be performed by a (second) accredited checking technician (see Section 4.3.5).

4.3.4 Dispense and label the item(s) as necessary

Unless the item is being dispensed as part of a dispensing for discharge scheme (see Section 4.2.2, in-patient orders do not usually have an additional or individual patient specific labels added. In some hospitals, they may be labelled with the patient's name and ward (so that the ward staff can easily identify who the medication is for when it arrives on the ward and then place it in the correct section of the ward drugs trolley) but not usually the dose or frequency of the medication.

For TTOs and out-patient prescriptions, they will be dispensed and labelled as for NHS prescriptions in the community (see Section 3.3.5). Remember that the label(s) will be generated first followed by the item(s) being dispensed.

The only difference when dispensing an item within a hospital compared with an NHS prescription form in a community setting is that all items (except in certain cases, for example, some sustained-release formulations) will be prescribed generically. Therefore the hospital pharmacy will, where possible, supply generic (and not the more expensive branded) versions of the drug(s) prescribed. Even if the items are prescribed by their proprietary name, where possible, generic items will be supplied. This is termed generic substitution and assists in reducing healthcare costs within secondary care.

4.3.5 Check the item(s) dispensed is/are correct and labelled appropriately.

As with items dispensed against NHS prescriptions within the community, once all the above points have been followed, it is important that the label(s) and dispensed item(s) are checked against the prescription form to ensure they are correct.

Ideally this check should be performed by a second competent colleague. However, there may be some situations where the pharmacist is working alone. In these cases, a second check still needs to take place and the pharmacist will need to perform this second check him- or herself.

In hospitals nowadays, many pharmacy technicians are qualified accredited checking technicians. This means that so long as the prescription has been clinically checked by a pharmacist and 'signed off' to indicate this, the item(s) can be dispensed by a pharmacy technician and then the dispensing check could be performed by a (second) accredited checking technician.

4.3.6 Pass the item(s) to the patient and counsel the patient in the use of the medication

As with items dispensed against NHS prescriptions within the community, once dispensed and checked, the item(s) may be passed to the patient or their representative. At this point, the pharmacist or pharmacy technician passing the medication to the patient or their representative needs to:

- confirm that the item(s) are going to the correct patient
- pass certain key information to the patient/patient's representative verbally
- verify that the patient/patient's representative understood what they have been told and check to see if they have any questions.

Further details on these three stages can be found in Section 3.3.7.

4.4 Worked examples

This section contains examples of hospital medication orders (an in-patient order, a TTO and an out-patient prescription) for dispensing in a hospital pharmacy.

4.4.1 Framework for systematic dispensing/supply of hospital prescriptions or medication orders

Although a number of different examples are used in this section, all orders can be addressed by using a standard systematic approach. This approach is summarised in Figure 4.6 overleaf.

4.4.2 Examples of hospital prescriptions and the dispensing process

The following section contains examples of prescriptions that may be encountered in a hospital pharmacy. In each case, the following sections have been completed to guide you through the dispensing process. Note that compared with the dispensing of NHS prescriptions (see Section 3.5.2) there is no need to check whether the item(s) are allowable on the NHS (unless the items are prescribed on a hospital NHS prescription form, in which case the prescription would be intended to be dispensed within the community):

1. Identity of order
2. Prescriber
3. Legally written?
4. Clinical check (complete the following table):

DRUG	INDICATIONS	DOSE CHECK	REFERENCE

5. Interactions
6. Suitability for patient
7. Records to be made (including copies of the record(s))
8. Process prescription (including example of label(s))
9. Endorse prescription
10. Destination of paperwork
11. Identity check/counselling.

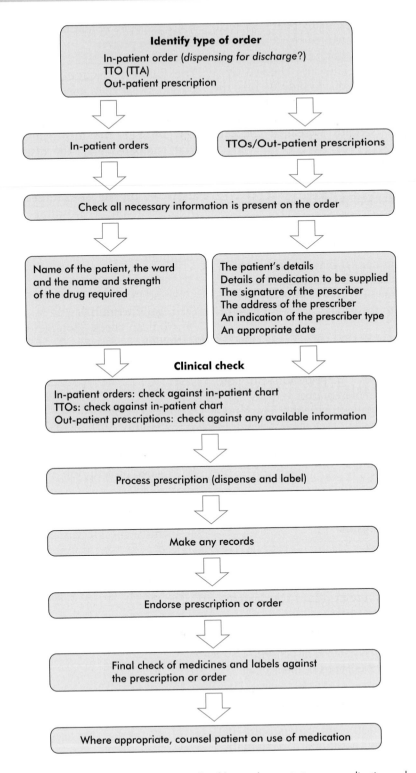

Figure 4.6   Framework for systematic dispensing/supply of hospital prescriptions or medication orders.

Example 4.1

This example is similar to Example 3.3 in Section 3.5.2, the difference being that instead of the item being prescribed by a GP on a standard FP10 NHS prescription form, the item has been prescribed as a TTO for a patient who is being discharged from a hospital ward. Note the differences between the dispensing process for this example and Example 3.3.

You receive the following TTO in your pharmacy.

ANYWHERE HOSPITAL

ANYWHERE

DISCHARGE MEDICATION

Patient's Name: Barbara Ache

Patient's address: 3 Pain Close, Anytown

Ward: Ward 7

Details of medication required:

Drug	Dosage and Instructions	Pharmacy
Fenbufen	300 mg om, 600 mg on	

Prescriber: Julie Timmins   **Bleep:** 3474

---

1. *Identity of order*: Hospital TTO (TTA) discharge prescription.
2. *Prescriber*: Doctor (hospital doctor).
3. *Legally written?* Yes.

Example 4.1 Continued

4. *Clinical check (complete the following table):*

DRUG	INDICATIONS	DOSE CHECK	REFERENCE
Fenbufen	Pain and inflammation	300 mg in the morning and 600 mg at night	*British National Formulary* 54th edition, section 10.1.1

5. *Interactions:* There is only one drug on the TTO. However, it would also be advisable for the pharmacist or pharmacy technician to check the patient's in-patient chart for any concurrent medication that could cause an interaction. Although a patient would need to continue to take all prescribed medication upon discharge, they may already have enough of some medication and therefore that medication may not appear on the TTO. This situation is especially likely to occur if the patient is part of a patients' own drugs scheme (see Section 4.2.2).

6. *Suitability for patient:* The item prescribed is safe and suitable for a patient of this age and the dose ordered on the prescription is within the recommended dose limits.

7. *Records to be made (including copies of the record(s)):* None.

8. *Process prescription (including example of label(s)):*

   - The quantity of medication to be supplied has not been stated. For most medication, the quantity supplied would be based on hospital policy (usually around 14 days). For 14 days' supply, you would need to supply 42 dosage units (1 × 300 mg in the morning and 2 × 300 mg in the evening).
   - The form of the medication to be supplied has not been stated. As the product comes as both tablets and capsules, it would be necessary for the pharmacist or pharmacy technician to check with the patient's in-patient chart to ascertain the form of the medication taken to date.
   - Check appendix 9 of *British National Formulary* for supplementary labelling requirements. Fenbufen: *British National Formulary* label number 21.
   - Select 42 fenbufen tablets or capsules (as appropriate), remembering to check the expiry date and taking care that the tablets or capsules are 300 mg (the packaging of other strengths/forms is very similar).
   - Perform final check of item, label and prescription.
   - Pack in a suitable bag ready to give to the patient or patient's representative.

   Labels (we have assumed that the name and address of the pharmacy and the words 'Keep out of the reach and sight of children' are pre-printed on the label):

Fenbufen 300 mg Capsules	**42**
Take ONE capsule in the morning and TWO at night.	
Take with or after food.	
Ms Barbara Ache	Date of dispensing

9. *Endorse prescription:* Endorse the pharmacy box on the TTO with the details of the medication supplied and initials of the pharmacist and pharmacy technician(s) involved in the dispensing process.

10. *Destination of paperwork:* Either the original or a copy of the TTO will be kept with the patient's hospital notes at the hospital. In addition, a copy may be supplied to the patient's GP.

Example 4.1 Continued

11. *Identity check/counselling*: The medication will need to be given to the patient. In most cases, the patient will either come down to the pharmacy and collect their medication as they are leaving the hospital, or the medication will be sent to the patient's ward and given to them by the ward pharmacist or a member of the nursing staff upon discharge. In both cases, the following information needs to be given to the patient or their representative.

- Check patient's name and address.
- Reinforce the dosage instructions; advise that the capsules are best taken with or after food to help prevent stomach irritation. Taking with milk will also 'protect' the stomach.
- Occasionally fenbufen causes skin to become more sensitive to sunlight. Use a sunscreen if affected and avoid sun beds.
- Initially some patients may experience dizziness. Do not drive or operate machinery if affected.
- Draw patient's attention to the patient information leaflet (PIL) and ask if she has any questions.

Example 4.2

This example is similar to Example 3.4 in Section 3.5.2, the difference being that instead of the item being prescribed by a GP on a standard FP10 NHS prescription form, the item has been prescribed as an out-patient prescription for a patient who has been seen by a consultant in an out-patient clinic. Note the differences between the dispensing process for this example and Example 3.4.

You receive the following out-patient prescription in your pharmacy:

ANYWHERE HOSPITAL

ANYWHERE

OUT-PATIENT PRESCRIPTION

Patient's Name: Sally ITCH

Patient's address: 7 Scratch Lane, Anytown

Details of medication required:

Betamethasone Cream 0.1%

Mitte 1 × OP

Sig apply qds

Prescriber: June Littlewood

---

1. *Identity of order*: Out-patient prescription.
2. *Prescriber*: Doctor (hospital consultant).
3. *Legally written?* Yes

Example 4.2 Continued

4. *Clinical check (complete the following table)*:

DRUG	INDICATIONS	DOSE CHECK	REFERENCE
Betamethasone valerate	Severe inflammatory skin disorders	Apply thinly once or twice a day	*British National Formulary* 54th edition, section 13.4

5. *Interactions*: There is only one item on the prescription form. However, it would also be advisable for the pharmacist or pharmacy technician to check, where possible, the patient's medication record for any concurrent medication that could cause an interaction. In this case, the patient's previous medication record indicated that she also used E45 cream (an emollient).

6. *Suitability for patient*: Item prescribed is safe and suitable for a patient of this age but the instructions for use on the prescription (i.e. to apply four times a day) is not within the recommended limits. Contact prescriber to check her intentions and arrange for the prescription to be changed to a more acceptable frequency (for example, twice a day).

7. *Records to be made (including copies of the record(s))*: Make a note of the intervention on a clinical intervention form (see Figure 1.5).

8. *Process prescription (including example of label(s))*:
   - Prepare label for product.
   - Check Appendix 9 of the *British National Formulary* for supplementary labelling requirements. Betamethasone valerate: *British National Formulary* label number 28.
   - Remember to add pharmaceutical cautions to label (For external use only).
   - Select tube of cream, remembering to check the expiry date and taking care that the cream and not the ointment has been selected (packaging of different forms may be very similar). As '1 × op' has been requested, the smallest pack size (30 g) should be supplied.
   - Label the primary container (i.e. the tube not the box).
   - Perform final check of item, label and prescription.
   - Pack in a suitable bag ready to give to patient/patient's representative.

   Labels (we have assumed that the name and address of the pharmacy and the words 'Keep out of the reach and sight of children' are pre-printed on the label):

Betamethasone Valerate 0.1% Cream	**30 g**
Apply TWICE a day. Spread thinly. For External Use Only.	
Miss Sally Itch	Date of dispensing

9. *Endorse prescription*: Endorse the out-patient prescription with the details of the medication supplied and initials of the pharmacist and pharmacy technician(s) involved in the dispensing process.

10. *Destination of paperwork*: File the prescription within the hospital according to local procedures.

Example 4.2 Continued

11. *Identity check/counselling*:
   - Check patient's name and address.
   - Advise patient of change in directions of use without alarming the patient.
   - Reinforce new dosage instructions and advice to apply the cream thinly and that it is for external use only.
   - Draw patient's attention to the patient information leaflet (PIL) and ask if she has any questions. The patient asks should she apply the cream before or after application of her E45 cream. What would be your answer? You should advise the patient to apply her steroid cream (the betamethasone valerate cream) first. Allow an hour before applying the emollient (the E45 cream) to prevent the emollient from diluting the steroid cream.

Example 4.3

This example is similar to Example 3.11 in Section 3.5.2, the difference being that instead of the item being prescribed by a GP on a standard FP10 NHS prescription form, the items have been requested for an in-patient on the ward. Note the differences between the dispensing process for this example and Example 3.11.

You are the ward pharmacist for Ward 18 and are asked by the nursing staff to order from the hospital pharmacy the antibiotics for June Bell that have just been written on the patient's drug chart by the doctor.

The chart looks as follows (only the page with entries on has been shown here. MH are the initials of the nurse administering the medication):

Surname:	BELL		Ward:		18					
First Name:	June Alice		Consultant:		Smith					
Patient Number:	123456		Date of Birth:		22/11/75					
Regular medication		Date:	2/5	3/5	4/5					
Drug name:	Frequency	(08.00)	MH	MH						
Pregaday	Daily	10.00								
Signature:	Route	12.00								
A Hardy	Oral	14.00								
Pharmacy	Date	18.00								
T Jones (Pts own)	1/5/07	22.00								
Drug name:	Frequency	08.00								
Trimethoprim	BD	(10.00)	X———┤							
Signature:	Route	12.00								
A Hardy	Oral	14.00								
Pharmacy	Date	18.00								
	3/5/07	(22.00)	X							
Drug name:	Frequency	08.00								
		10.00								
Signature:	Route	12.00								
		14.00								
Pharmacy	Date	18.00								
		22.00								

Example 4.3 Continued

Drug name:	Frequency	08.00							
		10.00							
Signature:	Route	12.00							
		14.00							
Pharmacy	Date	18.00							
		22.00							
Drug name:	Frequency	08.00							
		10.00							
Signature:	Route	12.00							
		14.00							
Pharmacy	Date	18.00							
		22.00							
Drug name:	Frequency	08.00							
		10.00							
Signature:	Route	12.00							
		14.00							
Pharmacy	Date	18.00							
		22.00							
Drugname:	Frequency	08.00							
		10.00							
Signature:	Route	12.00							
		14.00							
Pharmacy	Date	18.00							
		22.00							

1. *Identity of order*: In-patient drug chart.
2. *Prescriber*: Doctor (hospital doctor).
3. *Legally written?* Yes.

Example 4.3 Continued

4. *Clinical check (complete the following table):*

DRUG	INDICATIONS	DOSE	CHECK REFERENCE
Iron and folic acid	Prevention of iron and folate deficiency in pregnancy	1 tablet daily	*British National Formulary 54th edition, section 9.1.1.1*
Trimethoprim	Lower urinary tract infections	200 mg every 12 hours	*British National Formulary 54th edition, section 5.1.13*
Amoxicillin	Lower urinary tract infections	3 g repeated after 10–12 hours	*British National Formulary 54th edition, section 5.1.13*

5. *Interactions*: There is no interaction between the Pregaday tablets and the trimethoprim tablets. In addition, the ward pharmacist should check the other sections of the patient's in-patient drug chart for any additional concurrent medication that could cause an interaction. In this case, the other sections of the patient's in-patient drug chart did not contain the details of any other medication.

6. *Suitability for patient*: The use of the Pregaday suggests that the patient is pregnant and so the use of folate antagonists, like trimethoprim, is contraindicated. You will need to contact the prescriber with a suggested alternative. Amoxicillin is safe to use in pregnancy and therefore would be the drug of choice assuming the patient is not penicillin sensitive. Ask prescriber to change to amoxicillin sachets 3 g, 1 every 12 hours, mitte 2.

The patient's in-patient drug chart would need to be amended as follows:

Example 4.3 Continued

Surname:	BELL	Ward:		18
First Name:	June Alice	Consultant:		Smith
Patient Number:	123456	Date of Birth:		22/11/75

Regular medication		Date:	2/5	3/5	4/5				
Drug name:	Frequency	08.00	MH	MH					
Pregaday	Daily	10.00							
Signature:	Route	12.00							
A Hardy	Oral	14.00							
Pharmacy	Date	18.00							
T Jones (Pts own)	1/5/07	22.00							
Drug name:	Frequency	08.00							
Trimethoprim	BD	10.00	X						
Signature:	Route	12.00							
A Hardy	Oral	14.00							
Pharmacy	Date	18.00							
	3/5/07	22.00	X						
Drug name:	Frequency	08.00							
Amoxicillin	BD	10.00	X						
Signature:	Route	12.00							
A Hardy	Oral	14.00							
Pharmacy	Date	18.00							
T Jones	3/5/07	22.00	X						

Example 4.3 Continued

Drug name:	Frequency	08.00							
		10.00							
Signature:	Route	12.00							
		14.00							
Pharmacy	Date	18.00							
		22.00							
Drug name:	Frequency	08.00							
		10.00							
Signature:	Route	12.00							
		14.00							
Pharmacy	Date	18.00							
		22.00							
Drug name:	Frequency	08.00							
		10.00							
Signature:	Route	12.00							
		14.00							
Pharmacy	Date	18.00							
		22.00							
Drug name:	Frequency	08.00							
		10.00							
Signature:	Route	12.00							
		14.00							
Pharmacy	Date	18.00							
		22.00							

Once this change has been made, the ward pharmacist can order the amoxicillin sachets from the pharmacy via an in-patient order as follows:

Example 4.3 Continued

ANYWHERE HOSPITAL

ANYWHERE

Patient's Name: *Mrs June Bell*

Ward: *Ward 18*

Details of in-patient medication required:

Amoxicillin 3 g sachets x 2

Pharmacist: *Trevor Jones*   Bleep: *2134*

---

7. *Records to be made (including copies of the record(s))*: Make a note of the intervention on a clinical intervention form (see Figure 1.5).
8. *Process prescription (including example of label(s))*:
   - The in-patient order would be sent to the pharmacy and the pharmacy technician would dispense two amoxicillin 3 g sachets and send to the ward (once checked), labelled with the patient's name. As the medication will be administered by the ward's nursing staff according to the directions on the in-patient chart, it is not necessary to include administration details on the label.
   Labels (we have assumed that the name and address of the pharmacy and the words 'Keep out of the reach and sight of children' are pre-printed on the label):

Amoxicillin 3 g Sachets   **2**

Mrs June Bell (Ward 18)   Date of dispensing

---

9. *Endorse prescription*: Endorse the in-patient order with the details of the medication supplied.
10. *Destination of paperwork*: File the in-patient order within the hospital according to local procedures.
11. *Identity check/counselling*: Not necessary as the medication will be administered by the nursing staff to the patient on the ward.

4.5 Chapter summary

This chapter has covered the key points with which it is necessary to be familiar in order to supply medication to patients within a hospital setting. It is important that pharmacists and pharmacy technicians are familiar with the different types of hospital supply (in-patient orders, TTOs and out-patient prescriptions) and the new variants of these (for example, dispensing for discharge schemes or patient's own drugs schemes).

Finally, it should be remembered that in many cases, different rules apply to what may be supplied via an in-patient medication order or TTO/out-patient prescription compared with NHS supply in primary care. The main difference between these types of supply and NHS supply (see Chapters 2 and 3) is that the *Drug Tariff* rules do not apply.

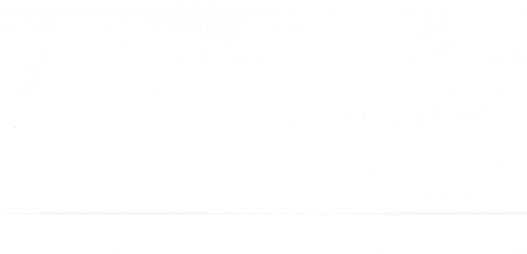

5

Non-NHS supply

Upon completion of this chapter, you should be able to:

- list which types of prescriber may prescribe items via a non-NHS (private) prescription form
- list which individuals may order drugs via written or oral requisitions and the restrictions placed on different healthcare professionals
- understand the general dispensing procedure for non-NHS (private) prescriptions in the community
- understand the general dispensing procedure for requisitions in the community
- complete a number of worked examples of non-NHS (private) prescriptions and the dispensing process
- complete a number of worked examples of requisitions and the dispensing process.

This chapter will cover all types of supply that are outside normal NHS supply. The following topics will be covered:

- the supply of medication via non-NHS (private) prescriptions
- the supply of medicinal products via written or oral requisitions.

The private supply of medication to patients within hospitals is similar to NHS hospital supply and has been covered in Chapter 4.

5.1 Non-NHS (private) prescription supply

Many patients who require medication will be supplied via the NHS either within the community (see Chapters 2 and 3) or in a hospital setting (see Chapter 4). However, an alternative to this would be to supply medication privately (i.e. outside the NHS). In these cases, the patient will be charged the cost of the item(s) plus a mark-up, and a fee levied by the pharmacist as payment for dispensing the item(s). This is clearly different from NHS supply, where patients are either exempt from paying the prescription charge or (currently in England, Northern Ireland and Scotland) simply pay a single fixed charge per item as a contribution to the cost (see Section 2.4.1, Part XVI for England; Section 2.4.2, Part VIII for Northern Ireland; and Section 2.4.3, Annex B for Scotland).

The dispensing procedure for non-NHS (private) prescriptions is similar to the dispensing procedure followed with NHS prescriptions (see Section 3.3). The main differences are that in most cases, an entry detailing the supply will always need to be made in the prescription-only medicines register (see Section 5.1.4) and that the pharmacist or pharmacy technician will not need to check that the item is allowed on the NHS. In summary, the procedure to be followed is as follows:

1. Check the legality of the non-NHS (private) prescription form (see Section 5.1.1).
2. Identify the prescriber (see Section 5.1.2).
3. Perform a clinical check on the prescription (see Section 5.1.3).
4. Dispense and label the item(s). This will include making a prescription-only medicines register entry (see Section 5.1.4).
5. Check the item(s) dispensed is/are correct and labelled appropriately. Ideally this check would be performed by a colleague (i.e. an independent check) but when working alone, the pharmacist will need to check the item(s) themselves (see Section 5.1.5).
6. Pass the item(s) to the patient and counsel the patient in the use of the medication (see Section 5.1.6)
7. Process the prescription form (see Section 5.1.7).

Key point 5.1

The dispensing procedure for non-NHS (private) prescriptions:

1. Check the legality of the non-NHS (private) prescription form.
2. Identify the prescriber.
3. Perform a clinical check on the prescription.
4. Dispense and label the item(s).
5. Check the item(s) dispensed is/are correct and labelled appropriately.
6. Pass the item(s) to the patient and counsel the patient in the use of the medication.
7. Process the prescription form.

5.1.1 Check the legality of the non-NHS (private) prescription form

Non-NHS (private) prescription form requirements

All prescription forms received by pharmacists or pharmacy technicians need to be checked to ensure that they are legally correct. Only prescriptions on forms that meet the requirements should be dispensed. If a prescription form is not legally correct, it should be referred to the prescriber for amendment before dispensing.

The requirements as to what needs to be present on a non-NHS (private) prescription form are similar to the requirements of an NHS prescription form (see Section 2.2.7). In summary, the necessary pieces of information are:

1. The patient's details. This must include the age or date of birth of the patient if they are under 12 years of age.
2. Sufficient details of the medication to be supplied. Except in the prescribing of controlled drugs (see Section 6.3.2) there is no legal requirement to provide particular information about the product. However, there will need to be sufficient information provided to enable the accurate and safe supply of medication to the patient and if there is insufficient information on the prescription, this must be queried with the prescriber before a supply can be made.
3. The signature of the prescriber.
4. The address of the prescriber.
5. An indication as to the prescriber type. On an NHS prescription form, the prescriber type is clearly identifiable. However, non-NHS (private) prescriptions will not be on specific prescription forms (except the private prescribing of Schedule 2 and Schedule 3 controlled drugs – see Section 6.3.3). Therefore, the identification of the prescriber is not always obvious. There needs to be something on the prescription to identify the prescriber type and usually, this will be the prescriber's qualifications (e.g. 'MB ChB' – see Appendix 1).
6. An appropriate date.

Key point 5.2

Non-NHS (private) prescription forms will need the following pieces of information to be present before the prescription can be dispensed:

- the patient's details
- details of the medication to be supplied
- the signature of the prescriber
- the address of the prescriber
- an indication of the prescriber type
- an appropriate date.

Repeatable non-NHS (private) prescription forms

Unlike NHS prescription forms, non-NHS (private) prescription forms may be repeatable (except in the case of non-NHS (private) prescription forms for Schedule 2 and Schedule 3 controlled drugs – see Section 6.3.3). In this situation, the prescriber will annotate the prescription form to indicate that the prescription may be dispensed more than once.

With repeat prescribing on a non-NHS (private) prescription form, the prescriber will annotate with the number of times that the prescription may be repeated (for example, 'repeat × 3'). In this example, the prescription may be dispensed a total of four times (i.e. one initial dispensing and then three repeats). On the first, second and third dispensing, the prescription may be returned to the patient as they are not obliged to receive subsequent supplies from the same pharmacy (see Section 5.1.7). However, many patients will return to the same pharmacy and so may ask you to hold the prescription on their behalf.

It is worth highlighting at this point that many patients (and even some healthcare professionals) will often discuss obtaining a 'repeat prescription' from their general practitioner (GP). This is where patients will request further supply of medication that they have been previously taking via an NHS prescription form. In this case, the GP will write a new NHS prescription form for the supply (the original NHS prescription form has been dispensed and passed by the pharmacy to the NHS Business Services Authority Prescription Pricing Division (or equivalent) for payment). However, this is often termed 'repeat prescribing' as the patient is obtaining a 'repeat' of the medication previous prescribed. Nonetheless, this is distinctly different from the 'repeats' described in this section as a new prescription form is being supplied each time.

In addition, it is important not to confuse repeatable non-NHS (private) prescriptions with instalment dispensing for addicts (see Section 6.3.5), where the NHS prescription is only dispensed once although the dispensing takes place in instalments.

Key point 5.3

If a non-NHS (private) prescription form stated that the medication may be repeated three times, the item may be supplied a total of four times (i.e. the one original dispensing, followed by three repeats).

After the last dispensing, the prescription will be retained by the dispensing pharmacy. The exception to this would be if there were, for example, two items on the prescription form and only one of those was repeatable. If the repeatable item were on the non-NHS (private) prescription form on its own, the form would be returned to the patient. However, as there is a non-repeatable item on the form, the form must be retained by the dispensing pharmacy. Therefore in rare cases such as these, the patient will have to return to the same pharmacy to obtain any repeats of the repeatable medication.

All supplies of medication will need to be entered in the prescription-only medicines register. However, if the supply is a repeat (and the pharmacy where the repeat is being dispensed has previously dispensed the medication), it is sufficient for the new entry in the prescription-only medicines register (which will have a new reference number) to refer to the details of the older entry (by referring to the older entry's reference number). Therefore, it is useful when stamping a non-NHS (private) prescription form following dispensing, to annotate the stamp with the prescription-only medicines register entry reference (see Section 5.1.7).

Please note that the prescription form, as with NHS prescription forms, is valid for six months (except in the case of prescription forms for some controlled drug; see Section 6.3.3). For repeatable non-NHS (private) prescription forms, the first dispensing must be within those six months. Although any repeats may then be made after the six months, it would be good practice for the pharmacist to make a professional judgement on the acceptability of supplying the medication if it had been originally prescribed a long time ago.

Finally, it is worth noting that if the prescriber just adds the word 'Repeat' to the prescription, it may be repeated once (i.e. one initial dispensing and one repeat dispensing). The exception to this is in the case of an oral contraceptive, where the supply may be repeated up to five times (i.e. a total of six supplies) within the six month validity of the prescription form. This regulation originated when all oral contraceptives were packed in one-month packs, the intention being to allow for six-month supplies. Nowadays, some oral contraceptives are packaged in three-month packs and therefore any more than one repeat (of three-month packs) should be questioned, even if within the six-month validity period.

Key point 5.4

Non-NHS (private) prescription forms may be repeatable. The first dispensing must take place within six months from the date on the prescription.

5.1.2 Identify the prescriber

As discussed above (Section 5.1.1) it is necessary to identify the prescriber to ensure that he or she is an individual who is legally allowed to prescribe item(s) on a non-NHS (private) prescription form. Non-NHS (private) prescription forms may be written by:

- doctors
- dentists
- community practitioner nurse prescribers
- supplementary prescribers (see Section 3.2.4).
- independent non-medical prescribers (currently only some nurses and some pharmacists; see Section 3.2.5).

Remember, that unlike prescribing on the NHS, prescribers are not limited to the items that they may prescribe on a non-NHS (private) prescription form. However, all prescribers are ethically obliged to only prescribe within their area of competence.

Therefore, it would not be uncommon for a dentist to prescribe analgesic medication on a non-NHS (private) prescription form for a patient under his care, even if that item was not in the Dental Practitioners' Formulary (see Section 3.2.2). However, it would be unusual for them to prescribe, for example, medication for the treatment of schizophrenia. If a pharmacist received a non-NHS (private) prescription form from a dentist for medication to treat schizophrenia, the pharmacist should query the supply with the prescribing dentist to confirm that the dentist is prescribing within their area of competence.

5.1.3 Perform a clinical check on the prescription

The process of clinical checking for a non-NHS (private) prescription is the same as for NHS prescriptions. This has been covered in Section 3.3.4. Remember that the following points will need to be covered:

- the patient
- the dose of the medication
- the patient's condition
- other medication the patient may be taking.

5.1.4 Dispense and label the item(s)

Once it has been established that the item(s) on the prescription form are safe and suitable for the patient, the label(s) can be generated and the item(s) dispensed. The same procedure can be followed when dispensing non-NHS (private) prescription items as for NHS prescription items (see Section 3.3.5).

In addition, an entry will need to be made of the supply in the prescription-only medicines register.

The prescription-only medicines register

Every community pharmacy will have a prescription-only medicines register, along with any other registered pharmacy (for example, a registered pharmacy within a hospital setting). Hospital pharmacies only need to keep such records if the supply of the prescription-only medicine requires registration as a pharmacy. Under the Medicines Act, medicines supplied in the course of the business of the hospital (see Chapter 4) do not need to be recorded.

The prescription-only medicines register usually takes the form of a bound book where the details of the supply of certain medicinal products are made, although nowadays computer records are permissible. The title of 'prescription-only medicines register' is a little misleading as there will be circumstances (either as legal requirements or as good practice requirements) where the supply of medicines other than prescription-only medicines (POMs) will be recorded.

It is a legal requirement to record the sale or supply of all prescription-only medicines (POMs) not supplied via the NHS (i.e. on an NHS prescription form) in the community unless:

- a separate record of the sale or supply is made in accordance with the Misuse of Drugs Regulations 2001 (see Section 6.3.7)
- a sale is by way of wholesale dealing if and so long as a copy of the order or invoice relating thereto is retained by the owner of the retail pharmacy business (see Section 5.2).

However, in both cases it is still considered good practice to make an entry (as it would be for non-NHS (private) prescriptions or wholesale dealing of non-prescription-only medicines (i.e. for GSL/P medicines)).

Records of medication supply are made in the prescription-only medicines register in the following instances:

- medication supply via a non-NHS (private) prescription (see Section 5.1)

- supply of medication via a written requisition (see Section 5.2)
- supply or medication in response to an oral requisition (see Section 5.3)
- emergency supply of medication at the request of a practitioner (see Section 7.1)
- emergency supply of prescription-only medication at the request of a patient (see Section 7.2).

Figure 5.1 shows a standard prescription-only medicines register page. The detail of what needs to be recorded in each of the sections in various different circumstances can be found in the relevant sections of this book. The prescription-only medicines register must be kept at the premises to which it relates during its period of use and for two years after the last entry. Each entry will have a unique reference number, usually made up of the page number and entry number on that page (for example, on page 12, the first entry is '12.1', the second '12.2', etc.).

Reference number	Details	Cost

Figure 5.1   An example of a standard prescription-only medicines register page.

Key point 5.5

Records of medication supply are made in the prescription-only medicines register in the following instances:

- medication supply via a non-NHS (private) prescription

→

- supply of medication via a written requisition
- supply or medication in response to an oral requisition
- emergency supply of medication at the request of a practitioner.
- emergency supply of prescription-only medication at the request of a patient.

The prescription-only medicines register must be kept at the premises to which it relates during its period of use and for two years after the last entry.

5.1.5 Check the item(s) dispensed is/are correct and labelled appropriately

Once all the above points have been followed, it is important that the label(s) and dispensed item(s) are checked against the prescription form to ensure they are correct.

Ideally, this check will be performed by a second competent colleague. However, there may be some situations where the pharmacist is working alone. In these cases, a second check still needs to take place and the pharmacist will need to perform this second check him- or herself.

5.1.6 Pass the item(s) to the patient and counsel the patient in the use of the medication

Once dispensed and checked, the item(s) will be passed to the patient or their representative. Remember, as with NHS prescriptions (see Section 3.3.7) at this point, three things need to happen:

1. The pharmacist or pharmacy technician passing the medication to the patient or their representative needs to confirm that the item(s) are going to the correct patient.
2. The pharmacist or pharmacy technician needs to pass certain key information to the patient or their representative verbally.
3. The pharmacist or pharmacy technician needs to verify that the patient or their representative understood what they have

been told and check to see if they have any questions.

For more information on these three points, see Section 3.3.7.

5.1.7 Process the prescription form

Unlike NHS prescription supply (see Section 3.3.8), the patient or the patient's representative will pay you for the entire cost of the medication (plus a mark-up cost and dispensing fee charged by the pharmacy to cover their costs). Therefore, non-NHS (private) prescription forms do not need to be sent off to the NHS Business Services Prescription Pricing Division (or equivalent) for reimbursement at the end of each month (except with the private prescribing of Schedule 2 and Schedule 3 controlled drugs; see Section 6.3.3).

For non-NHS (private) prescription supply, one of two things will happen with the prescription form. For non-repeatable prescriptions, the prescription will be kept by the pharmacy for two years. For repeatable non-NHS (private) prescriptions, unless it is the last repeat, the prescription will be returned to the patient or the patient's representative (the exception to this being if there were, for example, two items on the prescription form and only one of those was repeatable; see Section 5.1.1).

In both cases (for the supply of prescription-only medicines (POMs)), it is a legal requirement that an entry is made in the prescription-only medicines register (see Section 5.1.4).

For the last repeat of a repeatable prescription, this can be treated as if the prescription was not repeatable (i.e. the prescription form is kept in the pharmacy for two years and an entry will still be made in the prescription-only medicines register).

In both cases, the pharmacist or pharmacy technician will stamp the prescription with the pharmacy stamp and usually add the prescription-only medicines register reference number to the stamp. Please note that it is common practice to stamp the prescription form *above* the signature so as to prevent anyone cutting the bottom portion of the prescription form off, thus altering the apparent number of times the prescription has been dispensed (for repeatable prescriptions forms returned to the patient or their representative).

5.2 Written requisitions

In addition to the supply of medication on the NHS via individual prescription forms (see Chapters 2 and 3) or hospital order (see Chapter 4), and the supply of medication via non-NHS (private) prescription forms (see Section 5.1), it is also necessary to become familiar with other forms of supply. These are where a practitioner or other authorised individual requires a medicinal product for use during the course of their practice or business. This may not, at this stage, be for a named patient. This would include, for example, where a GP requests something for use during home visits or an optician requests a medicinal item for use during eye examinations.

This section is divided into the following parts:

* General requisition layout (see Section 5.2.1)
* Sale or supply of medicinal products to hospitals or health centres (see Section 5.2.2).
* Sale or supply of medicinal products to practitioners (see Section 5.2.3).
* Sale or supply of medicinal products to appropriate nurse prescribers (see Section 5.2.4).
* Sale or supply of medicinal products to midwives (see Section 5.2.5).
* Sale or supply of medicinal products to chiropodists (see Section 5.2.6).
* Sale or supply of medicinal products to opticians (see Section 5.2.7).
* Sale or supply of medicinal products to other individuals (see Section 5.2.8).

The sale or supply of medication is, under the Medicines Act 1968, classified as wholesale dealing, and individuals undertaking this activity would normally require a wholesale dealing licence. However, persons lawfully conducting a retail pharmacy business may undertake this activity without a licence so long as the activity constitutes no more than an inconsiderable part of the business. Although undefined, this is usu-ally taken to be less than 5% of the pharmacy's medicines trade.

Supplies of medication will normally take place via a written requisition (colloquially known as a 'signed order', although the term is somewhat misleading as most written requisitions do not actually need to be signed). However, it is also permissible for some individuals to request medication supply verbally. The oral requisition of medication is covered in Section 5.3.

5.2.1 General requisition layout

Except where detailed in the following section, for a written requisition for prescription-only medicines there are no legally defined details as to the content required. However, it would be reasonable to expect the requisition to provide enough information to make a prescription-only medicines register entry (see Section 5.1.4). We suggest, therefore, that the following list would be a good starting point:

* details of preparation (sufficient to be clear as to which product has been requested, i.e. name, quantity, form and strength as appropriate)
* name and address, trade business or profession of the person to whom the medicine is supplied
* the purpose for which the medicine is supplied
* signature of requisitioner.

An example of a requisition is shown in Figure 5.2.

It is worth noting at this point that requisitions for controlled drugs will have additional requirements (see Section 6.3.6).

When supplying medication via a written requisition, it should be noted that only complete packs (including any patient information leaflets) can be supplied. As the medication is usually not for a specific patient (at the point the requisition is made), there is no need to label the medication. If the medication were for a specific patient, it would be usual to issue a patient-specific prescription form (either an NHS or non-NHS (private) prescription form).

```
┌─────────────────────────────────────┐
│        Dr R U Better MBChB          │
│      ANYTOWN HEALTH CENTRE          │
│           ANYTOWN                   │
│            AN1 1RB                   │
│                                     │
│   Please supply for use in my practice │
│                                     │
│     100 Co-Dydramol Tablets         │
│                                     │
│                                     │
│    R U Better        Today's date   │
│                                     │
└─────────────────────────────────────┘
```

Figure 5.2   An example of a written requisition.

It is good practice to make an entry in the prescription-only medicines register at the time of supply; it is only a good practice requirement as the requisition will be retained within the pharmacy for two years from the date of supply (the exception to this is for Schedule 2 and Schedule 3 controlled drugs; see Section 6.3.6). However, if the request for the supply of a prescription-only medicine (POM) was an oral request (see Section 5.3) the prescription-only medicines register entry would be a legal requirement (as there is no paper requisition detailing the sale to keep for two years).

For completeness, it is also worth mentioning that it is not a legal requirement to make an entry in the prescription-only medicines register if a separate record of the sale or supply is made in the controlled drugs register (see Section 6.3.7). However, it is still good practice to make an entry in the prescription-only medicines register.

5.2.2 Sale or supply of medicinal products to hospitals or health centres

There are no restrictions in the supply of pre-scription-only medicines to hospitals and health centres provided that the prescription-only medicine is to be supplied either in response to a prescription that has been written by an appropriate practitioner or an order written by an appropriate practitioner. This applies to both hospitals and health centres within the NHS and private sector. The restrictions that apply to pharmacy-only medicines also do not apply if in response to an order from an appropriate practitioner.

5.2.3 Sale or supply of medicinal products to practitioners

For the sale or supply of medicinal products to practitioners the term practitioner refers to:

- medical practitioners
- dental practitioners
- veterinary practitioners/surgeons.

The controls over retail sale of medicines do not apply to the above practitioners. A doctor or dentist may offer to supply or sell prescription-only medicines to a patient or patient's carer (and similar arrangements apply to veterinary practitioners/surgeons for animals or herds under their care). Supplies may be obtained from pharmacies by way of wholesale dealing and requested via a written requisition.

Supplementary and independent prescribers at present do not have the exemptions available to the practitioners listed above.

5.2.4 Sale or supply of medicinal products to appropriate nurse prescribers

The restrictions that control the supply of medicines to nurses refers to registered nurses who are qualified to order drugs, medicines and appliances from the Nurse Prescribers' Formulary for Community Practitioners in current editions of the *British National Formulary* and *Drug Tariff*.

This distinction is noted on the Register of Nurses and shows who has the necessary additional qualification. Therefore the supply to and by these practitioners is limited to the items listed in the Nurse Prescribers' Formulary for Community Practitioners.

5.2.5 Sale or supply of medicinal products to midwives

Under the 'sale or supply' exemptions for midwives, a registered midwife may supply, but not offer for sale, the following:

- all general sale list (GSL) and pharmacy only (P) medicines
- prescription-only medicines containing the following:
  - chloral hydrate
  - ergometrine maleate (in preparations not for parenteral use)
  - pentazocine hydrochloride
  - phytomenadione
  - triclofos sodium.

In addition the following prescription-only medicines for parenteral administration are included in the exemptions:

- diamorphine
- ergometrine maleate
- lidocaine*
- lidocaine hydrochloride*
- morphine
- naloxone hydrochloride
- oxytocins natural and synthetic
- pentazocine lactate
- pethidine hydrochloride
- phytomenadione
- promazine hydrochloride.*

* These shall only be administered when attending on a woman in childbirth.

The administration shall only be in the course of their professional practice.

Midwives supply orders

Although controlled drugs are dealt with in Chapter 6, for completeness, it is worth mentioning midwives supply orders here. Midwives supply orders are needed for the lawful supply of certain controlled drugs to a midwife from a pharmacist (i.e. those items listed above that are Schedule 2 or Schedule 3 controlled drugs; diamorphine, morphine, pentazocine and pethidine). They are not required for the supply of other listed prescription-only medicines.

The supply orders enable the supply of controlled drugs to the midwife for use in his or her own professional practice. The midwife is not allowed to provide the controlled drug to a third party to administer.

Midwives supply orders must:

- be in writing

- include the name and occupation of the midwife obtaining the supply
- state the purpose for which the drug is required
- be signed by the appropriate medical officer who is a doctor authorised in writing by the local supervising authority or a supervisor of midwives.

In addition, although not legally required the following details would be desirable for audit purposes.

- the midwife's personal identification number (PIN)
- the name and contact details of the supervisor of midwives or approved medical officer authorising the supply
- the name and contact details of the midwife's named supervisor of midwives if it is different from the authorising supervisor of midwives
- the name of the woman to whom the drug is to be administered, if appropriate.

Currently, the pharmacist must retain the midwives supply order for two years (although this may change in line with other requisitions for controlled drugs; see Section 6.3.6).

The Royal Pharmaceutical Society of Great Britain (RPSGB) in *The Safe and Secure Handling of Medicines: a team approach* suggests that there should be a locally approved procedure for authorising the supply orders (for example, ensuring the quantity ordered is appropriate).

It would be good practice for the midwife to use a hospital pharmacy, a dispensing GP or a local community pharmacy in the territory in which he or she works and it is preferable that the midwife should be introduced to the pharmacist by the authorising medical officer so that the supply process can run smoothly.

5.2.6 Sale or supply of medicinal products to chiropodists

The Medicines Act 1968 uses the term chiropodist rather than the more accepted term podiatrist. Chiropodist is a term that was used in the UK; in other English speaking countries the term podiatrist was adopted, which is probably more accurate as chiropody refers to both hands and feet while podiatry is foot specific. In order to provide continuity the UK adopted the term podiatry in 1993.

The Act concerns 'state registered chiropodists' and provides a list of medicines that chiropodists may sell, supply and administer. However since the Act the registration process for podiatrists has changed. The terms 'chiropodist' and 'podiatrist' are now protected by law and can only be used by practitioners that are registered with the Health Professions Council.

Nowadays podiatrists need to complete a degree course of study to obtain a BSc (podiatry). Originally this course was a diploma course leading to a Diploma in Podiatric Medicine (DPodM).

The Act refers to 'state registered chiropodist' (SRCh) but this title has been out of use since 9 July 2003. It is still used by many podiatrists as it is seen by the general public as an indication that a podiatrist is fully qualified. What is required now is that they are registered with the Health Professions Council (HPC).

Other qualifications used by accredited podiatrists include:

- MChS – Member of the Society of Chiropodists and Podiatrists
- FChS – Fellow of the Society of Chiropodists and Podiatrists
- FCPods – Fellow of the College of Podiatrists of The Society of Chiropodists & Podiatrists.

Therefore it is important to check the qualifications of a podiatrist carefully before supplying medicines by way of wholesale dealing.

The Act states that state registered chiropodists can sell or supply certain medicinal products provided that:

> The sale or supply shall only be in the course of their professional practice and that the medicinal product has been made up for sale and supply in a container elsewhere than at the place at which it is sold or supplied.

The items that may be sold to chiropodists fall into two categories:

- items for sale or supply to patients
- items to be administered to patients.

The sale or supply of medicines by chiropodists

There are conditions laid down with regard to the sale or supply by chiropodists. A list of the items which chiropodist may sell or supply can be found in the most recent edition of *Medicines, Ethics and Practice – A Guide for Pharmacists and Pharmacy Technicians* or on the MHRA website.

The conditions imposed for sale or supply of listed medicines are:

- Prescription-only medicines (POMs):
  - podiatrist must be registered
  - the medicine must be pre-packed
  - the sale must be made in the course of professional practice
  - podiatrist must hold a certificate of competence in the use of the medicines.
- Pharmacy-only (P) medicines:
  - podiatrist must be registered
  - the medicine must be pre-packed
  - the sale must be made in the course of professional practice.
- General sale list (GSL) medicines:
  - the medicine must be pre-packed
  - the sale must be made in the course of professional practice.

The administration of medicines by chiropodists

State registered chiropodists who hold a certificate of competence in the use of analgesics issued by or with the approval of the Chiropodists Board or the Health Professions Council may administer parenterally in the course of their professional practice prescription-only medicines containing any of the following substances:

- adrenaline
- bupivacaine hydrochloride
- bupivacaine hydrochloride with adrenaline where the maximum strength of the adrenaline does not exceed 1 mg in 200 mL of bupivacaine hydrochloride
- levobupivacaine hydrochloride
- lidocaine hydrochloride
- lidocaine hydrochloride with adrenaline where the maximum strength of the adrenaline does not exceed 1 mg in 200 mL of lidocaine hydrochloride
- mepivacaine hydrochloride

- methylprednisolone
- prilocaine hydrochloride
- ropivacaine hydrochloride.

Any medicine that the chiropodist may sell, supply or administer can be purchased from a pharmacy by way of wholesale dealing.

5.2.7 Sale or supply of medicinal products to opticians

Registered optometrists are allowed to sell or supply all medicinal products on a general sale list (GSL) and all pharmacy-only medicines (P) providing that it is in the course of their professional practice.

They may also supply certain prescription-only medicines (POM) which are not for parenteral administration. Commonly, this includes the following prescription-only medicines:

- eye drops containing not more than 0.5% chloramphenicol*
- eye ointments containing not more than 1% chloramphenicol
- preparations containing cyclopentolate hydrochloride, fusidic acid or tropicamide.

*Chloramphenicol eye drops can be sold as pharmacy-only medicines (P) for limited conditions. The prescription-only medicines (POM) pack is for wider licensed use.

As these drugs may be purchased by optometrists from entry level registration and do not necessitate any further training to be undertaken the legislation allows for these medicines to be supplied to optometrists by retail pharmacies on provision of a signed order. A summary of the POMs that can be supplied to optometrists can be found in Table 5.1. Table 5.2 lists P medicines commonly used by optometrists.

Additional supply optometrists may sell or supply additional prescription-only medicines (POMs) provided it is in the course of their professional practice and in an emergency. Additional supply optometrists have undergone additional training and accreditation which is only available to optometrists who have completed at least two years in practice following registration.

Table 5.3 lists the common additions to make a more extensive formulary for additionally

qualified optometrists enabling them to manage more common non sight-threatening eye disorders, for example, infective conjunctivitis, allergic conjunctivitis, blepharitis, dry eye and superficial eye injuries.

All of the preparations listed in Table 5.3 are available for sale or supply by an optometrist in the course of their professional practice and in an emergency or available from a pharmacy on the presentation of an order signed by a registered ophthalmic optician. On occasion, the signed order may include the intended patient's details as they are the person purchasing the item on the authority of the signed order.

When optometrists present a signed order for a prescription-only medicine (POM) the following details are required:

1. the name and address of the optometrist
2. the date
3. the name and address of the patient (if applicable)
4. the purpose for the supply (e.g. 'For use in my practice')
5. name, quantity, strength and pharmaceutical form of medicine required
6. labelling directions (when applicable)
7. signature of the optometrist (this is one of the few times where a signature is actually a legal requirement on the written requisition).

The signed order may be hand-written, typewritten or computer-generated but it must be in indelible ink. The signature must be original (i.e. not a photocopy or a stamp).

The General Optical Council (GOC) code of ethics also states that the optometrist must include their GOC number to enable a pharmacist to check on the GOC register for opticians with the same name.

5.2.8 Sale or supply of medicinal products to other individuals

Other pharmacies

It is not uncommon for pharmacies to supply each other with medication from time to time. This would be classified as wholesale dealing

Table 5.1 Prescription-only medicines (POMs) that may be supplied to optometrists

Drug name	Proprietary name	Licensed indications	Use in practice
Antibacterials			
Chloramphenicol	Chloromycetin eye drops and ointment (also available as generic chloramphenicol eye drops and ointment)	Superficial eye infections	Sale or supply by optometrist in course of professional practice and in an emergency or available from a pharmacy on the presentation of an order signed by a registered ophthalmic optician
Fusidic acid	Fucithalmic eye drops M/R	Staphylococcal infections	Sale or supply by optometrist in course of professional practice and in an emergency or available from a pharmacy on the presentation of an order signed by a registered ophthalmic optician
Antimuscarinics			
Cyclopentolate hydrochloride	Mydrilate, Minims Cyclopentolate Hydrochloride	Cycloplegia	Sale or supply by optometrist in course of professional practice and in an emergency or available from a pharmacy on the presentation of an order signed by a registered ophthalmic optician
Tropicamide	Mydriacyl, Minims Tropicamide	Mydriasis	Sale or supply by optometrist in course of professional practice and in an emergency or available from a pharmacy on the presentation of an order signed by a registered ophthalmic optician
Local anaesthetics			
Lidocaine hydrochloride	Minims Lignocaine and Fluorescein	Local anaesthesia	POM medicine for administration (not for sale or supply)
Oxybuprocaine hydrochloride	Minims Oxybuprocaine Hydrochloride	Local anaesthesia	POM medicine for administration (not for sale or supply)
Proxymetacaine hydrochloride	Minims Proxymetacaine Minims Proxymetacaine and Fluorescein	Local anaesthesia	POM medicine for administration (not for sale or supply)
Tetracaine hydrochloride	Minims Amethocaine Hydrochloride	Local anaesthesia	POM medicine for administration (not for sale or supply)

and so would be done as with any other wholesale dealing transaction.

Supply to owners and masters of ships including foreign vessels

Fishing vessels and seagoing ships are required by law to carry medical stores which will include medicines, medical equipment and antidotes. The requirements vary with the size and type of the vessel and the distance it travels from port. Details of the requirements are laid out by the Merchant Shipping Act 1995 and the Merchant Shipping and Fishing Vessels (Medical Stores) Regulations 1995. Medical supplies may be obtained from shipping chemists and general retail pharmacies.

Under Merchant shipping (Ships' Doctors) Regulations 1995 all UK registered ships with more than 100 persons on board must carry a qualified medical practitioner. Other vessels may not carry a medical practitioner but the provision of medical attention on such ships is regulated and should be provided either by the

Table 5.2 Pharmacy-only (P) medicines commonly used by optometrists

Drug name	Proprietary name	Licensed indications
Antihistamines		
Antazoline sulphate	Otrivine-Antistin	Allergic conjunctivitis
Anti-infective preparations		
Chloramphenicol	Optrex Infected Eyes eye drops	Bacterial conjunctivitis
Propamidine isetionate	Brolene	Minor eye infections
Ocular diagnostic preparations		
Fluorescein sodium	Minims Fluorescein Sodium	Detection of lesions or foreign bodies in the eye
Rose Bengal	Minims Rose Bengal	Detection of lesions or foreign bodies in the eye
Ocular lubricants/artificial tears		
Carbomers	GelTears, Viscotears, Liposic	Treatment of tear deficiency
Carmellose sodium	Celluvisc	Dry eye conditions
Hydroxyethylcellulose	Minims Artificial Tears	Dry eye conditions/tear deficiency
Hypromellose	Isopto Alkaline, Isopto Plain, Tears Naturale	Treatment of tear deficiency
Liquid paraffin, yellow soft paraffin	Lubri-Tears, Lacri-Lube, Simple eye ointment	Dry eye conditions
Polyvinyl alcohol	Liquifilm Tears, Sno Tears	Treatment of tear deficiency
Other anti-inflammatory preparations		
Lodoxamide	Alomide Allergy Drops	Allergic conjunctivitis
Sodium cromoglicate	Clarityn Allergy Eye Drops, Hay-Crom Eye Drops, Opticrom Allergy Eye Drops (5 mL and 10 mL), Optrex Allergy Eye Drops, Vividrin Eye Drops	Allergic conjunctivitis

master of the ship or a person appointed by the master of the ship and operating under the supervision of the master of the ship. Medical training of officers of the merchant navy and fishing fleet consists of two levels of training:

1. First Aid at Sea Certificate
2. Ship's Captain's Medical Training Certificate.

The training courses are centred on the basic source of information regarding medical treatment and medicines aboard ship, *The Ship Captain's Medical Guide*, details of which can be found at the Maritime and Coastguard Agency website. The certificates are designed so that the officers will have a good working knowledge of *The Ship Captain's Medical Guide* and therefore can deal quickly and effectively with any medical emergency at sea. The owner of a vessel is legally responsible for ensuring that the correct medical equipment and stores are kept on their vessels. The master of the ship is responsible for the safekeeping and condition of the supplies.

Ships may also carry controlled drugs, usually morphine, which must be stored appropriately as laid out by the Misuse of Drugs Regulations (see Section 6.3.8). The regulations also state that a master of a foreign ship must in addition obtain a signed statement from the port health authority that the quantity of drug requested to be supplied is necessary for the equipment of his or her ship.

The master of a vessel registered in the UK will provide a signed order for the purchase of a controlled drug and will keep appropriate

Table 5.3 Preparations commonly available to additionally qualified optometrists for sale or supply by them in the course of their professional practice and in an emergency, or available from a pharmacy on the presentation of an order signed by a registered ophthalmic optician

Drug name	Proprietary name	Licensed indications
Antihistamines		
Azelastine hydrochloride	Optilast	Allergic conjunctivitis
Emedastine	Emadine	Seasonal allergic conjunctivitis
Ketotifen	Zaditen	Seasonal allergic conjunctivitis
Olopatadine	Opatanol	Seasonal allergic conjunctivitis
Anti-infective preparations		
Polymyxin B and Bacitracin	Polyfax	Superficial eye infections
Antimuscarinics		
Atropine sulphate	Minims Atropine Sulphate Isopto Atropine (also available as generic eye drops and ointment)	Cycloplegia for refraction in young children and treatment of anterior uveitis
Homatropine hydrobromide	Generic drops available	Treatment of anterior segment inflammation
Lubricants		
Acetylcysteine	Ilube	Tear deficiency or impaired or abnormal mucus production
Miotics		
Pilocarpine	Minims Pilocarpine Nitrate, Pilogel (also available as generic pilocarpine hydrochloride eye drops)	Treatment of glaucoma
Other anti-inflammatory preparations		
Lodoxamide	Alomide	Allergic conjunctivitis
Nedocromil sodium	Rapitil	Allergic conjunctivitis and seasonal keratoconjunctivitis
Sodium cromoglicate	Hay-Crom, Opticrom, Vividrin (also available as generic eye drops)	Allergic conjunctivitis and seasonal keratoconjunctivitis
Diclofenac sodium	Voltarol Ophtha Multidose Voltarol Ophtha	Seasonal allergic conjunctivitis, postoperative inflammation and pain in corneal epithelial defects

records on board ship to show the quantity carried and used by the vessel. Figure 5.3 shows a suggested requisition form for merchant ships. The order must be signed either by the vessel's owner or the master of the vessel.

It is not necessary for the master or owner of the vessel personally to collect the controlled drug from the supplier, but if the drugs are received by another person the requisition must also be endorsed as shown in Figure 5.4.

Occupational health schemes

Occupational health schemes are run by employers to provide facilities for employees for the treatment and prevention of disease. This can take a number of different forms, depending on the working environment, for example, monitoring for dermatitis in printing works, asthma in bakeries, providing travel medicines and information for employees travelling on behalf of the company, influenza vaccines for

Requisition

To _____ (name and address of authorised supplier)

From _____ (name of Master or Ship Owner)

Vessel name _____ (name of vessel)

Address_____ (address of Ship or the Ship Owner)

Please supply _____

_____

(name, strength and quantity of drugs in words and figures)

The above drugs are required for the Medical Stores of the above vessel in compliance with the Merchant Shipping and Fishing Vessels (Medical Stores) Regulations 1995

Signature _____

Name (capital letters) _____

Occupation _____

Date _____

Figure 5.3   An example of a requisition form for controlled drugs for use on a merchant ship.

I empower _____ to receive the above drugs on my behalf.

A specimen of their signature is provided below.

Specimen signature of person empowered

_____

Signature of Master or Owner

_____

Figure 5.4   An example of a form to allow another individual to collect any ordered controlled drugs for use on a merchant ship.

the workforce, eye tests for VDU (visual display unit) operators and health promotions schemes such as smoking cessation, etc. Prescription-only medicines may be sold to a person running an occupational health scheme only in response to a signed order written by a doctor or nurse.

In occupational health schemes if the person supplying the prescription-only medicine to the patient is not a doctor then they must be a registered nurse acting on instructions provided by a registered doctor. The supply may be made under Patient Group Directions (see Section 3.4). The prescriber must make clear when the use of a prescription-only medicine would be permissible, and the supply would only be made under the terms of the occupational health scheme.

If the prescription-only medicine is for parenteral use it must be administered by a registered nurse following written instruction from a medical practitioner.

Other individuals

There are a few other individuals who may be supplied medicines by a pharmacy. Supplies to these individuals are less common, and are listed here for completeness. In all cases, either a written requisition or oral request (see Section 5.3) will be required. These individuals are:

- ambulance paramedics (see the current edition of *Medicines, Ethics and Practice – A Guide for Pharmacists and Pharmacy Technicians* for further details)
- authorised individuals from the British Red Cross Society, St John Ambulance Association and Brigade, St Andrew's Ambulance Association and Order of Malta Ambulance Corps
- personnel from drug treatment services (ampoules of no more than 2 mL of sterile water)
- first aid personnel of offshore installations
- authorised individuals from the Royal National Lifeboat Institution
- authorised individuals from other organisations, for example, Primary Care Trusts (PCTs) and equivalent and police forces, prison services, etc. For further information on these and other additional individuals, see the current edition of *Medicines, Ethics and Practice – A Guide for Pharmacists and Pharmacy Technicians*.

Other exempted persons and organisations

The following persons or organisations can be sold or supplied medicinal products for certain specified purposes. Because they do not buy them for the purpose of selling or supplying them, or administering them in the course of their business, the sale to them does not fall within the definition of a wholesale transaction, and therefore is a retail transaction:

- dental schemes
- group authorities and licences
- marketing authorisation holders and holders of manufacturers' licences
- public analysts/sampling officers/NHS drug testing/British Standards Institution
- the operator or commander of an aircraft
- universities and other institutions
- unorthodox practitioners.

Medicines, Ethics and Practice – A Guide for Pharmacists and Pharmacy Technicians advises that any pharmacist who is approached to make a sale or supply to any of the above can check

with the Society's Fitness to Practise and Legal Affairs Directorate if any doubts exist as to the extent of the purchasers' authority.

5.3 Oral requests for medicines supply by practitioners

In addition to written requests by a variety of healthcare practitioners and other authorised individuals (see Section 5.2), some requests for the supply of medication do not have to be written down (i.e. via a written requisition). These are termed oral requisitions.

Oral requests may be made by any of the individuals listed in Section 5.2, except in the following cases:

- the supply of prescription-only medicines to an optician
- the supply of any Schedule 2 or Schedule 3 controlled drugs (see Section 6.3.6), including the supply of diamorphine, morphine, pentazocine and pethidine to midwives, which requires a midwives supply order (see Section 5.2.5).

Remember, in these situations there will be no written request for the supply and so it is a legal requirement (for the supply of POMs) that an entry is made in the prescription-only medicines register (see Section 5.1.4).

5.4 The dispensing procedure for non-NHS prescriptions

The dispensing procedure to be followed upon receipt of a non-NHS (private) prescription is similar to that of an NHS prescription (see Section 3.3). The main difference is that the pharmacist or pharmacy technician will not have to check whether the item is allowable on the NHS (as the prescribing is taking place outside the NHS).

Therefore, in summary, the following procedures should be followed:

1. Check the legality of the non-NHS (private) prescription form (see Section 5.1.1).

2. Identify the prescriber (see Section 5.1.2).
3. Perform a clinical check on the prescription (see Section 5.1.3).
4. Dispense and label the item(s) (see Section 5.1.4).
5. Check the item(s) dispensed is/are correct and labelled appropriately. Ideally this check would be performed by a colleague (i.e. an independent check) but when working alone, the pharmacist will need to check the item(s) themselves (see Section 5.1.5).
6. Pass the item(s) to the patient and counsel the patient in the use of the medication (see Section 5.1.6)
7. Process the prescription form (see Section 5.1.7).

Key point 5.6

The dispensing procedure for non-NHS (private) prescriptions:

1. Check the legality of the non-NHS (private) prescription form.
2. Identify the prescriber.
3. Perform a clinical check on the prescription.
4. Dispense and label the item(s).
5. Check the item(s) dispensed is/are correct and labelled appropriately.
6. Pass the item(s) to the patient and counsel the patient in the use of the medication.
7. Process the prescription form.

5.5 Worked examples

This section contains examples of non-NHS (private) prescription forms and requisitions for dispensing within a community pharmacy. Although a number of different examples are used in this section, from a variety of different prescribers, all prescription forms can be addressed by using a standard systematic approach (see Section 3.3 for NHS prescription forms, and Section 5.4 for non-NHS (private) prescription forms).

5.5.1 Framework for systematic dispensing/supply in the community

The approach is summarised in Figure 5.5 (this framework does not cover the supply of items from a pharmacy to non-practitioners; see Section 5.2.8).

5.5.2 Examples of non-NHS (private) prescriptions and the dispensing process

The following section contains examples of prescriptions that may be encountered in a community pharmacy. In each case, the following sections have been completed to guide you through the dispensing process (note that compared to the dispensing of NHS prescriptions (see Section 3.5.2). There is no need to check whether the item(s) is/are allowable on the NHS):

1. Identity of order
2. Prescriber
3. Legally written?
4. Clinical check (complete the following table):

DRUG	INDICATIONS	DOSE CHECK	REFERENCE

5. Interactions
6. Suitability for patient
7. Records to be made (including copies of the record(s))
8. Process prescription (including example of label(s))
9. Endorse prescription
10. Destination of paperwork
11. Identity check/counselling.

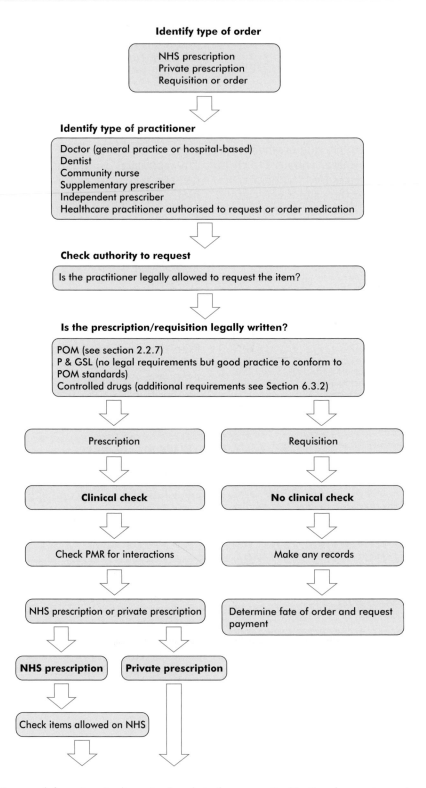

Figure 5.5   Framework for systematic dispensing/supply in the community. (Continued on next page.)

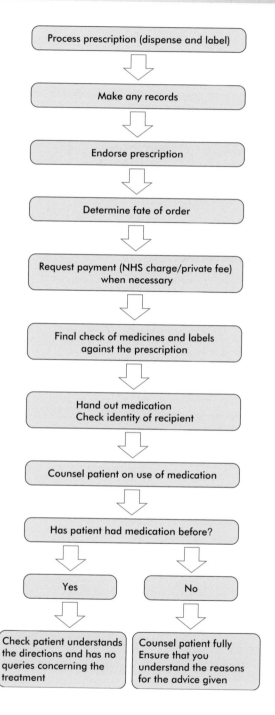

Figure 5.5   Continued

Example 5.1

You receive the following prescription in your pharmacy:

```
┌─────────────────────────────────────────┐
│         ANYTOWN HEALTH CENTRE            │
│               ANYTOWN                    │
│               AN1 1RB                     │
│   Mrs Jessica White                      │
│                                          │
│         Amoxicillin caps                 │
│            250mg tds 7/7                  │
│         Furosemide tabs                  │
│            40mg od. Mitte 28             │
│                                          │
│         R U Better                       │
│                          Today's date    │
└─────────────────────────────────────────┘
```

1. *Identity of order*: Private prescription.
2. *Prescriber*: Doctor (the prescriber is a local doctor).
3. *Legally written?* No. The doctor has failed to add the patient's address to the prescription and (although we may know from local knowledge) there is also no indication of type of prescriber on the prescription. This is usually indicated by the addition of qualifications to the prescription.

    Return the prescription to the prescriber for addition of address and indication of authority to prescriber (e.g. 'MB ChB') prior to dispensing.
4. *Clinical check (complete the following table)*:

DRUG	INDICATIONS	DOSE CHECK	REFERENCE
Amoxicillin	Urinary tract infections, otitis media, sinusitis, bronchitis	250 mg every 8 hours, doubled in severe infections	*British National Formulary* 54th edition, section 5.1.1.3
Furosemide	Oedema	Initially 40 mg in morning, maintenance 20–40 mg daily	*British National Formulary* 54th edition, section 2.2.2

5. *Interactions*: There is no interaction between amoxicillin and furosemide. However, it would also be advisable for the pharmacist or pharmacy technician to check the patient medication record (PMR) for any concurrent medication that could cause an interaction. In this case, the patient's PMR indicated that she usually takes an oral contraceptive.
6. *Suitability for patient*: The items prescribed are safe and suitable for an adult patient and the doses ordered on the prescription are within the recommended dose limits.
7. *Records to be made (including copies of the record(s))*: A prescription-only medicines register entry will be required.

Example 5.1 Continued

Reference number	Details	Cost
5.01	Mrs Jessica White	Cost
	7 Ash Grove Anytown	+
Date of		50%
supply	Amoxicillin 250 mg caps	+
	1 tds mitte 7/7 (21 caps)	Dispensing fee
	Furosemide tabs 40 mg	+
	1 od mitte 28	Container fee
	R U Better MB ChB	
	Anytown Health Centre	
	Anytown	
	Date on prescription: Today's	
	Prescriber contacted to add patient's address	
	and add his qualifications.	

8. *Process prescription (including example of label(s)).*
   - Prepare one label for each product.
   - Check Appendix 9 of the *British National Formulary* for supplementary labelling requirements. Amoxicillin: *British National Formulary* label number 9. Furosemide: no additional labels.
   - Perform final check of items, labels and prescription.
   - Pack in a suitable bag ready to give to patient/patient's representative.

   Labels (we have assumed that the name and address of the pharmacy and the words 'Keep out of the reach and sight of children' are pre-printed on the label):

Example 5.1 Continued

Amoxicillin 250 mg Capsules	**21**
Take ONE capsule THREE times a day.	
Take at regular intervals. Complete the prescribed	
course unless otherwise directed.	
Mrs Jessica White	Date of dispensing

Furosemide 40 mg Tablets	**28**
Take ONE tablet daily.	
Mrs Jessica White	Date of dispensing

---

9. *Endorse prescription*: Stamp with pharmacy stamp to indicate completion and annotate stamp with the prescription-only medicines register entry number (5.01).

10. *Destination of paperwork*: Retain prescription in pharmacy for two years.

11. *Identity check/counselling*:
   - Check patient's name and address.
   - Reinforce the dosage instructions.
   - Stress importance of taking amoxicillin regularly and completing the course.
   - Check patient is not penicillin sensitive and advise that there may be reduced efficacy of her oral contraceptive and therefore she may need to take extra precautions while taking the amoxicillin.
   - Advise that the furosemide is normally taken in the morning as may need to go to toilet more frequently within 2 hours of taking the medication.
   - Draw patient's attention to the patient information leaflets (PILs) and ask if she has any questions.

Example 5.2

You receive the following prescription in your pharmacy.

W. DRILLETT BDS
ANYTOWN DENTAL SURGERY
ANYTOWN
AN1 1RB

Mrs Julie Winter
34 Hill Road
Anytown

Clarithromycin Tablets

250 mg

1 bd for 7 days

W. Drillett

Today's date

---

1. *Identity of order*: Private prescription.
2. *Prescriber*: Dentist (the prescriber is a local dentist).
3. *Legally written?* Yes. The item (clarithromycin) is not listed within the Dental Practitioners' Formulary; however, as this is a private prescription form, the dentist is not limited to prescribing from within this list.

   Nevertheless, you should still ensure that the dentist is prescribing within his or her area of competence. As this prescription form is for an antibiotic, this prescribing is likely to be within the dentist's area of competence and so it would be acceptable to make the supply without any further information.
4. *Clinical check (complete the following table)*:

DRUG	INDICATIONS	DOSE CHECK	REFERENCE
Clarithromycin	Respiratory tract infections, skin and soft tissue infections	250–500 mg every 12 hours	*British National Formulary* 54th edition, section 5.1.5.

5. *Interactions*: There is only one item on the prescription form. However, it would also be advisable for the pharmacist or pharmacy technician to check the patient medication record (PMR) for any concurrent medication that could cause an interaction. In this case, the patient's PMR indicated that she usually takes an oral contraceptive.
6. *Suitability for patient*: The item prescribed is safe and suitable for an adult patient and the dose ordered on the prescription is within the recommended dose limits.
7. *Records to be made (including copies of the record(s))*: A prescription-only medicines register entry will be required:

Example 5.2 Continued

Reference number	Details	Cost
5.02	Mrs Julie Winter	Cost
	34 Hill Road	+
Date of	Anytown	50%
supply		+
	Clarithromycin Tablets	Dispensing fee
	250mg	+
		Container fee
	1 bd for 7 days (14 tablets)	
	W. Drillett BDS	
	Anytown Dental Surgery	
	Anytown	
	AN1 1RB	
	Date on prescription: Today's	

8. *Process prescription (including example of label(s))*:
   - Prepare produce label.
   - Check Appendix 9 of the *British National Formulary* for supplementary labelling requirements. Clarithromycin: *British National Formulary* label number 9.
   - Perform final check of item, label and prescription.
   - Pack in a suitable bag ready to give to patient/patient's representative.

Labels (we have assumed that the name and address of the pharmacy and the words 'Keep out of the reach and sight of children' are pre-printed on the label):

Clarithromycin 250 mg Tablets   **14**
Take ONE tablet TWICE a day.
Take at regular intervals. Complete the prescribed course
unless otherwise directed.
Mrs Julie Winter   Date of dispensing

Example 5.2 Continued

9. *Endorse prescription*: Stamp with pharmacy stamp to indicate completion and annotate stamp with the prescription-only medicines register entry number (5.02).
10. *Destination of paperwork*: Retain prescription in pharmacy for two years.
11. *Identity check/counselling*:
    - Check patient's name and address.
    - Reinforce the dosage instructions.
    - Stress importance of taking clarithromycin regularly and completing the course.
    - Advise the patient that there may be reduced efficacy of her oral contraceptive and therefore she may need to take extra precautions while taking the antibiotics.
    - Draw patient's attention to the patient information leaflet (PIL) and ask if she has any questions.

5.5.3 Examples of requisitions and the dispensing process

The following section contains examples of requisitions that may be encountered in a community pharmacy. In each case, the following sections have been completed to guide you through the dispensing process (note that compared to the dispensing of NHS prescriptions (see Section 3.5.2) and non-NHS (private) prescriptions (see Section 5.5.2), there is no need to perform a clinical check (except for some patient-specific written requests from optometrists), check for inter-

actions, check the suitability of the item(s) for the patient or check whether the item(s) are allowable on the NHS):

1. Identity of order
2. Prescriber
3. Legally written?
4. Records to be made (including copies of the record(s))
5. Process requisition
6. Endorse requisition
7. Destination of paperwork
8. Identity check/counselling.

Example 5.3

You receive the following requisition in your pharmacy:

W. DRILLETT BDS
ANYTOWN DENTAL SURGERY
ANYTOWN
AN1 1RB

Please supply

10 Amoxicillin Injections

W. Drillett   Today's date

Example 5.3 Continued

1. *Identity of order*: Written requisition.
2. *Prescriber*: Dentist (the prescriber is a local dentist).
3. *Legally written?* No. The prescriber needs to add the purpose of the supply to the requisition. 'For use in my practice' would be suitable. In addition the prescriber needs to clarify the strength of the injections required: 250 mg or 500 mg.
4. *Records to be made (including copies of the record(s))*: A prescription-only medicines register entry will be required, although as the requisition will be kept in the pharmacy, this entry is made as good practice rather than a legal requirement.

Reference number	Details	Cost
5.03	W. Drillett BDS	Cost
	Anytown Dental Surgery	+
Date of	Anytown	50%
supply	AN1 1RB	+
		Dispensing fee
	Please supply	+
	10 Amoxicillin Injections	Container fee
		+
	Date on requisition: Today's	VAT
	Dentist contacted for additions of purpose (For use in surgery) and for strength of injections required (250 mg).	

5. *Process requisition*:
   - Select a full original pack from shelf to sell to dentist without labelling.
   - Check expiry date. Make final check of item against the requisition.
   - Pack in a suitable bag ready to give to dentist.
6. *Endorse requisition*: Stamp with pharmacy stamp to indicate completion and annotate stamp with the prescription-only medicines register entry number (5.03).
7. *Destination of paperwork*: Retain requisition in pharmacy for two years.
8. *Identity check/counselling*: Check identity of person collecting.

Example 5.4

You receive the following requisition in your pharmacy:

> **Dr R U Better**
> **ANYTOWN HEALTH CENTRE**
> **ANYTOWN**
> **AN1 1RB**
>
> Please supply for use in my practice
>
> 50 Buccastem Tablets 3mg
>
> Today's date

1. *Identity of order*: Written requisition.
2. *Prescriber*: Doctor.
3. *Legally written?* The prescription-only medicines register entry must either state that the pharmacist knows Dr R U Better is an appropriate practitioner (so long as they do) or the pharmacist must ask for qualifications to be added and record these in the prescription-only medicines register. There is no signature on the order but this is not a legal requirement.
4. *Records to be made (including copies of the record(s))*: A prescription-only medicines register entry will be required, although as the requisition will be kept in the pharmacy, this entry is made as good practice rather than a legal requirement.

Reference number	Details	Cost
5.04 Date of supply	Dr R U Better Anytown Health Centre Anytown AN1 1RB Please supply 50 Buccastem Tablets 3mg For use in my practice Date on requisition: Today's Prescriber contacted for qualifications (MBChB). or Dr R .U. Better is a GP known to me.	Cost + 50% + Dispensing fee + Container fee + VAT

Example 5.4 Continued

5. *Process requisition*:
   - Select a full original pack from shelf to sell to doctor without labelling.
   - Check expiry date. Make final check of item against the requisition.
   - Pack in a suitable bag ready to give to doctor.
6. *Endorse requisition*: Stamp with pharmacy stamp to indicate completion and annotate stamp with the prescription-only medicines register entry number (5.04).
7. *Destination of paperwork*: Retain requisition in pharmacy for two years.
8. *Identity check/counselling*: Check identity of person collecting.

Example 5.5

You receive the following requisition in your pharmacy:

Miss C Ittall
Anytown Opticians
High Street
Anytown

Please supply:

Pilocarpine Hydrochloride
1% eye drops
1 × OP

C Ittall   Today's date

---

1. *Identity of order*: Written requisition.
2. *Prescriber*: Optometrist.
3. *Legally written?* No. The prescriber needs to add the purpose of the supply to the requisition. 'For use in my practice' would be suitable. Also the requisition needs to have the qualifications of the optometrist added. Pilocarpine can only be supplied to an additional supply optometrist and there-fore this would also have to be checked.
4. *Records to be made (including copies of the record(s))*: A prescription-only medicines register entry will be required, although as the requisition will be kept in the pharmacy, this entry is made as good practice rather than a legal requirement.

Example 5.5 Continued

Reference number	Details	Cost
5.05 Date of supply	Miss C Ittall Anytown Opticians High Street Anytown Please supply Pilocarpine Hydrochloride 1% eye drops 1 × OP Date on requisition: Today's Prescriber contacted for addition of qualification (Mcoptom) and confirmation that she is an additional supply optometrist. Also contacted for the purpose (for use in my practice).	Cost + 50% + Dispensing fee + Container fee + VAT

5. *Process requisition*:
   - Select a full original pack from shelf to sell to optometrist without labelling.
   - Check expiry date. Make final check of item against the requisition.
   - Pack in a suitable bag ready to give to optometrist.
6. *Endorse requisition*: Stamp with pharmacy stamp to indicate completion and annotate stamp with the prescription-only medicines register entry number (5.05).
7. *Destination of paperwork*: Retain requisition in pharmacy for two years.
8. *Identity check/counselling*: Check identity of person collecting.

Example 5.6

You receive the following requisition in your pharmacy:

> **Miss C Ittall MCOptom**
> **Anytown Opticians**
> **High Street**
> **Anytown**
>
> Please supply:
>
> Samantha Wright
> 3 The Grove   Anytown
>
> 1 OP Chloramphenicol eye ointment
> 1% for bacterial conjunctivitis
>
> Apply qds
>
> C Ittall   Today's date

1. *Identity of order*: Written requisition. Although this is a written requisition for a medicine, as it is from an optometrist for a specific patient (see Section 5.2.7), the pharmacists still has a professional obligation to ensure that the medicine is safe and suitable for the patient.
2. *Prescriber*: Optometrist.
3. *Legally written?* Yes.
4. *Records to be made (including copies of the record(s))*: A prescription-only medicines register entry will be required, although as the requisition will be kept in the pharmacy, this entry is made as good practice rather than a legal requirement.

Reference number	Details	Cost
5.06 Date of supply	Miss C Ittall MCOptom Anytown Opticians High Street Anytown Please supply Samantha Wright 3 The Grove Anytown 1 OP Chloramphenicol eye ointment 1% for bacterial conjunctivitis. Apply qds Date on requisition: Today's	Cost + 50% + Dispensing fee + Container fee + VAT

Example 5.6 Continued

5. *Process requisition*:
   - Select a full original pack from shelf and sell to patient.
   - Legally (as this is a signed order from an optician) we do not have to label the item. However, professionally we may feel obliged to pass on the dosage instructions from the optician.
   - Check expiry date. Make final check of item against the requisition.
   - Pack in a suitable bag ready to give to the patient.
6. *Endorse requisition*: Stamp with pharmacy stamp to indicate completion and annotate stamp with the prescription-only medicines register entry number (5.06).
7. *Destination of paperwork*: Retain requisition in pharmacy for two years.
8. *Identity check/counselling*:
   - Check patient's name and address.
   - Reinforce the dosage instructions (see Section 9.3).
     - Before applying ointment, wash your hands.
     - Sit in front of a mirror so you can see what you are doing.
     - Remove the cap of the ointment.
     - Tip your head back.
     - Gently pull down your lower eyelid and look up.
     - Hold the tube above the eye and gently squeeze a 1 cm line of ointment along the inside of the lower eyelid, taking care not to touch the eye or eyelashes with the tip of the tube.
     - Blink your eyes to spread the ointment over the surface of the eyeball.
     - Your vision may be blurred when you open your eyes – don't rub your eyes. The blurring will clear after a few moments if you keep blinking.
     - Wipe away any excess ointment with a clean tissue.
     - Repeat this procedure for the other eye if you have been advised to do so by your optician.
     - Replace the cap of the tube.
     - Take care not to touch the tip of the tube with your fingers.
   - Contact lenses: if you normally wear contact lenses, don't wear them while using eye ointment unless your optician has told you otherwise.
   - Eye ointments containing a preservative should be thrown away four weeks after opening. Write the date you open your eye ointment on the tube so you know when to throw it away.
   - Some people may find their eyes sting immediately after use. This will normally only be for a short time.
   - Eye ointments should only be used in the eyes and must not to be taken by mouth.
   - Draw patient's attention to the patient information leaflet (PIL) and ask if she has any questions.

Example 5.7

You receive the following requisition in your pharmacy:

> **MICHAEL FOOT MChS**
> **ANYTOWN HEALTH CENTRE**
> **ANYTOWN**
> **AN1 1RB**
>
> Please supply for use in my
> practice:
>
> 10 × 2 ml Lidocaine 1% injections
>
> Michael Foot   Today's date

1. *Identity of order*: Written requisition.
2. *Prescriber*: Chiropodist.
3. *Legally written?* Yes, but need to check certificate of competence in use of analgesia.
4. *Records to be made (including copies of the record(s))*: A prescription-only medicines register entry will be required, although as the requisition will be kept in the pharmacy, this entry is made as good practice rather than a legal requirement.

Reference number	Details	Cost
5.07	Michael Foot MChS Anytown Health Centre Anytown AN1 1RB	Cost
		+
Date of		50%
supply		+
	Please supply for use in my practice	Dispensing fee
	10 x 2 ml Lidocaine 1% injections	+
		Container fee
		+
	Date on requisition: Today's	VAT
	Checked that chiropodist had a certificate of competence in use of analgesia.	

Example 5.7 Continued

5. *Process requisition:*
   • Select a full original pack from shelf to sell to chiropodist without labelling.
   • Check expiry date. Make final check of item against the requisition.
   • Pack in a suitable bag ready to give to chiropodist.
6. *Endorse requisition:* Stamp with pharmacy stamp to indicate completion and annotate stamp with the prescription-only medicines register entry number (5.07).
7. *Destination of paperwork:* Retain requisition in pharmacy for two years.
8. *Identity check/counselling:* Check identity of person collecting.

5.6 Chapter summary

This chapter has covered the key points it is necessary to be familiar with in order to supply medication via non-NHS prescription forms (private prescriptions) and via both written and oral requisitions. This has included details on who may requisition medicines and the restrictions placed on different healthcare practitioners.

A collection of worked examples has been provided and it is suggested that the student pharmacist or pharmacy technician works though these examples and ensures that they are familiar with the key learning points.

6

Controlled drugs

Upon completion of this chapter, you should be able to:

- understand how controlled drugs are classified within pharmacy
- list authorised prescribers of controlled drugs
- be familiar with the different requirements for prescriptions for controlled drugs
- understand the purpose of specific non-NHS (private) prescription forms for controlled drugs
- be familiar with the dispensing procedure for controlled drugs, including the use of addict (instalment) prescriptions
- understand the procedures involved with the supply of controlled drugs via written requisitions
- appreciate the legislation relating to the record-keeping, storage and destruction of controlled drugs
- complete a number of worked examples of prescriptions containing controlled drugs and the dispensing process.

6.1 Introduction and the history of controlled drugs

Some drugs have increased measures placed upon them relating to possession and supply. Within pharmacy, these are termed controlled drugs or more commonly CDs. It is vital that pharmacists and pharmacy technicians become familiar with the additional requirements placed on controlled drugs as deviation from the legal requirements could lead to prosecution.

This chapter will highlight the key parts of the Misuse of Drugs Act 1971 and Misuse of Drugs Regulations 2001 (and subsequent amendments) that are relevant to current pharmaceutical practice. However, this is an area that at the time of writing is going through some key changes. Therefore, in a similar way to developments within clinical practice, it is the responsibility of individual pharmacists and pharmacy technicians to ensure that they are up-to-date with any changes to the legislation covering controlled drugs.

The aim of the Misuse of Drugs Act 1971 was to sort out the existing 'fragmentary, inadequate and inflexible legislation' that was controlling the supply of differing drugs at the time. In addition, the Act set up the Advisory Council on Misuse of Drugs, which is an independent expert body that advises Government on drug-related issues in the UK.

6.2 Classification of controlled drugs

The Misuse of Drugs Act 1971 classifies controlled drugs into three classes: Class A, Class B and Class C. These classes reflect the level of harm that the drug may do to individuals (with Class A being the highest level) but any classification is unlinked to whether the drug is used within medicine. The higher the class, the higher the penalties applied for possession and supply (i.e. dealing). Drugs may move between classes. One of the most contentious recent re-classifications was the move of cannabis from a Class B to a Class C drug in January 2004.

For day-to-day use in pharmacy, the classification of controlled drugs into different schedules is used. The schedules reflect more the use of the individual controlled drugs within medicine and is more useful. These schedules are set out in the Misuse of Drugs Regulations:

- Schedule 1 – Not used for medicinal purposes
- Schedule 2 – Opiates and stimulants
- Schedule 3 – Barbiturates and 'minor stimulants'
- Schedule 4
  - Part 1 Benzodiazepines
  - Part 2 Anabolic/androgenic steroids and polypeptide hormones
- Schedule 5 – Negligible risk/low strength.

Key point 6.1

Within pharmacy, controlled drugs are classified into five Schedules:

- Schedule 1 – Not used for medicinal purposes
- Schedule 2 – Opiates and stimulants
- Schedule 3 – Barbiturates and 'minor stimulants'

$\rightarrow$

- Schedule 4:
  - Part 1 Benzodiazepines
  - Part 2 Anabolic/androgenic steroids and polypeptide hormones
- Schedule 5 – Negligible risk/low strength.

The easiest way to identify which schedule of the Misuse of Drugs Act a drug is within is to refer to a current edition of *Medicines, Ethics and Practice – A Guide for Pharmacists and Pharmacy Technicians*. Within the 'Alphabetical list of medicines for human use', the list uses the following abbreviations to indicate the schedule(s) that apply to the drug:

- CD POM – Schedule 2
- CD No Reg POM – Schedule 3
- CD Benz POM – Schedule 4, Part I
- CD Anab POM – Schedule 4, Part II
- CD Inv POM or CD Inv P – Schedule 5.

Pharmacists and pharmacy technicians need to take care when using this list as one drug may appear in more than one schedule, depending on the strength of the drug within a particular preparation. For example, morphine sulphate is a schedule 2 controlled drug when it is in an injectable form. However, within kaolin and morphine mixture BP, the morphine is classified as a schedule 5 drug owing to the low concentration of morphine within the preparation.

It is important that pharmacists and pharmacy technicians become familiar with the different requirements of the different schedules. For example:

- Which schedule requires that controlled drugs need to be kept in a locked controlled drugs cupboard?
- Which schedule allows for some controlled drugs to be supplied in an emergency at the request of a patient?

Differing requirements apply to drugs in different schedules. This is further complicated as drugs in some schedules are exempt from some of the individual requirements. These requirements and how they are put into practice are covered in the next section.

6.3 Practical application of the Misuse of Drugs Act and Regulations

This section will cover the following requirements of the Misuse of Drugs Act and Regulations:

- prescribers of controlled drugs (see Section 6.3.1)
- prescription requirements (see Section 6.3.2)
- non-NHS (private) prescription forms for controlled drugs (see Section 6.3.3)
- dispensing controlled drugs (see Section 6.3.4)
- addict (instalment) prescriptions for controlled drugs (see Section 6.3.5)
- requisitions for controlled drugs (see Section 6.3.6)
- record-keeping (see Section 6.3.7)
- storage (see Section 6.3.8)
- destruction (see Section 6.3.9).

6.3.1 Prescribers of controlled drugs

Until recently, the numbers of individuals who may prescribe controlled drugs was fairly limited. However, with the onset of both supplementary and independent prescribing, the numbers of individuals who may prescribe controlled drugs has increased.

Currently, the following regulations apply:

- Doctors, dentists and vets may prescribe all Schedule 2 to 5 controlled drugs. Doctors can only prescribe diamorphine, dipipanone or cocaine for the treatment of addiction with a licence from the Home Office (although they can prescribe these drugs for any other medical purpose).
- Nurses who are independent non-medical prescribers (formerly extended formulary nurse prescribers) may prescribe certain controlled drugs for certain medical conditions (see Section 3.2.5). These drugs and the conditions which they may be prescribed within

are listed in Table 6.1. Currently the other group of independent non-medical prescribers, pharmacist independent prescribers, may not prescribe any controlled drugs (although this may change in the future).

- Some controlled drugs can be supplied or administered via Patient Group Directions (PGD) (see Section 3.4). These are:
  - diamorphine, but only for the treatment of cardiac pain by nurses working in coronary care units or hospital accident and emergency departments
  - all drugs listed in Schedule 4 of the Regulations, except anabolic steroids and injectable formulations for the purpose of treating a person who is addicted to a drug
  - all drugs listed in Schedule 5 of the Regulations
  - from 1 January 2008, midazolam became a Schedule 3 controlled drug and will be the only Schedule 3 controlled drug that can be included in a PGD.
- Supplementary prescribers (see Section 3.2.4) via clinical management plans:
  - Any supplementary prescriber may prescribe any controlled drug so long as it is in the clinical management plan specific to that patient and agreed between the independent prescriber, the supplementary prescriber and the patient.
  - Any person can administer any controlled drug in accordance with the directions of a supplementary prescriber (acting under and in accordance with the terms of a clinical management plan).
- Midwives can possess, supply and administer diamorphine, morphine, pethidine and pentazocine provided it is in the course of their professional midwifery practice (see Section 5.2.5).

6.3.2 Prescription requirements

Current prescription requirements for Schedule 2 and Schedule 3 controlled drugs

Prescriptions for Schedule 2 and Schedule 3 controlled drugs have additional requirements, above and beyond what would normally be

Table 6.1 The different controlled drugs, the conditions they may be prescribed for and the route they can be administered by nurse independent non-medical prescribers

Drug	Indication	Route of administration
Buprenorphine	Transdermal use in palliative care	Transdermal
Chlordiazepoxide hydrochloride	Treatment of initial or acute withdrawal symptoms caused by the withdrawal of alcohol from persons habituated to it	Oral
Codeine phosphate	N/A	Oral
Co-phenotrope	N/A	Oral
Diamorphine hydrochloride	Use in palliative care, pain relief in respect of suspected myocardial infarction or for relief of acute or severe pain after trauma, including in either case post-operative pain relief	Oral or parenteral
Diazepam	Use in palliative care, treatment of initial or acute withdrawal symptoms caused by the withdrawal of alcohol from persons habituated to it, tonic-clonic seizures	Oral, parenteral or rectal
Dihydrocodeine tartrate	N/A	Oral
Fentanyl	Transdermal use in palliative care	Transdermal
Lorazepam	Use in palliative care, tonic-clonic seizures	Oral or parenteral
Midazolam	Use in palliative care, tonic-clonic seizures	Parenteral or buccal
Morphine hydrochloride	Use in palliative care, pain relief in respect of suspected myocardial infarction or for relief of acute or severe pain after trauma, including in either case post-operative pain relief	Rectal
Morphine sulphate	Use in palliative care, pain relief in respect of suspected myocardial infarction or for relief of acute or severe pain after trauma, including in either case post-operative pain relief	Oral, parenteral or rectal
Oxycodone hydrochloride	Use in palliative care	Oral or parenteral administration in palliative care

required on a prescription for it to be legally dispensed. Prescriptions for Schedule 2 and Schedule 3 controlled drugs must:

- be signed by the prescriber
- be dated
- be written so as to be indelible
- specify the address of the prescriber and their prescriber's identifier: for Schedule 2 and Schedule 3 controlled drugs, the address of the prescriber must be within the UK. In addition, it is necessary for the prescriber's identifier to be present on the prescription form. For NHS prescriptions, this is the prescriber's NHS number and for private prescriptions (see below), this is a specific six-digit number starting with a '6'.

- for a private prescription (including temazepam) be written on a FP10PCD (or equivalent in Scotland and Wales) (see Section 6.3.3 below).
- specify the dose to be taken (e.g. 'MDU' is not acceptable, but '1 MDU' would be)
- specify the form of the preparation: prescriptions for Schedule 2 and Schedule 3 controlled drugs must specify the form of the preparation even if only one form is available
- specify, where appropriate, the strength of the preparation: prescriptions for Schedule 2 and Schedule 3 controlled drugs only need to specify the strength of the preparation if more than one strength is available (compare this with the requirement above for the form of the preparation always to be present)

- specify either the total quantity (in both words and figures) of the preparation or (in both words and figures) the number of dosage units
- have written on it, if for dental treatment, the words 'For dental treatment only'
- specify the name and address of the patient. In addition, it is currently good practice (and may become a legal requirement) for prescribers to include the patient's identifier on all prescriptions for controlled drugs. This is the patient's NHS number in England and the equivalent in other countries.

It is worth noting that although it is a Schedule 3 controlled drug, some of the requirements listed above do not apply to prescriptions for the drug temazepam.

Key point 6.2

Prescriptions for Schedule 2 and Schedule 3 controlled drugs must*:

- be signed by the prescriber
- be dated
- be written so as to be indelible
- specify the address of the prescriber
- for a private prescription (including temazepam) be written on a FP10PCD (see Section 6.3.3 below)
- specify the dose to be taken
- specify the form of the preparation
- specify, where appropriate, the strength of the preparation
- specify either the total quantity (in both words and figures) of the preparation or (in both words and figures) the number of dosage units
- have written on it, if for dental treatment, the words 'For dental treatment only'
- specify the name and address of the patient.

* Note that some of the requirements listed above do not apply to prescriptions for the drug temazepam.

Recent changes to the prescription requirements for Schedule 2 and Schedule 3 controlled drugs

The prescription requirements applicable to controlled drugs have recently changed. It is useful to be familiar with these recent changes. In summary they are as follows:

- Prescriptions no longer need to be in the prescriber's own handwriting. Previous regulations meant that most prescriptions for Schedule 2 and Schedule 3 controlled drugs needed to be in the prescriber's own handwriting. Recent changes to the regulations mean that this is no longer the case (except for the requirement that the prescriber's signature still needs to be in ink, i.e. written by the prescriber; not computer generated). The prescription can be written by someone else but the Department of Health have stated that this must be a prescriber authorised to write a controlled drug prescription.
- The validity of prescriptions for controlled drugs has been reduced from 13 weeks to 28 days. The 28 days is from the date the prescription was signed or from the specified start date (see instalment dispensing for addicts (Section 6.3.5)) and applies to Schedule 2, Schedule 3 and Schedule 4 controlled drugs.
- It is good practice for prescribers to limit their prescribing to 30 days' supply.
- It is good practice for prescribers not to prescribe controlled drugs for themselves or close family members unless in an emergency.

Key point 6.3

Recent key changes to prescription requirements applicable to Schedule 2 and Schedule 3 controlled drugs are as follows:

- Prescriptions no longer need to be in the prescriber's own handwriting.

- The validity of controlled drug prescriptions has been reduced from 13 weeks to 28 days.

$\rightarrow$

- It is good practice for prescribers to limit their prescribing to 30 days' supply.

- It is good practice for prescribers not to prescribe controlled drugs for themselves or close family members unless in an emergency.

Technical errors on prescription forms for Schedule 2 and Schedule 3 controlled drugs

Pharmacists will be able to supply Schedule 2 and 3 controlled drugs (except temazepam), against some prescriptions that have a minor technical error but where the prescriber's intention is clear. The only errors that pharmacists can currently amend are minor typographical errors or spelling mistakes or where the total quantity of the preparation of the controlled drug or the number of dosage units as the case may be is specified in either words or figures but not both (i.e. they can add the words *or* the figures to the controlled drug prescription if they have been omitted).

These technical errors may be corrected providing that:

- having exercised all due diligence, the pharmacist is satisfied on reasonable grounds that the prescription is genuine
- having exercised all due diligence, the pharmacist is satisfied on reasonable grounds that they are supplying the controlled drug in accordance with the intention of the prescriber
- the pharmacist amends the prescription in ink or otherwise indelibly to correct the minor typographical errors, spelling mistakes or adds the total quantity of drug or number of dosage units in either words *or* figures so that the prescription complies with the Misuse of Drugs controlled drug prescription requirements
- the pharmacist marks the prescription so that the amendment they have made is attributable to them (for example, annotate the amendment with the pharmacist's signature/ initials and registration number).

6.3.3 Non-NHS (private) prescription forms for controlled drugs

Recent changes to the legislation has meant that private prescriptions for Schedule 2 and Schedule 3 controlled drugs for dispensing within the community (for human use) must be on a specific form, known as an FP10PCD (England), PPCD(1) (Scotland) and WP10PCD/ WP10PCDSS (Wales). Although it resembles an NHS prescription, the FP10PCD (and equivalents) is a private prescription. After dispensing, these private prescription forms are sent to the Prescription Pricing Division (PPD) (or equivalent) at the end of the month (in a similar way to NHS prescriptions; see Section 3.3.8). However, this is not for reimbursement (as the pharmacist or pharmacy technician will have charged the patient to cover the cost of the medication and supply), but for monitoring purposes. In addition, repeats of medication (see Section 5.1.1) are not allowed for Schedule 2 and Schedule 3 controlled drugs.

The layout of an FP10PCD can be seen in Figures 6.1 and 6.2. The key difference from an ordinary FP10 (or equivalent) prescription form (see Section 2.2.6) is the absence on the rear of the form of the section for the patient to complete to indicate whether they are exempt from prescription charges. This is because the form is a private prescription form and as such the patient will be charged to cover the cost of the medication and supply.

6.3.4 Dispensing controlled drugs

The dispensing procedure

The dispensing procedure for a prescription form containing a controlled drug is the same as for any prescription except for the need for additional checks to be performed to ensure that the supply is legal. It is also worth mentioning that although pharmacists and pharmacy technicians will perform extra legal checks on a prescription, this does not negate the need for the usual full clinical checks to be performed. For example, a prescription can be legally written (when applying the requirements of the Misuse

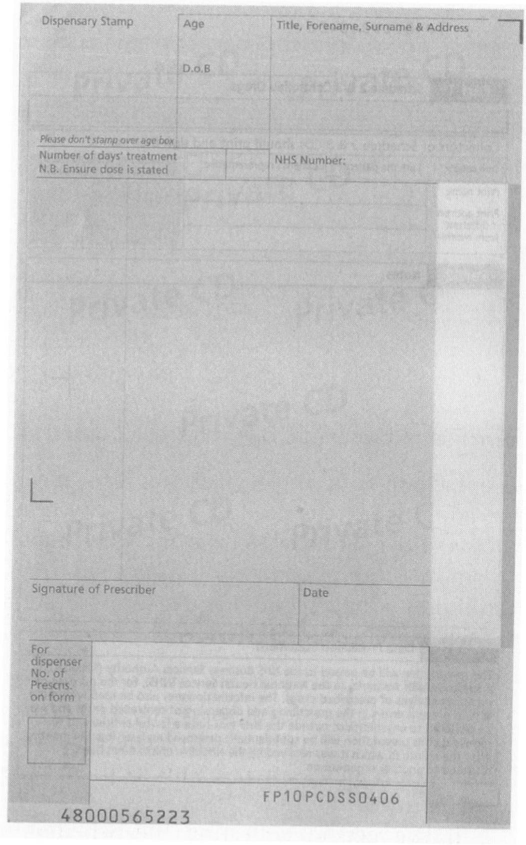
Dispensary Stamp
Age
Title, Forename, Surname & Address
D.o.B
Please don't stamp over age box
Number of days' treatment
N.B. Ensure dose is stated
NHS Number:
Signature of Prescriber
Date
For dispenser
No. of Prescns. on form
FP10PCDSS0406
48000565223

Figure 6.1 The front of an FP10PCD prescription form.

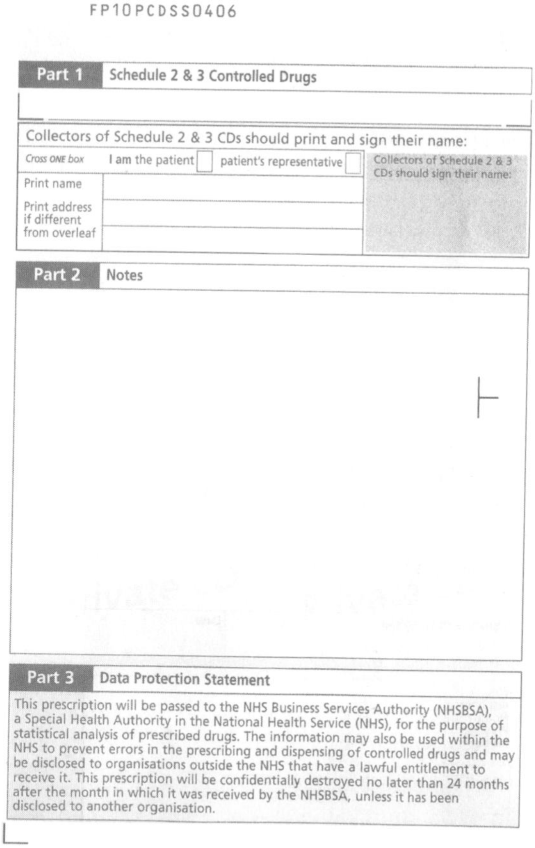
FP10PCDSS0406

Part 1 Schedule 2 & 3 Controlled Drugs

Collectors of Schedule 2 & 3 CDs should print and sign their name:

Cross ONE box — I am the patient ☐ — patient's representative ☐ — Collectors of Schedule 2 & 3 CDs should sign their name:

Print name

Print address if different from overleaf

Part 2 Notes

Part 3 Data Protection Statement

This prescription will be passed to the NHS Business Services Authority (NHSBSA), a Special Health Authority in the National Health Service (NHS), for the purpose of statistical analysis of prescribed drugs. The information may also be used within the NHS to prevent errors in the prescribing and dispensing of controlled drugs and may be disclosed to organisations outside the NHS that have a lawful entitlement to receive it. This prescription will be confidentially destroyed no later than 24 months after the month in which it was received by the NHSBSA, unless it has been disclosed to another organisation.

Figure 6.2 The back of an FP10PCD prescription form.

of Drugs Act and Regulations) but may still contain an overdose that the pharmacist or pharmacy technician would be expected to identify.

The regulations state that the prescription must not be dispensed:

- unless it complies with the requirements (i.e. the additional requirements that apply to prescriptions for controlled drugs listed in Section 6.3.2)
- if the prescriber's address given on the prescription is not within the UK (for Schedule 2 and Schedule 3 controlled drugs)
- unless the prescriber's signature is genuine
- before the date specified on the prescription
- more than 28 days after the date on the prescription (or specified start date) for Schedule 2, Schedule 3 and Schedule 4 controlled drugs.

Further points relating to the dispensing of prescriptions for controlled drugs:

- The date of each supply must be marked on the prescription.
  - If only part of a supply can be made due to lack of stock, the quantity and date of the original supply must be noted on the prescription (and for a Schedule 2 controlled drug, entered in the controlled drugs register; see Section 6.3.7).
  - For any subsequent supply to complete the prescription, the quantity and date of supply must be noted on the prescription

(and for a Schedule 2 controlled drug, entered in the controlled drugs register). The remaining quantity must be supplied within the 28-day validity period of the prescription (see Section 6.3.2).

- Repeats of Schedule 2 and Schedule 3 drugs are not allowed, but instalments are (this is particularly useful with addicts' prescriptions; see Section 6.3.5).
- For supply against a non-NHS (private) prescription form, a prescription-only medicines register entry is not legally required if a controlled drugs register entry is made (see Section 6.3.7), but it is still good practice to do so.
- Emergency supplies (see Chapter 7) of Schedule 2 and Schedule 3 controlled drugs are not allowed except phenobarbital for the treatment of epilepsy.

Key point 6.4

When dispensing a prescription for a controlled drug, pharmacists and pharmacy technicians need to take the following points into consideration. A prescription for a controlled drug must not be dispensed:

- unless it complies with the requirements
- if the prescriber's address given on the prescription is not within the UK (for Schedule 2 and Schedule 3 controlled drugs)
- unless the prescriber's signature is genuine
- before the date specified on the prescription
- more than 28 days after the date on the prescription (or specified start date).

In addition:

- The date of each supply must be marked on the prescription.
- Repeats of Schedule 2 and 3 drugs are not allowed, but instalments are.

→

- For private prescriptions, a prescription-only medicines register entry is not legally required if a controlled drugs register entry is made, but it is still good practice to do so.
- Emergency supplies of Schedule 2 and Schedule 3 controlled drugs are not allowed except phenobarbital for the treatment of epilepsy.

Collection of prescriptions for controlled drugs

Recent changes to the regulations have meant that additional steps need to be taken by pharmacists and pharmacy technicians when handing out medication containing controlled drugs. These additional requirements can be summarised as follows:

- Pharmacists must ascertain whether the person collecting a Schedule 2 controlled drug is the patient, the patient's representative or a healthcare professional acting in their capacity as such.
  - If the person collecting the Schedule 2 controlled drug is a healthcare professional acting in their professional capacity on behalf of the patient, the pharmacist must obtain the name and address of the healthcare professional and, unless they are already acquainted with that person, they should request evidence of that person's identity (however, even if identification is not provided the pharmacist may still supply the controlled drug).
- Pharmacists are expected to ask for identification upon collection of Schedule 2 controlled drug and to obtain a signature on the back of prescription (see Figure 6.3).
  - Pharmacists have the discretion not to ask for identification but this must be recorded in the controlled drug register (see Section 6.3.7).
- The collection of Schedule 3 controlled drugs does not require identification, but the collector is still expected to sign back of prescription (see Figure 6.3).

Collectors of Schedule 2 & 3
CDs should sign their name:

Figure 6.3   The box on the rear of a prescription form for collectors of Schedule 2 and Schedule 3 controlled drugs to sign.

6.3.5 Addict (instalment) prescriptions for controlled drugs

The treatment of addiction to certain drugs utilises substitution therapy. This is where the drug that the patient is addicted to is substituted for another drug that may be prescribed on a prescription form. Drugs allowed as substitutes are (most commonly) methadone, buprenorphine, dextromoramide, morphine and pethidine. In addition, it is possible for prescribers to prescribe diazepam on instalment prescriptions for the management of side-effects to addiction treatment.

As it may not be desirable to supply patients addicted to drugs with a large quantity of a drug substitute, it is possible to supply the drug in instalments via specific instalment prescription forms. These prescription forms are similar to standard NHS prescription forms; however, they contain an extra portion for the pharmacist or pharmacy technician to record the details of each instalment. Details of the different instalment prescription forms can be found in Section 2.2 (note that in Scotland, general practitioners can prescribe in instalments on a GP10 or GP10SS). An example of an NHS prescription form used for instalment dispensing in England is shown in Figure 6.4.

Any pattern of instalments on an instalment prescription is permitted, although (for England and Wales) prescribers should limit their supply to 14 days (30 days for Scotland). For details of the different drugs which may be prescribed in instalments for England, Scotland and Wales, see *Medicines, Ethics and Practice – A Guide for Pharmacists and Pharmacy Technicians*.

A specific start date may be specified; if it is, then it must be followed. If no start date is specified then the prescription may legally be started any time within the 28 days, but professionally we would be concerned if there was a gap in treatment.

Until recently there was a strict rule that instalments could only be collected on the day specified. However, if the prescriber includes the following wording (or similar wording approved by the Home Office) on the prescription then exceptions can be made:

> Instalment prescriptions covering more than one day should be collected on the specified day; if this collection is missed the remainder of the instalment (i.e. the instalment less the amount prescribed for the day(s) missed) may be supplied.

Therefore if, for example, a patient collected his instalments on Monday (for Monday and Tuesday), Wednesday (for Wednesday and Thursday) and Friday (for Friday, Saturday and Sunday), but failed to collect the instalments on a Friday, he would have to either wait until Monday to collect the next set of instalments, or visit the prescriber (on Saturday or Sunday) to gain a prescription to cover the intervening days. However, if the instalment prescription contained the wording as detailed above and if the patient failed to collect his instalments on Friday but came to the pharmacy on Saturday, he would still be able to collect Saturday's and Sunday's instalments (although not Friday's).

6.3.6 Requisitions for controlled drugs

Requisitions for controlled drugs follow the same basic format as for other written requisitions (see Section 5.2). The following individuals may be supplied with a Schedule 2 or Schedule 3 controlled drug via a written requisition (remember that prescribers cannot normally obtain or prescribe Schedule 1 controlled drugs without the authority of a Home Office licence):

- a practitioner (doctor, dentist or vet)

Pharmacy Stamp	Age	Title, Forename, Surname & Address		Date	Item	Quantity supplied	Pharmacist's initials
	D.o.B						
Please don't stamp over age box							
Number of days' treatment N.B. Ensure dose is stated		NHS Number:					
Endorsements							
Signature of Prescriber		Date					
For dispenser No. of Prescns. on form	Prescriber's name and address						
NHS	FP10MDA0406						
42144580006				NOTE Details of items supplied - see notes overleaf			

Figure 6.4   An example of a prescription form used for the instalment supply of substitution therapy to patients suffering from drug addiction in England (FP10MDA).

- the matron or acting matron of a hospital or nursing home
  - the requisition must be signed by a doctor or dentist employed there
- a sister or acting sister in charge of a ward, theatre or other hospital or nursing home
- a person in charge of a laboratory used for scientific education or research
- the owner or master of a British ship where there is no doctor employed on board (see Figure 5.3 and Figure 5.4)
- the installation manager of an offshore installation
- the master of a foreign ship in a port in Great Britain (N.B. extra requirements apply)
- a supplementary prescriber.

The following requirements apply to requisitions for Schedule 2 or Schedule 3 controlled drugs. They must:

- be signed by the recipient (i.e. the person authorised to be supplied)
- state name, address, and profession or occupation
- specify total quantity of drug and purpose for which it is required.

The supplier must also be satisfied that both the signature and qualification are genuine.

Key point 6.5

The following requirements apply to requisitions for Schedule 2 or Schedule 3 controlled drugs:

→

- They must be signed by the recipient (i.e. the person authorised to be supplied).
- They should state name, address, and profession or occupation.
- They must specify total quantity of drug and purpose for which it is required.
- The supplier must be satisfied that signature and qualification are genuine.

Requisitions for controlled drugs within the community

All requisitions for Schedule 2 and Schedule 3 controlled drugs against which supplies are made by pharmacists from a community pharmacy are now sent to the PPD (or equivalent) at the end of the month (in a similar way to NHS prescriptions; see Section 3.3.8). However, this is not for reimbursement (as the pharmacist or pharmacy technician will have charged the recipient to cover the cost of the medication and supply), but for monitoring purposes. In addition, the pharmacy should keep a photocopy of the requisition. This requirement does not apply to requisitions by veterinary practitioners or veterinary surgeons.

Once the requisition has been fulfilled, the pharmacist or pharmacy technician should mark the requisition with the name and address of supplying pharmacy (for example, stamp the requisition with the pharmacy stamp) and the date of supply.

The recording of the supply of Schedule 2 controlled drugs in the prescription-only medicines register against a written requisition is only a good practice requirement as an entry will be made detailing the supply in the controlled drugs register (see Section 6.3.7). In addition, although you will be sending the original requisition to the PPD (or equivalent) at the end of the month, you would still have a photocopy. For Schedule 3 controlled drugs, a prescription-only medicines register entry is also only good practice as you will also keep a photocopy of the original requisition form.

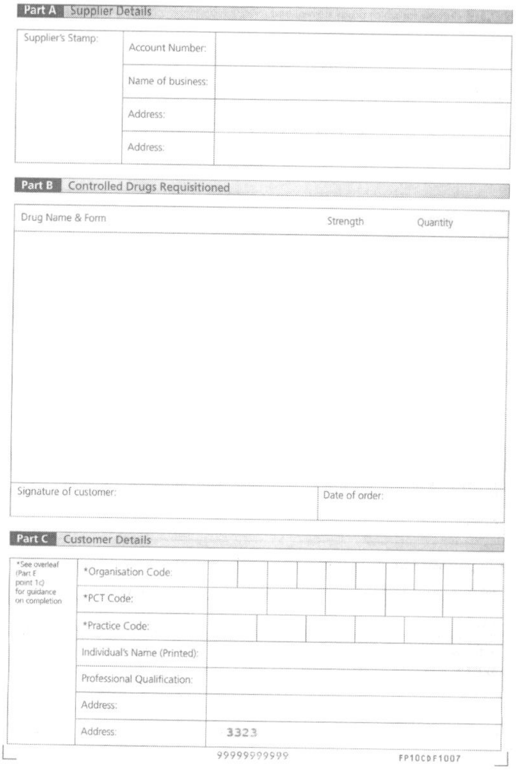
Part A Supplier Details

Supplier's Stamp:

Account Number:	
Name of business:	
Address:	
Address:	

Part B Controlled Drugs Requisitioned

Drug Name & Form	Strength	Quantity

Signature of customer:	Date of order:

Part C Customer Details

*See overleaf (Part E point 1c) for guidance on completion

*Organisation Code:	
*PCT Code:	
*Practice Code:	
Individual's Name (Printed):	
Professional Qualification:	
Address:	
Address:	3323

99999999999 FP10CDF1007

Figure 6.5 The front of a controlled drugs requisition form for England (FP10CDF).

From 1 January 2008, standardised requisition forms were introduced in England, (FP10CDF; see Figures 6.5 and 6.6), Scotland (CDRF) and Wales (WP10CDF) for the ordering of Schedule 2 and 3 controlled drugs and it is good practice for practitioners to use these forms when requisitioning Schedule 2 and 3 controlled drugs for human use from a community pharmacy. In exceptional circumstances, where a form other than the standardised requisition is used, there is still a legal requirement to submit the original requisition to the PPD (or equivalent) and to retain a copy.

Although it is not a legal requirement to provide a requisition where one community pharmacy supplies another community pharmacy, as good practice, a written requisition should be obtained. This requisition should also be submitted to the PPD (or equivalent) for processing.

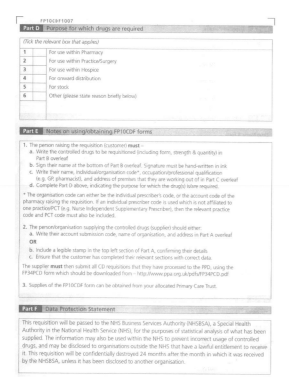

Figure 6.6 The back of a controlled drugs requisition form for England (FP10CDF).

In Scotland, a specific form for use by one community pharmacy to obtain stock from another community pharmacy has been developed and should be used for this purpose.

A pharmacist may supply a controlled drug to a practitioner in advance of requisition in an emergency. The pharmacist must receive the requisition within 24 hours of the supply. A messenger (for example, a receptionist from the surgery) must have a letter of authorisation in order to be in legal possession of the drugs.

A midwife's supply order is a particular type of requisition for specific controlled drugs and has been discussed in Section 5.2.5.

6.3.7 Record-keeping

Receipts and supplies of all Schedule 2 controlled drugs need to be recorded in the controlled drugs register. Currently in most pharmacies, the controlled drugs register is in the form of a bound book. Recent changes to the legislation have enabled the legal use of electronic controlled drugs registers, although suitable computer software is only just being developed. In the future, all controlled drugs registers will be electronic (as this facilitates audit of the use of controlled drugs).

The regulations surrounding controlled drugs and their recording in the controlled drugs register state the following:

- Entries must be in ink or otherwise indelible.
- Entries must be in date order (i.e. chronological).
- Entries must be made on day of transaction or next day following.
- No cancellation, alteration or obliteration. If a pharmacist or pharmacy technician makes a mistake when completing an entry in the controlled drugs register, they should annotate the entry (by the inclusion of an asterisk) and make a dated marginal note or footnote detailing the error. It is considered good practice for the pharmacist or pharmacy technician to sign the footnote and detail their registration number to provide a transparent audit trail.
- The register entry must be made for each quantity supplied. Therefore, if a Schedule 2 controlled drug is supplied in parts (for example, if it is supplied in instalments (see Section 6.3.5) then each supply will need to be recorded as a separate entry in the controlled drugs register.
- The register must be kept at the premises at all times during use and for two years from the last date of entry.
- A separate register/part of the register is used for each class of drugs, and the class must be specified at the top of each page (although see below for recent changes and additional requirements).
- Register, documents and stocks of drugs must be available for inspection (for example, by the RPSGB Inspector or Drug Squad Officer).

Key point 6.6

The regulations surrounding controlled drugs and their recording in the controlled drugs register state the following:

- Entries must be in ink or otherwise indelible.
- Entries must be in date order (i.e. chronological).
- Entries must be made on day of transaction or next day following.
- No cancellation, alteration or obliteration.
- The register entry must be made for each quantity supplied.
- The register must be kept at the premises at all times during use and for two years from the last date of entry.
- A separate register/part of the register is used for each class of drugs, and the class must be specified at the top of each page (although see below in the recent changes section for additional requirements).
- Register, documents and stocks of drugs must be available for inspection.

Recent changes to the regulations surrounding the controlled drugs register include the following:

- As discussed above, controlled drugs registers can be electronic, so long as they comply with national guidance.
- A record of whether the collector was the patient, the patient's representative or a healthcare professional (name and address needs to be recorded) should be noted in the controlled drugs register (see Section 6.3.4).
- Pharmacists should make a record of whether or not they asked for proof of identity of individuals collecting Schedule 2 controlled drugs and whether proof of identity was provided (see Section 6.3.4).
- All controlled drugs registers should contain a running balance.

These recent changes to the regulations surrounding the controlled drugs register has resulted in a change to the design of the pages of the register. Previously, receipts of each drug type (irrespective of presentation) were recorded in one part of the register and supplies (again, irrespective of presentation) were recorded in another. To enable running balances to be recorded, each presentation of a particular drug needs to be recorded on separate pages and both receipts and supplies need to be recorded on the same page. This means that each different drug, form and strength needs to be recorded on its own separate page.

An example of a page from a controlled drugs register is shown in Figure 6.7. This example contains columns for the minimum amount of information that needs to be recorded. However, it should be noted that the regulations do not prevent additional information being recorded (for example, the details of the supplying pharmacist).

6.3.8 Storage

Some controlled drugs need, according to the regulations, to be stored within a controlled drugs cupboard. The Misuse of Drugs regulations

Key point 6.7

The parts of the Misuse of Drugs regulations relating to the storage of controlled drugs within pharmacies are as follows:

- A cabinet built to specification in the regulations.
- Safe custody regulations apply to all Schedule 1 and 2 controlled drugs, except quinalbarbitone.
- Safe custody regulations also apply to Schedule 3 controlled drugs but all drugs used are exempt, apart from buprenorphine, diethylpropion, flunitrazepam and temazepam.

MISUSE OF DRUGS ACT
REGISTER OF:

DRUGS CLASS _____

NAME (brand, strength, form) _____

Date	Obtained		Supplied							Balance
					Person collecting					
Supply received or date supplied	Name, address of person or firm from whom obtained	Amount obtained	Name, address of person or firm supplied	Authority to possess – prescriber or licence holder details	Patient/Representative or Healthcare Professional (name and address)	Proof of identity requested Yes/No	Proof of identity provided Yes/No	Amount supplied		Carried over:

Figure 6.7   An example of a page from the controlled drugs register.

relating to the storage of controlled drugs within pharmacies are as follows:

- A cabinet built to the specification in the regulations must be provided (or the pharmacist can obtain police consent to use the pharmacy safe).
- Safe custody regulations apply to all Schedule 1 and 2 controlled drugs, except quinalbarbitone (however the RPSGB has stated that pharmacists may still wish to keep quinalbarbitone in the controlled drugs cabinet).
- Safe custody regulations also apply to Schedule 3 controlled drugs but all drugs used are exempt, apart from buprenorphine, diethylpropion, flunitrazepam and temazepam (i.e. these four drugs must be kept in the controlled drugs cupboard).

6.3.9 Destruction

The regulations regarding the destruction of controlled drugs are separated into those applied to pharmacy stock and those applied to patient-returned controlled drugs.

Destruction of controlled drugs as part of the pharmacy stock

Schedule 2 controlled drugs can only be destroyed in the presence of an appropriate person. Appropriate people currently include RPSGB Inspectors, some police officers (for example, controlled drugs liaison officers), chief executives of NHS trusts and some other individuals. This also applies to pharmacies who produce (i.e. manufacture or compound) Schedule 3 and Schedule 4 controlled drugs (as the pharmacy would be required to keep records relating to this activity).

A record of the destruction would need to be made in the controlled drugs register (see Section 6.3.7) and be signed by the authorised person.

Destruction of patient-returned controlled drugs

Currently, a pharmacist may destroy controlled drugs returned to pharmacies by patients. It is advised that patient-returned controlled drugs are destroyed as soon as possible and that a record of the destruction is made. Specific forms are available for this record, but pharmacists can currently record the information anywhere so long as it is not in the controlled drugs register (for example, a record could be kept on the back page of the prescription-only medicines register).

Specific denaturing kits are available for use and further guidance on the disposal of patient-returned controlled drugs can be found in the current edition of *Medicines, Ethics and Practice – A Guide for Pharmacists and Pharmacy Technicians*.

6.4 Worked examples

This section contains a number of worked examples of prescriptions forms containing controlled drugs. The same standard systematic approach will be followed as for other prescription forms (i.e. those which do not contain controlled drugs; see Section 3.3 for NHS prescription forms, and Section 5.4 for private prescription forms). This approach is summarised in Section 3.5.1.

As before, complete the following sections to guide you through the dispensing process:

1. Identity of order
2. Prescriber
3. Legally written?
4. Clinical check (complete the following table):

DRUG	INDICATIONS	DOSE CHECK	REFERENCE

5. Interactions
6. Suitability for patient
7. Item(s) allowable on the NHS
8. Records to be made (including copies of the record(s))
9. Process prescription (including example of label(s))
10. Endorse prescription
11. Destination of paperwork
12. Identity check/counselling.

Example 6.1

You receive the following prescription in your pharmacy:

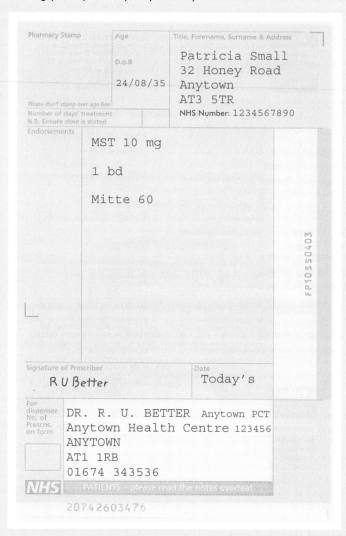

1. *Identity of order*: NHS prescription (FP10SS). The prescription is for a drug which is classified as a Schedule 2 controlled drug. Therefore the additional requirements relating to Schedule 2 controlled drugs need to be met before the prescription can be dispensed.
2. *Prescriber*: Doctor (general practitioner).

Example 6.1 Continued

3. *Legally written?* No. As the prescription is for a Schedule 2 controlled drug, additional prescription requirements need to be met before the prescription can be dispensed (see Section 6.3.2). In this case, the form of the prescription item and the quantity of drug to be supplied in both words and figures are missing. Return the prescription form to the prescriber for the addition of the pharmaceutical form and the quantity in words (note, if the only omission was the total quantity in words, the pharmacist could amend this without the need to send the prescription back to the prescriber; see Section 6.3.2).

4. *Clinical check (complete the following table):*

DRUG	INDICATIONS	DOSE CHECK	REFERENCE
Morphine (MST)	Acute pain	10 mg every 12 hours adjusted according to response	*British National Formulary* 54th edition, 'Prescribing in palliative care' and section 4.7.2

5. *Interactions:* There is only one drug on the prescription. However, it would also be advisable for the pharmacist or pharmacy technician to check the patient medication record (PMR) for any concurrent medication that could cause an interaction.

6. *Suitability for patient:* Item prescribed is safe and suitable for a patient of this age and the dose ordered on the prescription is within the recommended dose limits.

7. *Item(s) allowable on the NHS:* Yes (see *Drug Tariff*).

8. *Records to be made (including copies of the record(s)):* An entry would need to be made in the relevant section of the controlled drugs register detailing the supply. In addition a note of the intervention on a clinical intervention form would be made (see Figure 1.5).

DRUG CLASS *Morphine sulphate*

NAME (brand, strength, form) *MST 10 mg tablets*

Date supply received or date supplied	Obtained		Supplied							Balance
	Name, address of person or firm from whom obtained	Amount Obtained	Name, address of person or firm supplied	Authority to possess-presciber or licence holder details	Person collecting / Patient/Representative or Healthcare Professional (name and address)	Proof of identity requested Yes/No	Proof of identity provided Yes/No	Amount supplied		Carried over: 180
Today's			*Patricia Small 32 Honey Road Anytown*	*Dr R U Better FP10*	*Patient*	*Yes*	*Yes*	*60*		*120*

9. *Process prescription (including example of label(s)):*
   - Prepare label for product.
   - Check Appendix 9 of *British National Formulary* for supplementary labelling requirements. MST: *British National Formulary* label number 2 and 25.

Example 6.1 Continued

- Select pack of MST from the controlled drugs cupboard, remembering to check the expiry date and taking care that the correct strength of drug has been selected (the packaging of other strengths is very similar).
- Perform final check of item, label and prescription.
- Pack in a suitable bag ready to give to the patient or patient's representative (as this is a Schedule 2 controlled drug, it should be kept in the controlled drugs cupboard until it is collected by the patient or patient's representative).

Labels (we have assumed that the name and address of the pharmacy and the words 'Keep out of the reach and sight of children' are pre-printed on the label):

MST Continus 10 mg Tablets	**60**
Take ONE tablet TWICE a day swallowed whole, not chewed. Warning: May cause drowsiness. If affected do not drive or operate machinery. Avoid alcoholic drink.	
Ms Patricia Small	Date of dispensing

10. *Endorse prescription*: Stamp with pharmacy stamp to indicate completion and mark the date of supply.
11. *Destination of paperwork*: Send to the PPD at the end of the month. The controlled drugs register in which the details of the supply were made must be kept at the premises at all times during use and for two years from the last date of entry.
12. *Identity check/counselling*:
    - Check patient's name and address.
    - The pharmacist or pharmacy technician must identify whether the collector is the patient, patient's representative or a healthcare professional. This information (including the name and professional address if the collector is a healthcare professional) must be recorded in the controlled drugs register (see Section 6.3.4).
    - The pharmacist or pharmacy technician must note in the controlled drugs register whether the ID was requested from the collector and whether it was produced (see Section 6.3.4).
    - The collector should be asked to sign the rear of the prescription (see Section 6.3.4).
    - Reinforce the dosage instructions; advise that the tablets are best taken 12 hours apart, with or after food, and may cause drowsiness.
    - Draw patient's attention to the patient information leaflet (PIL) and ask if she has any questions.

Example 6.2

You receive the following prescription in your pharmacy:

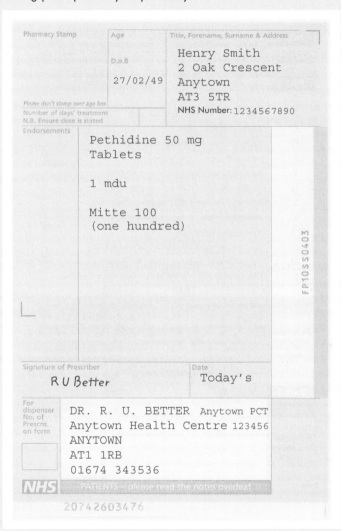

Pharmacy Stamp

Age

Title, Forename, Surname & Address

D.o.B

27/02/49

Henry Smith
2 Oak Crescent
Anytown
AT3 5TR

NHS Number: 1234567890

Please don't stamp over age box
Number of days' treatment
N.B. Ensure dose is stated

Endorsements

Pethidine 50 mg
Tablets

1 mdu

Mitte 100
(one hundred)

FP10SS0403

Signature of Prescriber

R U Better

Date

Today's

For dispenser
No. of
Prescns.
on form

DR. R. U. BETTER Anytown PCT
Anytown Health Centre 123456
ANYTOWN
AT1 1RB
01674 343536

NHS PATIENTS – please read the notes overleaf

20742603476

1. *Identity of order*: NHS prescription (FP10SS). The prescription is for a drug which is classified as a Schedule 2 controlled drug. Therefore the additional requirements relating to Schedule 2 controlled drugs need to be met before the prescription can be dispensed.
2. *Prescriber*: Doctor (general practitioner).
3. *Legally written?* Yes. As the prescription is for a Schedule 2 controlled drug, additional prescription requirements need to be met before the prescription can be dispensed (see Section 6.3.2). In this case, all the additional legal requirements for a prescription for a Schedule 2 controlled drug have been met.

Example 6.2 Continued

However, it is good practice for the prescriber to limit the supply of Schedule 2 and Schedule 3 controlled drugs to 30 days (see Section 6.3.2). Although the dosage instruction is legal for a prescription for a Schedule 2 controlled drug (1 mdu), it is not clear from the prescription the duration of treatment the requested supply will cover.

In this case, it would be a good idea to check with the patient what frequency of administration they have been informed to follow by the prescriber and then use this information to check the length of treatment the prescription quantity would cover. If this were greater than 30 days, the pharmacist should give consideration to querying the quantity requested with the prescriber.

4. *Clinical check (complete the following table)*:

DRUG	INDICATIONS	DOSE CHECK	REFERENCE
Pethidine	Acute pain	50–150 mg every 4 hours	*British National Formulary* 54th edition, section 4.7.2

5. *Interactions*: There is only one drug on the prescription. However, it would also be advisable for the pharmacist or pharmacy technician to check the patient medication record (PMR) for any concurrent medication that could cause an interaction.

6. *Suitability for patient*: Item prescribed is safe and suitable for a patient of this age and the dose ordered on the prescription is within the recommended dose limits.

7. *Item(s) allowable on the NHS*: Yes (see *Drug Tariff*).

8. *Records to be made (including copies of the record(s))*: An entry would need to be made in the relevant section of the controlled drugs register detailing the supply. In addition a note of the intervention on a clinical intervention form would be made (see Figure 1.5).

MISUSE OF DRUGS ACT
REGISTER OF:

DRUG CLASS *Pethidine*

NAME (brand, strength, form) *Pethidine hydrochloride 50 mg tablets*

Date supply received or date supplied	Obtained		Supplied						Balance
	Name, address of person or firm from whom obtained	Amount Obtained	Name, address of person or firm supplied	Authority to possess-prescriber or licence holder details	Person collecting / Patient/Representative or Healthcare Professional (name and address)	Proof of identity requested Yes/No	Proof of identity provided Yes/No	Amount supplied	Carried over: 300
Today's			Henry Smith 2 Oak Crescent Anytown	Dr R U Better FP10	Representative	Yes	Yes	100	200

Example 6.2 Continued

9. *Process prescription (including example of label(s)):*
   - Prepare label for product.
   - Check Appendix 9 of *British National Formulary* for supplementary labelling requirements. Pethidine: *British National Formulary* label number 2.
   - Select pack of pethidine from the controlled drugs cupboard, remembering to check the expiry date.
   - Perform final check of item, label and prescription.
   - Pack in a suitable bag ready to give to the patient or patient's representative (as this is a Schedule 2 controlled drug, it should be kept in the controlled drugs cupboard until it is collected by the patient or patient's representative).

   Labels (we have assumed that the name and address of the pharmacy and the words 'Keep out of the reach and sight of children' are pre-printed on the label):

Pethidine hydrochloride 50 mg Tablets	**100**
Take ONE tablet as directed.	
Warning. May cause drowsiness. If affected do not drive or operate machinery. Avoid alcoholic drink	
Mr Henry Smith	Date of dispensing

10. *Endorse prescription*: Stamp with pharmacy stamp to indicate completion and mark the date of supply.
11. *Destination of paperwork*: Send to the PPD at the end of the month. The controlled drugs register in which the details of the supply were made must be kept at the premises at all times during use and for two years from the last date of entry.
12. *Identity check/counselling*:
    - Check patient's name and address.
    - The pharmacist or pharmacy technician must identify whether the collector is the patient, patient's representative or a healthcare professional. This information (including the name and professional address if the collector is a healthcare professional) must be recorded in the controlled drugs register (see Section 6.3.4).
    - The pharmacist or pharmacy technician must note in the controlled drugs register whether the ID was requested from the collector and whether it was produced (see Section 6.3.4).
    - The collector should be asked to sign the rear of the prescription (see Section 6.3.4).
    - Reinforce the dosage instructions; advise that the tablets may cause drowsiness.
    - Draw patient's attention to the patient information leaflet (PIL) and ask if he has any questions.

Example 6.3

You receive the following prescription in your pharmacy:

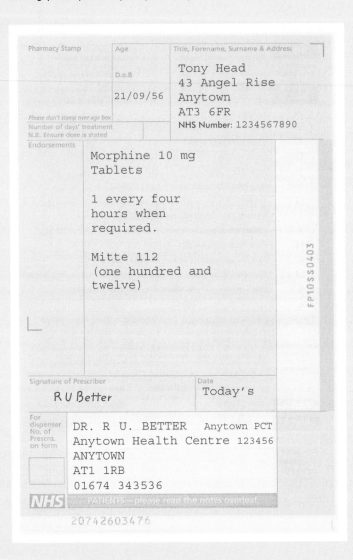

Pharmacy Stamp	Age	Title, Forename, Surname & Address
	D.o.B	Tony Head
	21/09/56	43 Angel Rise
		Anytown
		AT3 6FR
Please don't stamp over age box		NHS Number: 1234567890

Number of days' treatment
N.B. Ensure dose is stated

Endorsements

Morphine 10 mg
Tablets

1 every four
hours when
required.

Mitte 112
(one hundred and
twelve)

FP10SS0403

Signature of Prescriber

R U Better

Date
Today's

For dispenser
No. of
Prescns.
on form

DR. R U. BETTER   Anytown PCT
Anytown Health Centre 123456
ANYTOWN
AT1 1RB
01674 343536

NHS   PATIENTS – please read the notes overleaf

20742603476

1. *Identity of order*: NHS prescription (FP10SS). The prescription is for a drug which is classified as a Schedule 2 controlled drug. Therefore the additional requirements relating to Schedule 2 controlled drugs need to be met before the prescription can be dispensed.
2. *Prescriber*: Doctor (general practitioner).
3. *Legally written?* Yes.

Example 6.3 Continued

4. *Clinical check (complete the following table)*:

DRUG	INDICATIONS	DOSE CHECK	REFERENCE
Morphine	Acute pain	10 mg every 4 hours adjusted according to response	*British National Formulary* 54th edition, 'Prescribing in palliative care' and section 4.7.2

5. *Interactions*: There is only one drug on the prescription. However, it would also be advisable for the pharmacist or pharmacy technician to check the patient medication record (PMR) for any concurrent medication that could cause an interaction.
6. *Suitability for patient*: Item prescribed is safe and suitable for a patient of this age and the dose ordered on the prescription is within the recommended dose limits.
7. *Item(s) allowable on the NHS*: Yes (see *Drug Tariff*).
8. *Records to be made (including copies of the record(s))*: An entry would need to be made in the relevant section of the controlled drugs register detailing the supply.

   In this case, upon checking your stock, it is noted that you only have 56 tablets available. Therefore, you would need to supply 56 now and inform the patient or the patient's representative that you will order the remainder of the prescription for collection when it arrives. The supply of the remaining 56 tablets would need to be made within the 28-day validity period of the prescription.

   You will need to make an entry in the controlled drugs register for each supply made and mark the date of each supply on the prescription.

**MISUSE OF DRUGS ACT
REGISTER OF:**

DRUG CLASS   *Morphine*

NAME (brand, strength, form)   *Sevredol 10 mg tablets*

Date supply received or date supplied	Obtained		Supplied						Balance
	Name, address of person or firm from whom obtained	Amount Obtained	Name, address of person or firm supplied	Authority to possess- presciber or licence holder details	Person collecting / Patient/Representative or Healthcare Professional (name and address)	Proof of identity requested Yes/No	Proof of identity provided Yes/No	Amount supplied	Carried over: 56
Today's			Tony Head 43 Angel Rise Anytown	Dr R U Better FP10	Patient	Yes	Yes	56	0
Date stock arrives	A Wholesaler 2 Supply Road Anytown	112							112
Date of supply			Tony Head 43 Angel Rise Anytown	Dr R U Better FP10	Patient	No	No	56	56

Example 6.3 Continued

9. *Process prescription (including example of label(s))*:
   - Prepare label for product.
   - Check Appendix 9 of *British National Formulary* for supplementary labelling requirements. Sevredol: *British National Formulary* label number 2.
   - Select pack of Sevredol from the controlled drugs cupboard, remembering to check the expiry date and taking care that the correct strength of drug has been selected (the packaging of other strengths is very similar).
   - Perform final check of item, label and prescription.
   - Pack in a suitable bag ready to give to the patient or patient's representative (as this is a Schedule 2 controlled drug, it should be kept in the controlled drugs cupboard until it is collected by the patient or patient's representative).

   Labels (we have assumed that the name and address of the pharmacy and the words 'Keep out of the reach and sight of children' are pre-printed on the label):

Morphine sulphate 10 mg Tablets	**56**
Take ONE tablet every FOUR hours when required.	
Warning. May cause drowsiness. If affected do not drive	
or operate machinery. Avoid alcoholic drink.	
Mr Tony Head	Date of dispensing

10. *Endorse prescription*: The date of the original supply (i.e. 56) needs to be marked on the prescription. If the patient or patient's representative collects the remainder of the prescription (remember, they may not), then the date of this subsequent supply also needs to be marked on the prescription. In addition, before submission to the PPD (see part 11 below), the prescription needs to be stamped with the pharmacy stamp to indicate completion.
11. *Destination of paperwork*: Send to the PPD at the end of the month. The controlled drugs register in which the details of the supply was made must be kept at the premises at all times during use and for two years from the last date of entry.
12. *Identity check/counselling*:
    - Check patient's name and address.
    - The pharmacist or pharmacy technician must identify whether the collector is the patient, patient's representative or a healthcare professional. This information (including the name and professional address if the collector is a healthcare professional) must be recorded in the controlled drugs register (see Section 6.3.4).
    - The pharmacist or pharmacy technician must note in the controlled drugs register whether the ID was requested from the collector and whether it was produced (see Section 6.3.4). In this example, the patient has collected both the original and subsequent supplies. Therefore, it was not necessary to request identification for the second supply as the pharmacist was already familiar with the patient (assuming that it was the same pharmacist who made the original supply).
    - The collector should be asked to sign the rear of the prescription (see Section 6.3.4).
    - Reinforce the dosage instructions; advise that the tablets are best taken every 4 hours as required and may cause drowsiness.
    - Draw patient's attention to the patient information leaflet (PIL) and ask if he has any questions.

6.5 Chapter summary

This chapter has covered all the key parts of the legislation relating to the use of controlled drugs within pharmacy. It is important that all pharmacists and pharmacy technicians become familiar with the different requirements relating to how controlled drugs are handled within the pharmacy as any deviation from the requirements could result in prosecution.

In addition, it is important that pharmacists and pharmacy technicians are aware of any developments or changes to the regulations that may be made in the future. Details of any updates or changes in the management of controlled drugs will be published via the Royal Pharmaceutical Society's website and in the pages of the *Pharmaceutical Journal*. In addition, new editions of *Medicines, Ethics and Practice – A Guide for Pharmacists and Pharmacy Technicians* will collate all the recent changes. Pharmacies are expected to have standard operating procedures (see Section 1.4) in place for all aspects of the management of controlled drugs and it is important that any changes in the regulations are also reflected in any standard operating procedures in place.

7

Emergency supply

Upon completion of this chapter, you should be able to:

- understand the role of the pharmacist in the emergency supply of medication to both practitioners and patients
- make a legal emergency supply of a medicinal product at the request of a practitioner
- make a legal emergency supply of a prescription-only medicine at the request of a patient
- understand the role of Patient Group Directions in the urgent supply of medication to patients in Scotland.

In addition to the supply of medication to patients against both NHS prescription forms in the community (see Chapters 2 and 3) and in a hospital setting (see Chapter 4), and against private prescription forms (see Section 5.1), it may be necessary for pharmacists to supply medicines to patients, in an emergency, without a prescription form being present.

There are two types of emergency supply. Although colloquially they are both termed 'emergency supply', they are essentially very different. The two different forms are emergency supply at the request of a practitioner (see Section 7.1) and emergency supply at the request of a patient (see Section 7.2).

In addition, Scotland has implemented a system whereby Patient Group Direction (see Section 3.4) can be used in the urgent supply of medication to patients (see Section 7.3).

7.1 Emergency supply at the request of a practitioner

When we are dealing with emergency supply at the request of a practitioner, the term 'practitioner' is currently applied to one of the following:

- doctors
- community practitioner nurse prescribers
- supplementary prescribers
- nurse independent prescribers
- pharmacist independent prescribers.

This means that an emergency supply at the request of any other health professional, including dentists, would be unlawful. In addition, the requesting practitioner must be registered within the UK.

Essentially, this form of emergency supply is supply of medication in advance of a prescription form being supplied. It is the responsibility of the practitioner requesting the emergency supply to furnish the supplying pharmacist with a prescription form within 72 hours.

Key point 7.1

Currently, emergency supplies at the request of a practitioner can only be made by one of the following UK registered practitioners:

- doctors
- community practitioner nurse prescribers
- supplementary prescribers
- nurse independent prescribers
- pharmacist independent prescribers.

Pharmacists must ensure that they are satisfied that the request is genuine and has originated from one of the practitioners listed above (it would be usual for the pharmacist to know the practitioner personally, although this is not a legal requirement). Although it is the practitioner's responsibility to furnish the supplying pharmacist with a prescription form within 72 hours, the supplying pharmacist would be advised to remind the practitioner of this requirement.

All prescription-only medicines may be supplied by emergency supply at the request of a practitioner, except controlled drugs in Schedules 1, 2 and 3 of the Misuse of Drugs Regulations (apart from phenobarbital or phenobarbital sodium for the treatment of epilepsy). Please note that the emergency supply of phenobarbital or phenobarbital sodium for the treatment of a medical condition other than epilepsy would therefore be unlawful.

The procedure to be followed to make an emergency supply at the request of a practitioner is as follows:

1. The pharmacist must be satisfied that the supply is being requested by a doctor, community practitioner nurse prescriber, supplementary prescriber, nurse independent prescriber or pharmacist independent prescriber.

2. The pharmacist should remind the practitioner that it is their responsibility to furnish him or her with a prescription form within 72 hours.

3. The item must not be a controlled drug in Schedule 1, 2 or 3 of the Misuse of Drugs Regulations (the only exception to this being phenobarbital or phenobarbital sodium for the treatment of epilepsy).

4. The item should be dispensed and labelled, as for any other supply against a prescription form, according to the directions of the practitioner.

5. An entry should be made in the prescription-only medicines register stating the following:
   (a) The date on which the emergency supply was made.
   (b) The name, quantity and, except where it is apparent from the name, the pharmaceutical form and strength of the medicine. It is also good practice to record the dose and frequency of the medication.
   (c) The name and address of the practitioner.
   (d) The name and address of the patient.

When the prescription form is received, the pharmacist should add both the date on the prescription form and the date the prescription form was received.

Therefore, all entries in the prescription-only medicines register relating to emergency supplies at the request of a practitioner will contain three dates:

1. the date the emergency supply was made (i.e. supplied to the patient)
2. the date on the prescription form (once it has been received)
3. the date the prescription form was received in the pharmacy.

All three dates should be present in the prescription-only medicines register, even if all three are the same.

It is also good practice, unless the medication is for a patient with whom you are familiar, to ask the practitioner for the age of the patient. This will enable you to perform a suitable dose check. Remember, just because the medication

Reference number	Details		Cost
7.01

Date of supply | Emergency supply at the request of Dr Smith

John Fulbright
27 Station Road
Anytown

21 Amoxicillin 250 mg capsules
1 TDS

Date on prescription form:
Date prescription form received: | Dr Smith
The Health Centre
Anytown | Prescription charge (NHS or private) or details of exemption (NHS). |

Figure 7.1 An example of a prescription-only medicines register entry for an emergency supply made at the request of a practitioner.

is being requested by a practitioner as an emergency supply, this does not negate the need for you to perform a suitable clinical check.

An example of a prescription-only medicines register entry for an emergency supply at the request of a practitioner is shown in Figure 7.1.

The label for this supply would look as shown in Figure 7.2 (we have assumed that the name and address of the pharmacy and the words 'Keep out of the reach and sight of children' are pre-printed on the label).

the dose and frequency of the medication
- the name and address of the practitioner
- the name and address of the patient.

When the prescription form is received, the pharmacist should add:

- the date on the prescription form
- the date the prescription form was received.

Key point 7.2

The prescription-only medicines register entry for an emergency supply at the request of a practitioner will need to include the following pieces of information:

- the date on which the emergency supply was made
- the name, quantity and, except where it is apparent from the name, the pharmaceutical form and strength of the medicine. It is also good practice to record

Amoxicillin 250 mg Capsules   21

Take ONE capsule THREE times a day.

Take at regular intervals. Complete the prescribed course unless otherwise directed.

Mr John Fulbright   Date of dispensing

Figure 7.2 An example of the label for the emergency supply in Figure 7.1.

The patient may need to pay for the medication, but this will depend on the type of prescription form to be supplied. If the prescription form that will follow is an NHS prescription form, there will be either no charge to the patient for the supply (if the patient is exempt from prescription charges) or the standard prescription charge amount will be levied. If the prescription form that will follow is a private prescription form, this will be charged as for any private prescription form (see Section 5.1).

Although patients who are exempt from payment of prescription charges are entitled to receive their medication without charge, in normal circumstances when they present their prescription form at the pharmacy they will sign the reverse of the prescription form to claim the relevant exemption (see Figure 2.2). With an emergency supply at the request of a prescriber, although a prescription form will follow, it is not possible for the patient to sign the reverse of the prescription form at the time of supply as the prescription form will not arrive at the pharmacy until sometime within the next 72 hours.

Once the prescription form has arrived at the pharmacy, it would be possible for the pharmacist or pharmacy technician to sign the reverse of the prescription form as the patient's representative; however, apart from age-related exemptions (which are easy to verify), it would not be appropriate for the pharmacist to claim the relevant exemption on behalf of the patient. This is because if the exemption then turned out to be claimed falsely, it could be the pharmacist who was prosecuted (as it was the pharmacist who claimed the exemption on behalf of the patient). Therefore, in these circumstances, it is usual practice to charge the patient the equivalent prescription charge(s) and then ask them to return to the pharmacy a few days later to complete the reverse of the prescription form and receive a refund.

Alternatively, the patient can pay the charge(s) and then subsequently complete a prescription charge receipt and refund claim form (FP57 (England and Scotland), PS7 (Northern Ireland) or WP57 (Wales)) to receive a refund of the prescription charge(s) paid. A prescription charge receipt and refund claim form is usually only issued where there is doubt as to whether an exemption exists or not, for example, where a patient who pays the charge has applied for medical exemption, but has not yet received a medical exemption certificate. This enables a patient to identify at a later date the reason why a prescription charge should not have been paid and claim a refund (the refund may be claimed from any community pharmacy, not necessarily the one that took the original charge(s)).

In this case, the patient could simply complete the form in the pharmacy. Then, when the prescription form arrives, the pharmacist can indicate that a charge was collected (for each item) and refunded by processing the form as usual, along with the prescription charge receipt and refund claim form.

---

e.g.   Example 7.1

It is Friday afternoon at around 16.00. You receive a call in your pharmacy from a local doctor, Dr Smith, with whom you are familiar. He informs you that he is just visiting a patient under his care who requires a course of antibiotics. Unfortunately, he has forgotten his prescription form pad and so is unable to write a prescription form for the supply. He is not returning to his surgery until Monday morning and so requests that you make an emergency supply of the antibiotics. He will write a prescription form for the supply of the antibiotics on Monday morning and place the prescription form in the post to you on Monday evening. Should you make the emergency supply?

The request is from a practitioner (Dr Smith) with whom you are familiar. Therefore, it is a reasonable request for you to supply the medication in this situation. You will need to know the following:

Example 7.1 Continued

- the name and address (and if appropriate, the age) of the patient
- the name and address of the practitioner (although as you are familiar with Dr Smith you should have these details)
- details of the medication that the practitioner wishes the patient to take, including the name, form, strength, dose and frequency of the medication.

An entry will need to be made in the prescription-only medicines register stating the following:

- The date on which the emergency supply was made.
- The name, quantity and, except where it is apparent from the name, the pharmaceutical form and strength of the medicine. It is also good practice to record the dose and frequency of the medication.
- The name and address of the practitioner.
- The name and address of the patient.

A space should be left for (i) the date on the prescription form and (ii) the date the prescription form was received in the pharmacy.

In addition, it should be pointed out to Dr Smith that if the prescription form is not posted to the pharmacy until Monday evening, even using first-class post it may not arrive until Wednesday (if it is posted Monday evening, the post may not be collected until the following morning). This is longer than the 72 hours allowed for the prescriber to furnish you with a prescription form for the emergency supply. Although it is the prescriber's responsibility to ensure that you have the prescription form within 72 hours, it would be advisable for you to remind the prescriber of his responsibility at this point.

The prescription-only medicines register entry for this supply would appear in the register as follows:

Reference number	Details		Cost
7.02	Emergency supply at the request of Dr Smith		Prescription charge (NHS or private) or details of exemption (NHS).
Date of supply	Mary Jones 13 High Street Anytown	Dr Smith The Health Centre Anytown	
	28 Erythromycin 250 mg tablets 1 QDS		
	Date on prescription form:		
	Date prescription form received:		

Example 7.1 Continued

The label for this supply would look as follows (we have assumed that the name and address of the pharmacy and the words 'Keep out of the reach and sight of children' are pre-printed on the label):

Erythromycin 250 mg Tablets	**28**
Take ONE tablet FOUR times a day.	
Do not take indigestion remedies at the same time	
of day as this medicine.	
Take at regular intervals. Complete the prescribed	
course unless otherwise directed.	
Swallow whole, do not chew.	
Ms Mary Jones	Date of dispensing

Exercise 7.1

It is Saturday lunchtime. You receive a call in your pharmacy from an individual who identifies himself as a locum doctor, Dr Jones, who is working in the local surgery. He informs you that he is just visiting a patient under his care who requires a further supply of diazepam. Unfortunately, he had forgotten his prescription form pad and so was unable to write a prescription form for the supply. He is not returning to the local surgery until Monday morning and so requests that you make an emergency supply of the diazepam. He will write a prescription form for the supply of the diazepam on Monday morning and drop the form straight round to the pharmacy. Should you make the emergency supply?

7.2 Emergency supply at the request of a patient

Emergency supply at the request of a patient is very different to emergency supply at the request of a practitioner (see Section 7.1). In this case, as with emergency supply at the request of a practitioner, there is no prescription form present at the time of supply of the prescription-only medication. However, unlike emergency supply at the request of a practitioner, there will not be a prescription form to cover the supply provided at a later date. Remember that emergency supply of medication other than prescription-only medicines (POMs) (i.e. general sale list (GSL) items or pharmacy-only (P) items) is not necessary as patients would be able to purchase these items from the pharmacy (so long as there was a clinical need).

The pharmacist making the emergency supply must have interviewed the patient making the request and be satisfied that:

1. there is an immediate need for the prescription-only medicine and that the patient is unable to obtain a prescription form for the item within a reasonable time
2. the item has been previously prescribed by a doctor, community practitioner nurse prescriber, supplementary prescriber, nurse independent prescriber or pharmacist independent prescriber
3. the dose the patient is stating they use would be appropriate for him or her to take
4. any other medication the patient may be taking will not adversely interact with the requested emergency supply.

Normally the pharmacist would interview the patient in person in the pharmacy. However, in certain circumstances it may be impractical to do so and on exceptional occasions, a telephone conversation, with any subsequent supply made via the patient's representative, may be appropriate.

If the emergency supply is for a child, it would be usual for the pharmacist to interview a responsible adult (i.e. the child's parent or guardian), instead of the child.

If the pharmacist is satisfied that an emergency supply should be made, no more than five days' supply of the medication can be made, except in the following circumstances:

1. Where it would be impractical to split a package (so long as the package has been made up in a container elsewhere than at the place of sale or supply), for example, an emergency supply of an asthma inhaler.
2. An oral contraceptive, where a full cycle may be supplied.
3. An antibiotic in liquid form for oral administration where the smallest quantity that will provide a full course of treatment may be supplied.

Although the pharmacist can supply up to five days' treatment, consideration should be given to when the patient may be able realistically to obtain a prescription form and it may be appropriate to supply less than five days' treatment.

An entry must be made in the prescription-only medicines register stating the following:

1. The date on which the emergency supply was made.
2. The name, quantity and, except where it is apparent from the name, the pharmaceutical form and strength of the medicine. It is also good practice to include the dose and frequency of the medication and details of the patient's GP's name and address.
3. The name and address of the patient and his or her temporary address if appropriate.
4. The nature of the emergency (i.e. why the patient requested the prescription-only medicine and why they were unable to obtain a prescription form).

The medication should be dispensed and labelled as normal, but in addition should include the words 'Emergency supply' on the label (often with the reference number of the prescription-only medicines register entry relating to the emergency supply). This prevents patients from using old pharmaceutical packaging (with a suitable label) as evidence of previous supply (see Exercise 7.2) or from using an emergency supply from one community pharmacy to obtain a subsequent emergency supply from a different community pharmacy.

As for emergency supplies at the request of a practitioner, emergency supplies at the request of a patient may not be for any controlled dugs in Schedules 1, 2 and 3 of the Misuse of Drugs Regulations (except phenobarbital or phenobarbital sodium for the treatment of epilepsy) (see Chapter 6). Please note that the emergency supply of phenobarbital or phenobarbital sodium for the treatment of a medical condition other than epilepsy would therefore be unlawful.

An example of a prescription-only medicines register entry for an emergency supply at the request of a patient is shown in Figure 7.3. In addition, for a case such as the one in Figure 7.3,

---

Key point 7.3

The prescription-only medicines register entry for an emergency supply at the request of a patient will need to include the following pieces of information:

- The date on which the emergency supply was made.
- The name, quantity and, except where it is apparent from the name, the pharmaceutical form and strength of the medicine. It is also good practice to include the dose and frequency of the medication and details of the patient's GP's name and address.
- The name and address of the patient.
- The nature of the emergency (i.e. why the patient requested the prescription-only medicine and why they were unable to obtain a prescription form).

Reference number	Details		Cost
7.04	Emergency supply at the request of Dr Smith		Cost of drug + % Mark–up + Professional Fee + VAT.
Date of supply	Sue Taylor 4 Laurel Close Southampton	Dr Philip Roberts Main Surgery Southampton	
	Residing at: The Grand Hotel Anytown		
	1 sabutamol 100 micrograms inhaler 1 puff to be inhaled pm		
	The patient is on holiday and has left her inhaler at home. The request was made on Saturday afternoon and it is impractical for the patient to obtain a prescription form before Monday morning.		

Figure 7.3 An example of a prescription-only medicines register entry for an emergency supply made at the request of a patient.

Salbutamol 100 mcg inhaler	1
Inhale ONE puff when required	
Emergency Supply (7.04)	
Ms Sue Taylor	Date of dispensing

Figure 7.4 An example of the label for the emergency supply in Figure 7.3.

it would also be good practice to record the patient's temporary (i.e. holiday) address.

The label for this supply would look as shown in Figure 7.4 (we have assumed that the name and address of the pharmacy and the words 'Keep out of the reach and sight of children' are pre-printed on the label).

In addition to the restrictions on emergency supplies at the request of a patient of any controlled drugs in Schedules 1, 2 and 3 of the Misuse of Drugs Regulations (except phenobarbital or phenobarbital sodium for the treatment of epilepsy), emergency supplies at the request of a patient may not also be for medicines containing any of the following substances:

- ammonium bromide
- calcium bromide
- calcium bromidolactobionate
- embutramide
- fencamfamin hydrochloride
- fluanisone
- hexobarbitone
- hexobarbitone sodium
- hydrobromic acid
- meclofenoxate hydrochloride
- methohexitone sodium
- pemoline
- phenylmethylbarbituric acid
- piracetam
- potassium bromide
- prolintane hydrochloride
- quinidine phenylethylbarbiturate
- sodium bromide
- strychnine hydrochloride

- tacrine hydrochloride
- thiopentone sodium.

It should always be remembered that if a pharmacist is not able to make a supply, he or she should do everything possible to advise the patient how to obtain essential medical care (i.e. signpost to local out-of-hours care etc.).

It is usual to charge patients for the emergency supply. This will comprise the cost of the medication (possibly with a mark-up), plus a dispensing fee and VAT. The charge is there to cover the cost of the medication because, unlike emergency supply at the request of a practitioner, emergency supply at the request of a patient will not involve the subsequent supply of a prescription form.

It is common for patients to follow any emergency supply with a new prescription form. An emergency supply at the request of a patient will normally be for up to five days' supply. Therefore for the administration of the medication to continue, a new prescription form will usually be required. If this is going to be the case, some pharmacies will not charge the patient for the emergency supply and then subtract the supplied number of dosage units from the subsequent prescription form. Although this may be common practice in some pharmacies, strictly speaking this situation should be treated as two separate transactions. Just because a patient requests an emergency supply from your pharmacy does not mean that he or she is obliged to bring any subsequent prescription forms to your pharmacy.

 Example 7.2

It is Saturday morning at around 11.00 am. A patient with whom you are familiar comes into the pharmacy and asks for your assistance. She has epilepsy and has run out of her medication. Her doctor's surgery is closed at the weekend and she cannot obtain a prescription form until Monday morning. Should you make the emergency supply?

The request is from a patient with whom you are familiar. She is a regular patient of your pharmacy and upon examining her patient medication record (PMR) you notice regular supplies of phenobarbital. You will also be aware of the opening times of the local surgery and will be able to confirm that the surgery is closed until Monday morning. Therefore, it is a reasonable request for you to supply the medication in this situation. You will need to interview the patient and ascertain that:

1. there is an immediate need for the prescription-only medicine and that the patient is unable to obtain a prescription form for the item
2. the item has been previously prescribed by a doctor, or other suitably qualified practitioner
3. the dose and frequency the patient is saying she uses would be appropriate for her to take
4. the requested emergency supply does not interact with any other medication the patient is currently taking.

The patient states that she takes one 60 mg tablet at night for the treatment of epilepsy. Although phenobarbital is a Schedule 3 controlled drug, it may be supplied in an emergency (both at the request of a patient and at the request of a practitioner) for the treatment of epilepsy. The patient cannot get a prescription form from her GP until Monday morning. Therefore, she requires an emergency supply for tonight (Saturday) and tomorrow night (Sunday) (i.e. two doses).

An entry will need to be made in the prescription-only medicines register stating the following:

Example 7.2 Continued

- The date on which the emergency supply was made.
- The name, quantity and, except where it is apparent from the name, the pharmaceutical form and strength of the medicine. It is also good practice to include the dose and frequency of the medication and details of the patient's GP's name and address.
- The name and address of the patient.
- The nature of the emergency (i.e. why the patient requested the prescription-only medicine and why they were unable to obtain a prescription form).

The prescription-only medicines register entry for this supply would appear in the register as follows:

Reference number	Details		Cost
7.05	Emergency supply at the request of a patient		Cost of drug + % Mark–up + Professional Fee + VAT
Date of supply	Janet Baker 56 High Street Anytown	Dr RU Better The Health Centre Anytown	
	2 phenobarbital 60 mg tablets 1 to be taken at night		
	The patient suffers from epilepsy and has run out of medication. The request was made on Saturday morning and it is impractical for the patient to obtain a prescription form before Monday morning.		

The label for this supply would look as follows (we have assumed that the name and address of the pharmacy and the words 'Keep out of the reach and sight of children' are pre-printed on the label):

Phenobarbital 60 mg Tablets   **2**
Take ONE tablet at night.
Emergency Supply (7.05)
Warning. May cause drowsiness. If affected do not drive
or operate machinery. Avoid alcoholic drink.
Do not stop taking this medicine except on your doctor's
advice.
Mrs Janet Baker   Date of dispensing

Exercise 7.2

It is Saturday afternoon at around 16.00. A young lady with whom you are not familiar comes into the pharmacy and asks for your assistance. She has come to your town to visit relatives but has forgotten her 'pills'. Upon further questioning you ascertain that the young lady is referring to her oral contraceptive. Obviously, she is not registered with the local doctor's surgery and the surgery is closed at the weekend anyway. Should you make the emergency supply?

7.3 The urgent supply of medicines or appliances to patients via Patient Group Direction in Scotland

In Scotland another way of dealing with the urgent supply of medicines or appliances at the request of a patient, in addition to the emergency supply detailed in Section 7.2, has been implemented using a Patient Group Direction (for details of Patient Group Directions, see Section 3.4).

As with emergency supply of prescription-only medicines in England and Wales, this Patient Group Direction allows for the urgent supply of previously prescribed medicines that would normally be prescribed again once a supply had been exhausted. The main difference in this case from the emergency supply outlined in Section 7.2 is that it allows for the full amount that would normally be prescribed to be supplied (rather than in most cases being limited to five days). The urgent supply Patient Group Direction was implemented in Scotland to allow patients to obtain supplies of routine medicines out of hours without having to contact out-of-hours services, especially over holiday periods.

In England and Wales, in most cases up to five days' treatment can be supplied to the patient (see Section 7.2). This is becoming less practical when considering the move towards patient pack dispensing, with many items supplied in calendar packs. Cutting strips of tablets or capsules to accommodate the five-day supply rule results in a less professional appearance of the supply and the problem of what to do with the remaining tablets or capsules in the split pack. The urgent supply Patient Group Direction in place in Scotland also helps to minimise this problem.

The similarities continue with regard to when and why an urgent supply can be made under the Patient Group Direction. In order to use a Patient Group Direction the following criteria must be met:

1. The patient's GP must be unavailable (either the surgery is closed or an out-of-hours system is operating).
2. As the Patient Group Direction applies solely to NHS patients in Scotland, the patient must be registered with a Scottish GP.
3. The patient must show that they have received the medication or appliance requested before and it should be a medication or appliance that would be prescribed again.
4. The pharmacist must be satisfied that the patient's clinical condition has not changed since the most recent dispensing (if the condition is suspected to have changed a supply could not be made under the Patient Group Direction).
5. The most recent previous supply of the medication cannot have been made under the Patient Group Direction (a patient is not allowed two successive supplies under the rules of the emergency supply Patient Group Direction).
6. The item requested must not be one that is excluded from being supplied under the Patient Group Direction.

Patients may come into the pharmacy and request a supply as with the standard emergency supply or they may be referred to the pharmacy either by an out-of-hours service (for example, NHS 24 which provides health information and self-care advice in Scotland), a GP or an accident and emergency department of a hospital.

The medicines and appliances covered by the Patient Group Direction are set into sections that mirror the chapters of the *British National Formulary*. The Patient Group Direction gives explicit instructions as to what may or may not be provided.

For example, chapter 1 of the *British National Formulary* contains drugs used to treat conditions relating to the gastro-intestinal system.

- Part A of the Patient Group Direction will list the conditions that can be treated by use of this Patient Group Direction (for example, anal fissures, inflammatory bowel disease, management of colostomy/ileostomy patients, etc.).
- Part B lists the medicines in chapter 1 of the *British National Formulary* that may not be supplied to a patient under this Patient Group Direction (for example, items not intended for repeat use, items only intended for acute use or items not intended for primary care use). This is repeated for each chapter of the *British National Formulary*.

In addition, all Schedule 2 and 3 controlled drugs are excluded from supply under the Patient Group Direction and even though morphine 10 mg/5 mL is not a Schedule 2 or 3 controlled drug, this is also outside the limits of the Patient Group Direction. Schedule 4 controlled drugs such as benzodiazepines may be supplied at the pharmacist's discretion and the quantity supplied may be restricted and the amount supplied may be less than would have been the case via a prescription form (this is particularly important when dealing with unfamiliar patients).

In order to complete the CP(US) form (community pharmacy urgent supply form) to be able to make the supply, the pharmacist will need the following information:

- patient's name
- patient's address
- patient's Community Health Index (CHI) number (if not available, their date of birth should be entered into the first six boxes of the CHI number) (The CHI number is a ten-digit number created from the patient's date of birth and four other numbers. It is allo-

cated to all patients registered with a GP in Scotland and is unique number for any health communication related to a given patient both in primary and secondary care.)
- the pharmacy contractor's code
- the RPSGB number of the pharmacist completing the CP(US) form
- the patient's prescriber reference number.

If the patient does not know his or her CHI number it can be obtained from the surgery when it is next open; but it must be added before forwarding the form to the Practitioner Services Division (PSD) for processing (see Section 3.3.8).

The pharmacist completes the CP(US) form by adding the quantity, the name of drug and pharmaceutical form and the appropriate dosage instructions. The medicine or appliance is then dispensed and labelled as normal. It is good practice (although not mandatory) to mark the patient's patient medication record (PMR) to indicate that this supply has been made under the Patient Group Direction.

Once dispensed, the item is given to the patient or patient's representative who may pay the normal prescription levy (although this may be abolished in Scotland in time; see Section 2.4.3) or if claiming exemption the patient or the patient's representative will be required to indicate the reason for exemption and sign the CP(US) form. Patients must also be advised of the normal procedure to obtain additional prescriptions and informed that they will not be able to receive a second successive supply of the medicine provided under this Patient Group Direction. The CP(US) form will then be endorsed and stamped as required.

After the patient has left the pharmacy a copy of the CP(US) form should be sent to the prescriber to allow staff to update the patient notes and also destroy any repeats for the item that are at the surgery awaiting collection. The completed CP(US) form should be sent to the Practitioner Services Division (PSD) for processing.

The provision of the urgent supply Patient Group Direction does not mean that pharmacies in Scotland can no longer make an emergency supply as outlined in Section 7.2; nor does it mean that a pharmacist may no longer use their professional judgement with regard to supply. Pharmacists are not obliged to make urgent supplies but as with standard emergency supplies they are required to consider the consequences should they not supply. The Patient Group Direction recognises that there may be times when a supply using the Patient Group Direction may be inappropriate and therefore allows for the pharmacist to exercise their professional judgement and either supply under standard emergency supply mechanisms or redirect the patient to an out-of-hours doctors service.

In order to use the Patient Group Direction the relevant Health Board must have authorised its use in their area. Pharmacists in turn must sign up for the Patient Group Direction for each Health Board they work within.

7.4 Chapter summary

In summary, the following key points relate to emergency supply:

1. There are two distinctly different types of emergency supply: (a) emergency supply at the request of a practitioner (in effect, supply of medication in advance of a pre-scription form) and (b) emergency supply (of prescription-only medication) at the request of a patient (where no prescription form will be provided). Although both are termed 'emergency supply' they are essentially very different and it is important that pharmacists and pharmacy technicians become familiar with both types.

2. In both cases, an entry in the prescription-only medicines register will be made. This will provide details of, and reason for, the supply.

3. The emergency supply of Schedule 1, 2 and 3 controlled dugs is prohibited, except phenobarbital and phenobarbital sodium for the treatment of epilepsy.

4. For emergency supply at the request of a patient, up to five days' supply may be made (except in certain circumstances) (also see point 5 below). However, consideration should be given to supplying less than five days. Emergency supply at the request of a practitioner has no supply limit, although professional judgement should be exercised if the requested quantity appears excessive.

5. In addition to the traditional emergency supply, additional arrangements exist within Scotland to allow the urgent supply of medicines or appliances to patients via Patient Group Direction.

8

Patient counselling and communication 1 – The basics of patient communication

Upon completion of this chapter, you should be able to:

- understand the key points behind effective interpersonal communication
- learn how to undertake successful verbal communication
- appreciate the importance of non-verbal communication
- realise the role of body language in both verbal and non-verbal communication
- understand the different types of questioning that can be used
- be aware of the role that questioning mnemonics can play in effective patient communication
- learn how important listening and clear explanation can be
- learn about patient compliance and concordance and the role of both verbal and written communication
- understand the importance of clear communication with other healthcare professionals
- examine some communication case studies.

The supply of medication to a patient is an important role for pharmacy. However, in addition to the actual supply, sufficient information needs to be given to the patient or the patient's representative to enable them to use the medicine safely and effectively. Although it is important to supply the correct medication to the patient, if it is not used correctly by the patient it may be ineffectual. In extreme cases, this can lead to patient harm or even death.

In addition to information being supplied to the patient in a printed format (i.e. via the medicine's label and via the patient information leaflet), information is often needed in the form of verbal instructions and demonstration. It is sometimes the role of the pharmacist or pharmacy technician to verbally counsel the patient or the patient's carer and demonstrate the use of the medication. It is therefore vital that pharmacists and pharmacy technicians develop effective communication skills.

This chapter will cover the basics of patient communication. Chapter 9 will provide specific detail of the important counselling points which need to be considered for specific dosage forms.

8.1 Interpersonal communication

Because pharmacists and pharmacy technicians communicate with patients, carers and other healthcare professionals on a regular basis, communication skills are an essential part of any pharmacist's or pharmacy technician's skill set.

The Royal Pharmaceutical Society of Great Britain's Code of Ethics for Pharmacists and Pharmacy Technicians is based on seven principles. A pharmacist or technician must endeavour to:

- make the care of patients their primary concern
- apply professional judgement in the interests of patients and the public
- show respect for others
- encourage patients to participate in decisions about their care
- develop their professional knowledge and competence
- be honest and trustworthy
- take responsibility for their working practices.

As illustrated in Figure 8.1, communication is a two-way process.

The essence of good communication is that the message received is the same as the message sent. The well-known children's game 'Chinese Whispers' can be used to demonstrate this point effectively. To play the game, everyone sits in a circle. One person whispers a long phrase to their neighbour, who, in turn, whispers what they

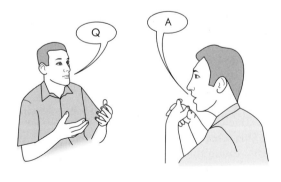

Figure 8.1   Communication is a two-way process.

heard to the next person, and so on. The last person in the circle announces what they heard.

According to the famous anecdote demonstrating the massive changes that can occur, the original message 'Send reinforcements we're going to advance' at the end of the chain turned into 'Send three and four-pence we're going to a dance'.

The number of people in the chain can significantly affect the final outcome as the number of opportunities for misinterpretation increases.

The *Chinese Whispers* effect could have serious consequences in a pharmacy environment. In a worse case scenario there could be seven or eight possible interactions involved. Consider the scenario below, a not unusual occurrence in a community pharmacy:

Mrs Jones brings her husband's prescription into the pharmacy. The pharmacist enters the details of the patient into the computer and realises there is a patient medication record. The prescription is for a new item that is not already on the PMR. The item ordered is timolol eye drops but there is no indication of the strength required nor are there any directions for use for the patient.

The pharmacist asks Mrs Jones if she knows the strength of the eye drops her husband normally uses. She replies that her husband has been to the doctor this morning but she was unable to go with him and as far as she was aware he had never been given eye drops before. The pharmacist tries to phone the surgery but the phone is engaged. The pharmacy is very busy and therefore the pharmacist explains the problem to the pharmacy technician.

The technician then phones the surgery and speaks to the receptionist, the receptionist then speaks to the doctor, the doctor tells the receptionist, the receptionist tells the technician and the technician tells the pharmacist. The pharmacist then dispenses the item and passes on the information to the patient's wife who then in turn passes on the information to the patient.

There is plenty of opportunity for misinterpretation at any point. In the above scenario, there are at least eight possibilities for misinterpretation.

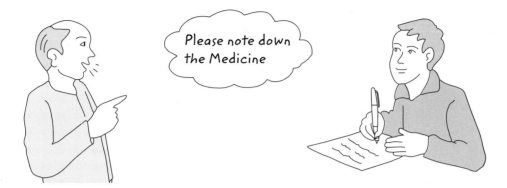

Figure 8.2 Communication involves three elements: sender, receiver and message.

As illustrated in Figure 8.2, communication involves three elements: the sender, the receiver and the message.

The sender

The sender can try to make sure the message is received correctly by:

- speaking clearly
- speaking slowly
- using appropriate language
- checking understanding.

The receiver

The receiver can make sure the message is received correctly by:

- listening carefully
- asking for clarification
- writing it down
- repeating the message back in order to check the message received is the one given.

Key point 8.1

Sending a message – in order to ensure that a message is received correctly, the message sender needs to:

- speak clearly
- speak slowly
- use appropriate language
- check understanding.

→

Receiving a message – in order to ensure that a message is received correctly, the message receiver needs to:

- listen carefully
- ask for clarification
- write it down
- repeat the message back in order to check the message received is the one given.

The message

When we communicate we send a message but what makes up the message? The message we send normally consists of factual information and 'feeling' information and this is transmitted both verbally and non-verbally.

A message is sent from the sender to the receiver but there is usually some feedback from the receiver and this feedback will influence the action of the sender. This can be verbal or non-verbal (see Figure 8.3).

Key point 8.2

A message consists of:

- *factual* information transmitted *verbally*
- *feeling* information transmitted *non-verbally*.

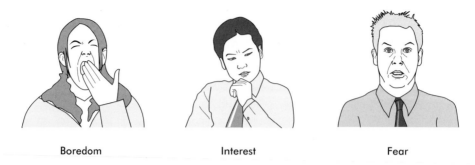

| Boredom | Interest | Fear |

Figure 8.3 Examples of different non-verbal communications.

8.1.1 Verbal communication

Verbal communication is purely the linguistic element of the message. It is affected by the vocabulary employed and the use of language.

The use of appropriate vocabulary and avoidance of jargon is important. Often words that are second nature to the pharmacist may be totally alien to the patient. For example, if a pharmacist or pharmacy technician advised a patient that there is a 'PIL' enclosed with their medication, instead of saying there is a 'patient information leaflet' enclosed, it may lead to confusion. To a patient the term 'PIL' is likely to mean a pharmaceutical form (a pill) and they will probably think of a tablet or more likely the contraceptive pill.

Try to avoid what has been referred to as 'restricted language code'. This makes use of colloquial expressions, very short and simple sentences, repetitive use of conjunctions (but, because, so . . .) and the use of statements phrased as questions 'Know what I mean?', ' . . . you know?', ' . . . isn't it?', etc. In most patient interactions the use of restricted language code is undesirable; however, occasionally you may need to apply it when interacting with certain patients to ensure the information is clearly understood.

8.1.2 Non-verbal communication

Everything we do is communication. Non-verbal communication could be defined as all forms of human communication except for the purely verbal message, i.e. the words used themselves.

Vocal non-verbal communication includes the tone, pitch, volume, accent, speed, etc. and this is known as paralanguage. In other words 'it ain't what you say it's the way that you say it'.

A meaning of a phrase can be altered by changing the emphasis placed on the words. Consider the following phrase: 'Dr Better told me to buy tablets' and see how the meaning changes depending on the emphasis (as indicated by the underlined word or words):

- 'Dr Better told me to buy tablets' (i.e. he was the one who told me, no-one else).
- 'Dr Better told me to buy tablets' (i.e. he didn't ask or request, he told me).
- 'Dr Better told me to buy tablets' (i.e. he told me, not you or anyone else).
- 'Dr Better told me to buy tablets' (i.e. I don't expect them for nothing; I want you to sell them to me).
- 'Dr Better told me to buy tablets' (i.e. not capsules or liquid, but tablets).

Your voice can also be used to infer emotional states and your inner feelings. The message a patient coming into the pharmacy receives can be quite different depending on your demeanour and tone of voice. For example, the greeting 'Good afternoon, I'm Jane the pharmacist. How may I help you?' accompanied by an attentive look, a smile and clear diction will give the right message. But imagine the difference if there is no eye contact, no smile and a mumbled question. This more likely gives the message 'Not another customer, my feet are killing me and I want to go home'. Pharmacists and pharmacy technicians must be aware of how tone of voice can alter the message given out.

8.1.3 Body language

Body language used in transmitting a message also affects communication. In fact, tone of voice and body language combined contribute more towards communication than the words in the message.

There are five main areas of body language: gaze or eye contact, facial expression, proximity and orientation, posture, and touch.

Gaze or eye contact

The presence or lack of eye contact can be significant. In a two-way conversation:

- the speaker often looks away from the listener when talking (because they are concentrating on what they are saying) and then will look directly at the listener if trying to elicit a response
- the listener will look straight into the eye of the speaker while paying attention, but will look away if attention wanders.

It is very important when listening to look at the speaker because if the speaker looks up and notices the listener's gaze is elsewhere, he or she will assume your attention is elsewhere. Therefore when listening to a patient it is important to maintain eye contact in order to show attentiveness.

Facial expression

Judgements are often made about the emotional state of someone just by the interpretation of facial expressions, particularly movements of the eyebrows and mouth, which signal different types of emotion. This has led to the popularity of 'emoticons' when conversing on-line or via mobile telephone text messages (Figure 8.4).

Proximity and orientation

Table 8.1 outlines the approximate distances relating to the proximity we generally accept in our day-to-day life.

The orientation and level of the individuals during a conversation is also important. Consider the differences when the patient is seated and the pharmacist is standing; or if the pharmacist is speaking from a raised dispensary down to the patient in the pharmacy (or to a patient in a wheelchair); or the patient is one side of the counter and the pharmacist is the other (a physical barrier).

Positioning can be very important if a patient is asking for recommended treatment for a rash

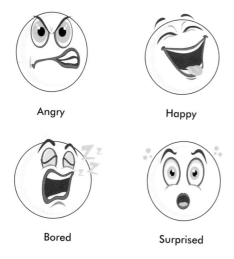

Angry   Happy

Bored   Surprised

Figure 8.4   Examples of computer emoticons.

Table 8.1   Approximate distances of the proximity we generally accept in our day to day life

Distance	Appropriate relationships and activities
Less than 46 cm	Intimate contacts, e.g. physical sports
Personal distance: 46 cm to 1.22 m	Close friends or acquaintances
Social distance: 1.22 m to 3.66 m	Impersonal, businesslike contacts
Public distance: greater than 3.66 m	Formal contacts, e.g. in a lecture theatre

for example. If the pharmacist moves across or out from behind the counter to examine the condition this shows interest in the patient. Similarly if a patient requests a pregnancy test and the pharmacist gets close to the patient to give the results this shows empathy with the patient; the pharmacist demonstrates sensitivity to the need for confidentiality.

Posture

How people sit, stand or lie can communicate feelings to others. Upright or slouched, arms crossed or not. A forward sloping stance suggests a wish to dominate. This could be made worse if accompanied by invasion of the personal space. A slouched or bent posture suggests lack of interest and conviction in what is being said, while an upright posture demonstrates assertive behaviour without any hidden meanings and shows that a speaker has confidence in what they are saying. Body movements such as clenched fists, fidgeting hands, tapping feet are all indicators of stress or tension, while still, open hands suggest a relaxed frame of mind. The position of the head and shoulders further conveys non-verbal messages: tension, anger, anxiety, excitement, happiness and approach-ability can all be conveyed non-verbally by the posture adopted.

Touch

There are many different types of touch, for example:

- social touch such as a handshake
- consoling touch, usually on arm or hand used to calm a distressed person
- occupational touch, such as, for a pharmacist, simple examination, minor first aid, measuring and fitting hosiery/trusses or demonstration of use of medication or appliances (e.g. asthma inhalers).

You should be aware that while most UK citizens will be happy with the physical contact involved in our examinations, etc., different cultures will have different expectations of what is acceptable and what is taboo.

> **Key point 8.3**
>
> There are five main areas of body language:
>
> - gaze or eye contact
> - facial expression
> - proximity and orientation
> - posture
> - touch.

You should be aware that physical appearance may be very deceptive; there is truth to the saying 'don't judge a book by its cover'. Try not to be judgemental about a person's appearance and always remember that when communicating, the way the message is delivered affects the way the message is received.

Communication consists of three main parts, questioning, listening and explaining. All are required for successful communication to occur. These three concepts will be discussed in the next three sections.

8.2 Questioning

There are different styles of questioning and different question types that may be used to elicit a response, but what is a question? By definition it is a request for information. The amount and quality of information received may well be affected by the questioning style.

A number of styles of question have been identified by psychologists and linguists, but there are six basic types that will be used by pharmacists: closed, open, leading/biased, probing, prompting and multiple questions.

Closed questions

Closed questions require short factual, often one-word answers. They place restrictions on the responder by closing down the number of options available. There are three categories that are useful in pharmacy:

- Selection questions – the patient is asked to choose one from two or more alternatives, e.g. 'Would you prefer tablets or capsules?' 'Would you like aspirin or paracetamol?'
- Yes/no questions – these simply require a yes or no answer, e.g. 'Have you had this pain before?' 'Did you get on OK with the medicine I gave you last week?'
- Identification questions – the patient provides a piece of factual information as a response to the question, e.g. 'What is your name?' 'How old is your baby?'

Open questions

Open questions give a patient the opportunity to give full answers and there is a greater degree of freedom in deciding how to respond. Open questions are generally broad in nature and require more than a one- or two-word answer. Words such as 'how', 'what', 'feel' and 'think' are useful for encouraging a full response, e.g. 'How did you get on at the doctor's today?' 'What exactly are the symptoms?' 'What do you think about trying to do these exercises once a day?'

Leading/biased questions

These questions always have an expectation attached to them. They indicate to the listener the answer the questioner wants to hear. Therefore the patient is led in the direction of a certain answer. They may be used in a positive manner to stimulate the flow of conversation. The idea here is that they should anticipate a likely response to show a common understanding and therefore help to develop a rapport, e.g. 'It's a lovely day today, isn't it?

Leading questions may be simple in style, leading the patient in the direction that the pharmacist wants them to go or placing pressure on the patient to concur, e.g. 'You don't drive while your taking these tablets, do you?' 'You have been using the cream as we discussed, haven't you?'

More complex leads exert more pressure on a patient to reply in the expected manner. This can be a problem as it can affect the evaluation of information and eventual diagnosis. The patient may be afraid to disagree or alternatively agree in order to please you, the questioner, e.g. 'Like most conscientious parents, wouldn't you want to give your children fluoride supplements to strengthen their teeth?'

Probing questions

Probing questions are add-on questions or follow-up questions used to build upon an initial response. They may be open, closed or leading in nature. They are of value because they indicate attention to and interest in the patient. The problem is that they may become interrogative in nature if used too frequently. They may be used in different situations. Consider the following questions and how they differ:

- 'What do you mean?' 'Can you explain that?' 'In what way?' These questions are asking for previously received information to be clarified.
- 'Why do you say that?' Here the patient is being asked to justify a statement they have previously made.
- 'Can you remember anything else?' 'Go on?' These questions encourage the patient to give further information to extend the information they have given earlier.
- 'What type of pain?' This question asks for more detail to illustrate the meaning of previous information.
- 'Are you sure you took one twice a day?' This question reaffirms information received and checks the accuracy of information provided by the patient.

Finally there are parroting or echoing styles of questioning which are considered probing. For example:

Patient: I don't like tablets, I prefer syrup.
Pharmacist: You prefer syrup?

Prompting questions

These are useful if a patient fails to answer the original question or gives an inadequate answer. They may be necessary because the original question posed was not sufficiently specific. For example, following the original question and answer:

Pharmacist: How often do you take the tablets?

Patient: Fairly often.

could be followed with the prompt:

Pharmacist: How many do you take each day?

Patient: Four.

Sometimes the question posed may confuse the patient or unintentionally use words with which the patient is unfamiliar. Therefore a simpler question needs to be posed.

For example, the original question and answer:

Pharmacist: Do you have any gastro-intestinal symptoms?

Patient: (*Perplexed silence, puzzled expression*)

could be followed by a simpler question:

Pharmacist: Do you have a stomach upset?

Patient: Yes I get heartburn if I eat late at night.

Multiple questions

The use of multiple questions is not recommended. Consider the following two examples:

- 'Do you know how to take them? Would you like me to explain again?'
- 'Have you had the pain long? Is it worse in the morning? Are your joints stiff?'

The first example is not too bad but can lead to

misunderstanding. The patient might just answer 'Yes' but do they mean 'Yes, I know how to take them' or 'Yes, I would like you to explain again'?

The second could result in confusion because the patient does not know which question to answer first and will probably be unable to remember all the questions that have been fired at them.

It will not always be the pharmacist or pharmacy technician who will ask questions. You should also encourage patients to ask you questions. When patients are comfortable asking you questions, you know you have rapport and that you have good communication skills.

Read the following scenario and decide if the questions posed by the pharmacist are open, closed, leading, prompting or multiple.

Pharmacist: Hello, How can I help you? (Question 1)

Patient: I want something for a stomach upset.

Pharmacist: Stomach upset? (Question 2)

Patient: Yes, I've had it for over a week.

Pharmacist: How does it affect you? What are your symptoms? (Question 3)

Patient: Sickness and diarrhoea.

Pharmacist: When did it start? (Question 4)

Patient: Just after I came back from holiday with the family.

Pharmacist: Too much of the good life eating and drinking while you were away? (Question 5)

Patient: NO!

Pharmacist: How long have you been back? (Question 6)

Patient: Two weeks.

Pharmacist: It's been really bad all that time? Have you taken anything for it or been to the doctor? (Question 7)

Patient: Yes.

Pharmacist: What did he say? (Question 8)

Patient: No. I had kaolin and morphine in the house so I took that for diarrhoea.

Pharmacist: But have you seen the doctor? (Question 9)

Patient: No.

Pharmacist: Is your temperature raised? (Question 10)

Key point 8.4

There are six types of questions:

- closed questions
- open questions
- leading/biased questions
- probing questions
- prompting questions
- multiple questions.

It is important to use the right type of question to elicit the information required.

Patient: Yes I get hot at times.

Pharmacist: Have you had this before or is this the first time? (Question 11)

Patient: I've had sickness and diarrhoea before but never for as long as this.

Pharmacist: Do any other members of your family have gastroenteritis? (Question 12)

Patient: Pardon. What's that?

Pharmacist: Do they have diarrhoea and vomiting as well? (Question 13)

Patient: My wife had it but it seems to have cleared up.

The questions vary in style:

- Question 1 is an *open question*. Almost a greeting question.
- Question 2 is a *probing question*, asking the patient to further explain what they mean by 'stomach upset'. This could mean different things to different people. It could indicate gastroenteritis as in this case, or it may just be sickness or just diarrhoea.
- Question 3 is a *multiple question*. This offers an open question and then immediately qualifies that with a probing question. Consider whether it would be better to just ask the one probing question. In this case the multiple question is reinforcing the information required.
- Question 4 is an *open question*.
- Question 5 is a *leading question*, perhaps suggesting that the condition was somehow self-inflicted, causing possible offence and hostility in the patient.
- Question 6 is a *closed question*, allowing the pharmacist to identify the duration of the problem.
- Question 7 is a *multiple question*. Note the patient only responds with a simple yes. The real question is 'yes' to which question? It is obvious from the next question that the response is not to the question that the pharmacist thought they had posed.
- Question 8 is a *probing question* trying to gain more information but, because the original question was part of a multiple question some confusion sets in as the patient tries to tie in this question with the previous one.
- Question 9 is a *closed question* that finally elicits the response required from question 7.

- Question 10 is a *closed question* obtaining specific information.
- Question 11 is a *multiple question*. In this case the patient was helpful. 'Yes' could easily have been the answer, which would have left the pharmacist wondering whether he meant 'Yes, I have had it before' or 'Yes, it was the first time'. An answer 'No' could have meant 'No, I have not had it before' or 'No, it was the first time'. A closed multiple question allows for misinterpretation.
- Question 12 clearly shows how the use of language must be kept simple in order not to confuse or embarrass the patient. Using the term 'gastroenteritis' in this setting assumes the patient has knowledge of the disease and will understand. This patient clearly does not understand. How will that patient feel? Stupid? How would this be likely to affect their relationship with the pharmacist?
- Question 13 is a *prompting question*, but the use of diarrhoea and vomiting rather than the patient's terminology of sickness and diarrhoea may serve to further alienate the patient.

Consider the following scenario: Mrs Smith is a regular customer, and she wants you to give her something for indigestion. Some suggested questions have been given below. Try to think of your own questions and identify the types of questions used. Consider the strengths and weaknesses of the questions asked and the styles used.

- Question 1: 'Tell me about your symptoms.'
- Question 2: 'Do you get pain at night?'
- Question 3: 'So you want to buy some indigestion mixture?'
- Question 4: 'Would you prefer liquid or tablets.'
- Question 5: 'Is the main problem pain or are you getting wind as well?'

8.2.1 Questioning mnemonics

The importance of questioning patients correctly cannot be underestimated. The information from the patient is vital when 'responding to symptoms'. Therefore the interaction needs to be structured in order to ensure all the relevant details are obtained.

How do you ensure that your interview with a patient is unbiased and thorough? How do you make sure that you do not forget to ask something? Your decision with regards to counter prescribing or referral to a GP will be based on the information you manage to obtain from the patient.

Because of the importance of remembering all of the information a number of mnemonics are used. These are valuable as a starting point. All the information is valid and you can build upon the framework to obtain further information from a patient. It is important to bear in mind, however, that no mnemonic is fully comprehensive.

WWHAM

- Who is the medicine for?
- What are the symptoms?
- How long have you been ill?
- Action taken so far?
- Medicines being taken at the moment?

This system of questioning will establish the presenting complaint and will also give information about what the patient has already done about the symptoms. However it fails to consider family history, previous symptoms, general appearance or any social or lifestyle factors associated with the presenting symptoms.

For example, if these were the only questions used to differentiate between patients, a young mum presenting with indigestion/heartburn caused by hectic lifestyle with poor eating habits ('eating on the go') might be given the same treatment as an elderly man presenting with similar symptoms but with a greater chance of the symptoms being caused by a disease state rather than poor eating habits.

ENCORE

- Explore
- No medication?
- Care
- Observe
- Refer
- Explain.

Explore
This gives the opportunity to obtain information regarding the nature of the symptoms, discover any other associated symptoms or any other medication being taken by the patient and hence any other pre-existing medical conditions. As a result of our 'exploration' we may exclude possibility of serious disease. It also enables the questioner to obtain the identity of the patient.

No medication
This is a reminder that medication is not always the answer and lifestyle changes may be more advisable – there is not necessarily 'a pill for all ills'.

Care
This is to remind us that different patients have different needs. Some patients' needs are greater, for example paediatric and geriatric patients may be special cases as would be pregnant or breast-feeding women. These factors may well influence the recommendations made by pharmacists or pharmacy technicians.

Observe
This is particularly important when attempting diagnosis.

Refer
This is to remind you that you can refer a patient for a second opinion. Usually referral is advised if the patients are at increased risk, for example, paediatric patients, geriatric patients, etc., if the symptoms are persistent or if the symptoms suggest a potentially serious condition.

Explain
This is to remind us to fully explain decisions to patients. If a course of action is clearly explained the patient is more likely to be compliant.

This system of questioning takes into account the appearance of the patient. Careful observation of a patient can reveal a lot. If a patient presenting with symptoms is seriously ill, they will rarely look well. If you define what you think are observable symptoms of ill health you could include flushing, sweating, dilated pupils or smell. 'N' and 'R', although they are relevant, do not really help towards making differential diagnosis. Once again no social or lifestyle factors are considered; nor is family history taken into account.

ASMETTHOD

- Age of the patient?
- Self or someone else?
- Medicines the patient is taking?
- Exactly what does the patient mean by the symptom?
- Time/duration of the symptom?
- Taken anything for it or seen the doctor?
- History of any disease or condition?
- Other symptoms being experienced?
- Doing anything to aggravate or alleviate the condition?

This system establishes the presenting complaint and whether or not the patient has had it before. It can be used to find the necessary information for making a diagnosis. Remember that not all questions will necessarily need to be asked and that the order of questioning is not that critical. Use the mnemonic as a checklist or aide memoir.

SIT DOWN SIR

- Site or location?
- Intensity or severity?
- Type or nature?
- Duration?
- Onset?
- With? (Other symptoms)
- N annoyed or aggravated by?
- Spread or radiation?
- Incidence or frequency pattern?
- Relieved by?

This mnemonic may help to elicit more information. It establishes severity, nature of symptoms and previous history but again the importance of social or lifestyle factors is ignored, as is the general appearance of the patient.

Try using these mnemonics in the scenario above that demonstrated the use of different types of questions. Were all the points covered?

While these mnemonics are a useful aid or memory jogger they are not a replacement for clinical consultation. They should aid your decision making but not constrain it.

8.3 Listening

Listening involves both verbal and non-verbal communication. There are different levels of listening and, as explained earlier, what we say is not always what is heard and, conversely, we do not always hear what is said to us.

There are various different modes of listening:

- 'Half an ear listening' is background noise listening. We can hear the radio in the background but are we really listening to it?
- In 'passive listening', also known as 'stunned mullet listening' (an Australian term), the listener shows a vacant expression, a completely blank look and gives the speaker no feedback. This can be useful for calming people down but is not generally the type of listening we would want to see in a pharmacy.
- In 'reflective listening' the listener reflects the statements back to the speaker to encourage them to carry on with the thread of conversation. This is the type of listening employed by psychiatrists and counsellors.
- 'Active listening' is the main type of listening used in pharmacy when responding to symptoms.

Listening can be divided into six distinct processes:

1. Concentrating, organising and analysing what is said. This may seem obvious but the process can be hindered in a number of ways through, for example:
   - distractions from other demands within the pharmacy
   - tiredness at the end of the day resulting in simple inattentiveness
   - the 'I've heard this all before' syndrome.
2. Processing the information provided. As you do this you may find you need to alter the pattern of the consultation to accommodate any new issues that arise. Words do

not always paint a true picture: Listen to the underlying message that is conveyed by 'feelings'.

3.   Approaching the conversation with an open mind and avoiding preconceptions. This can be difficult to achieve when dealing with regular patients who may be known at the pharmacy as 'That nice Mr Jones' or 'That nuisance Mrs Smith'. If you listen to a person having already stereotyped them you are likely to only hear what you expect to hear and may therefore miss a vital piece of information. Remember also that patients may make snap judgements about the pharmacist that may hinder communication.

4.   Listening with eyes as well as ears. Maintain eye contact as this will help to maintain interest and show interest. More than two-thirds of communication can be non-verbal (see Section 8.1.2). Look at the patient's facial expression and posture and be aware of your own posture.

5.   Keeping quiet while the other person is speaking. Do not interrupt a patient: let them finish before you speak.

6.   Acknowledging the other person and showing them that you are listening. When listening to a patient:

   • make encouraging gestures, for example, nod occasionally
   • encourage verbally by prompts: 'And ...', for example, and reinforce your understanding by summarising information given to you: 'Now let me see if I've got that right?' 'You say that . . .'
   • repeat certain significant or 'loaded' phrases or words or paraphrase some of the things the patient has said.

   If you are listening actively to a patient you should be able to repeat back in your own words what has been said by the patient. You do not necessarily have to agree with what they are saying!

Remember, all the benefits of effective communication will be lost if the pharmacist then fails to explain the use of the recommended treatment.

8.4 Explanation

When responding to symptoms in the pharmacy it is important to explain any decisions made to the patient clearly. Perhaps even more crucial is explanation of the purpose and use of prescribed or over-the-counter medicines. Pharmacists and pharmacy technicians are the last link in the prescribing chain. We are responsible for ensuring the correct medicine is dispensed and it is important that we make certain the patient knows how to take it correctly. Part of the pharmacist's and pharmacy technician's role is to help patients overcome any confusion they may have with respect to their medication.

It has been said that 'Good explanations, like good bikinis, should be brief, appealing, yet cover the essential features'! A mnemonic to help remember this is 'KISSER':

• Keep
• It
• Simple
• Short
• Empathetic
• Relevant.

There are three parts to a good explanation: planning, presentation and feedback.

Planning

Identify the information to be given and link your explanation to the individual to ensure understanding.

At a basic level the information can just be provided to the patient but if the information can be linked to the individual, the relevance of the information will be understood and the information will more likely be taken on board by the patient.

Presentation

This refers to the clarity of the message given, including the use of appropriate language. Tips for successful presentation include:

• use analogies, examples and illustrations

- use pauses for effect, breaking down the information into bite-sized chunks
- emphasise important points, use words or phrases such as 'important', 'essential' or 'the main thing to remember is'
- if appropriate, do not just explain verbally, demonstrate (e.g. the use of an inhaler)
- summarise key points, e.g. 'KISSER' (see above).

Feedback

Check that the listener has understood by:

- asking if they have any questions
- getting them to summarise what they have been told or demonstrate their understanding
- looking for non-verbal feedback, for example looking puzzled or confused
- asking questions in order to check understanding.

Key point 8.5

Remember, there are three parts to a good explanation:

- planning
- presentation
- feedback.

Consider these two explanations about how to take indometacin MR capsules:

1. 'These are the capsules for your arthritis. Take one capsule in the morning and one at night before going to bed. They should be swallowed whole and always taken with food.'
2. 'These are the capsules for your arthritis. Take one capsule in the morning and one at night before going to bed. You should find that the night time dose will help relieve the morning stiffness you have been experiencing. It is important to take the capsules with food to help reduce or prevent any stomach upset. Also the capsules have been designed to have a long lasting effect, so they must be swallowed whole. Have you any further questions? If you have any

concerns do not hesitate to come back and see me.'

Which explanation do you think will help the patient to remember? It is a fact that if a patient understands the reasons for doing something they are far more likely to be compliant. It is human nature. The pharmacist had planned what was to be said to the patient and the comment regarding morning stiffness showed that this pharmacist had taken the time to develop a rapport with the patient previously.

When do we use explanations in pharmacy?

- When responding to a patient's symptoms. In this case we need to explain/justify our actions.
- When dispensing prescriptions. Here we need to clearly explain the prescriber's directions and any associated cautions that apply to a particular medicine. We need to ensure that patients understand complex dosage instructions, such as a reducing dosage for a course or oral steroids, or the importance of completing a course of antibiotics.
- When demonstrating the use of a dosage form or appliance. Often it is better to explain verbally before doing the actual demonstration as the act of demonstrating may detract from the art of listening.
- When discussing side-effects and their prevalence. The rare but serious side-effects associated with some drugs need to be explained.
- When explaining possible medication and/or food interactions, for example the importance of avoiding alcohol with certain drugs such metronidazole or cheese with monoamine oxidase inhibitors (MAOIs).
- When explaining public health issues, such as the reasons to give up smoking, reduce cholesterol or blood pressure or the benefits of a healthy diet and lifestyle.
- When correcting mistaken beliefs. Patients often believe firmly in old wives tales, such as:
  - 'Feed a cold and starve a fever' – It is highly unlikely if a patient has a fever that they will want to eat but with the help of an antipyretic, their temperature will come down and subsequently their appetite will return.

– 'Colds cause ear infections' – This is unlikely since colds are caused by viruses and most ear infections by bacteria, however the build up of fluids in the ears associated with a cold is a fertile breeding ground for bacteria so the two can seem to go hand in hand.

• When providing advice. Pharmacists and pharmacy technicians advise patients in response to their symptoms on a daily basis. For example:

– Advising a patient with a blocked nose: 'Have you tried an inhalation? Karvol Capsules or Friar's Balsam can help.'

– Advising against the purchase of an old-fashioned medicine and guiding towards a better, evidence-based treatment. For example liquid paraffin is not considered to be the best treatment for constipation. Lactulose is the preferred treatment nowadays.

– Advising the choice of one medicine rather than another, such as an expectorant rather than a cough suppressant for a patient requesting a cough medicine. In this case a logical explanation may be required. For example, 'An expectorant will help clear your lungs of the phlegm as it will thin the phlegm and you will be able to cough it up yourself. A suppressant, while it will stop you coughing, will leave the phlegm sitting on your lungs, which is not advised.'

8.5 Case studies responding to symptoms or over-the-counter requests

Consider the following scenarios. For each, decide what questions you would need to ask and whether you would be likely to counter prescribe for the patient and what if anything you would be likely to give. The first scenario is laid out to help you.

Example 8.1

A woman aged approximately 20 years old complains of having had a cough for the last week. She is on her lunch hour and does not want to take time off to go to see the doctor.

Using the WWHAM mnemonic elicits the following information:

• Who is the medicine for? – It is for the patient herself.
• What are the symptoms? – Loose chesty cough that 'rattles'.
• How long have you been ill? – About a week.
• Action taken so far? – None.
• Medication being taken at the moment? – None.

This system discovers the basics but does not encourage elaboration. This is an easily remembered mnemonic often used by pharmacy assistants for their initial assessment of a patient before asking for further advice from the pharmacist.

Using the ENCORE mnemonic elicits the following information:

• Explore – It is for a young girl who has a loose chesty cough that 'rattles'.
• No medication? – Not an option in this case.
• Care – Could she be pregnant? – No, she is not.
• Observe – She seems a bit 'snuffly' and has a cold.

Example 8.1 Continued

- Refer – Symptoms suggest a simple chesty cough associated with a cold; probably viral in nature therefore no necessity to refer.
- Explain – Simple chesty cough and that she needs an expectorant to help 'cough it up' so advise she purchases an expectorant such as guaifenesin or an expectorant with a decongestant, such as pseudoephedrine. If symptoms persist for more than five days with treatment she should consult her GP.

This system did not elicit all symptoms but did take care to discover whether pregnancy could be a possibility. Observation showed evidence that she had a cold accompanying her symptoms. The course of action was clearly explained to the patient. The prompt 'No medication?' refers to the option of not giving medicine, just advice, but could also be adapted to use as a reminder to find out if she is taking any other medication prescribed or purchased.

This is the only mnemonic that emphasises the importance of explaining your decision about treatment. The patient needs to feel involved in the treatment programme and this in turn will mean that the patient will be happy to take your advice and get the best from the medicine they purchase.

Using the ASMETTHOD mnemonic elicits the following information:

- Age of the patient? – Approximately 20 years old.
- Self or someone else? – For herself.
- Medicines the patient is taking? – None at present.
- Exactly what does the patient mean by the symptom? – Loose 'rattly' cough, phlegm is clear but finds it difficult to 'cough it up'.
- Time/duration of the symptom? – About a week.
- Taken anything for it or seen the doctor? – No.
- History of any disease or condition? – No other health problems.
- Other symptoms being experienced? – Sore throat and cold.
- Doing anything to aggravate or alleviate the condition? – Not taken anything other than a couple of paracetamol. Avoiding smokey rooms, tending to sip lots of water to stop my throat feeling so 'scratchy'.

This system identified the patient and the age of the patient and elicited more details of the symptoms, associated symptoms and the duration of symptoms than the previous methods. Indirectly the question of pregnancy was addressed (in 'History of other disease or condition') as was what the patient had already done if anything to try and alleviate the symptoms. Again the question of whether or not she is a smoker was not addressed directly.

Using the SIT DOWN SIR mnemonic elicits the following information:

- Site or location? – Chest.
- Intensity or severity? – Seems to be lingering and causing distress.
- Type or nature? – Chesty cough that is loose with clear phlegm but she cannot 'cough it up'.
- Duration? – About a week.
- Onset? – Gradually getting worse.
- With? (Other symptoms) – Sore throat and cold symptoms.
- N annoyed or aggravated by? – Smoke-filled rooms.
- Spread or radiation? – Not really applicable.
- Incidence or frequency pattern? – Seem to be coughing all the time.
- Relieved by? – Hoping you can give me something to relieve it so far been sipping water to try and alleviate the problem.

Example 8.1 Continued

This system does not address the question 'who is it for?' nor the age or pregnancy issue. There was no check to see if the patient was on any other medication or suffers from any other medical conditions, nor was there any attempt to find out if she had tried any other treatment for the condition. Details of the symptoms were expanded upon and the onset and duration of the symptoms obtained.

The main information that you would need to discover is that the medication is for her and that she has had a chesty cough for about a week. The cough is loose and 'rattly'. There is clear phlegm but she is having difficulty coughing it up. She also has a sore throat and cold symptoms. She does not smoke.

These symptoms indicate that it is a simple chesty cough associated with a cold. It is probably viral in nature, it would be highly unlikely that a secondary bacterial infection would be present, and therefore the type of product to advise would be an expectorant-containing cough medicine such as guaifenesin or a cough medicine containing both an expectorant and a decongestant such as pseudoephedrine.

An alternative would be to recommend a steam inhalation such as Menthol and Eucalyptus Inhalation BP and to advise drinking plenty of fluids. If the symptoms persist after five days she should be advised to go to see her GP.

Look at the different levels of information each mnemonic obtains in the above example and decide which you feel gave the most information. None of them cover all the information needed. None asked outright, for example, whether or not she smoked; the patient had to volunteer the information that smoky rooms affected her cough (a smoker would be unlikely to say this).

This demonstrates that no mnemonic is all inclusive. They are there as reminders and all the time you must use your own clinical judgement and probe for more details when needed.

 Example 8.2

A mother is asking which cough medicine you would recommend for her son who is three years old. He has a tickly cough that tends to keep him awake at night.

In this case you need to establish the type of cough: it is dry without any phlegm and it affects him only at night. Other associated symptoms/history include that the child had a cold last week. There is no wheezing but the mother volunteers the information that his brother does wheeze. He has had no shortness of breath and has no other medical conditions and has only taken paracetamol when he had the cold.

This is probably a viral infection and a soothing linctus would help, but because of the absence of cough during the day and the brother with wheezing problems a visit to the GP to eliminate the possibility of asthma would be advised. (Remember: do not alarm the mother when giving this last piece of advice.)

Example 8.3

A man aged approximately 60 years complains of having a persistent cough. He says 'I just can't seem to get rid of it'. He is pale and appears to be rather tired. Your pharmacy assistant mentions the fact that he was made redundant from the local roofing factory about 12 months ago.

On questioning the patient you discover that he has a productive cough and the sputum is a yellowish colour and there have been tinges of blood apparent. The coughing has been evident for about six months. He is tired and has lost his appetite and with it some weight too. He also complains of shortness of breath. He is a smoker who smokes about 40 cigarettes a day and has done since he was a teenager. He has already tried Benylin Expectorant but that has not worked.

This patient needs to be referred to his GP urgently as the symptoms could suggest carcinoma of the bronchus or an industrial-related disease, for example, pneumoconiosis or chronic bronchitis or emphysema.

Example 8.4

A woman aged approximately 50 years asks for a different indigestion mixture, she seems to have 'got used to' the one she usually takes.

Anyone who has tried an antacid and 'gets used to it' such that it no longer provides the relief that it did should be referred to the doctor. An improvement in symptoms should be expected not a worsening. On questioning the customer you discover that the pain is in the upper abdomen and that she has been self-treating for about six months. She feels uncomfortable and occasionally nauseous. She has lost her appetite and is losing weight. She has been sick a couple of times this week. She takes no other medication either prescribed or purchased; she thinks the mixture she used to take was magnesium trisilicate mixture – 'the white indigestion mixture'.

By this time it is obvious that immediate referral to the doctor is the only option. The symptoms could suggest gastric cancer or pancreatic cancer. The patient needs to be advised to make an urgent appointment with her GP, but try not to alarm her. Explain for example that there are tests the doctor could do to discover the cause of the indigestion and therefore make the treatment more specific, or suggest the doctor may be able to prescribe something that is 'stronger' than the over-the-counter medicines and therefore she would be best to see her GP.

Example 8.5

A man aged approximately 40 years complains of indigestion. You know that he holds an executive position in a large company whose offices are across the road from your pharmacy.

On questioning you find that the pain is in the upper abdomen, the pain is worse after eating and he often feels nauseous. He cannot pin it down to certain foods, it does not get worse when he exercises at

Example 8.5 Continued

the gym and the pain does not seem to move. He has had the problem for the past two weeks on and off. He has lost his appetite because he dreads eating just in case the pain comes back, but he has not lost any weight. He has no other medical conditions and is taking no other medication. He has not tried antacids to see if they will alleviate the symptoms. He is a smoker (about 20 cigarettes a day) and also drinks alcohol (a gin and tonic to wind down and half a bottle of wine with dinner) and lives on snacks during the day with a large evening meal.

His indigestion is probably due to poor dietary habits. He should try to have small, regular meals and reduce his alcohol consumption. Now might also be a good time to consider giving up smoking

Example 8.6

A woman, aged about 30 years, complains of having a burning sensation in her chest that afternoon. She is the mother of three young children.

On questioning you find that the burning sensation gets worse on bending and it feels as though it 'moves upwards'. She has just had lunch with friends and this has just 'come on'. She has also found herself belching quite a lot. She is not nauseous and has no shortness of breath. She has not tried anything as yet to treat the pain and assures you she is not pregnant and not taking any other medication. She admits that her lifestyle is rather rushed, and that she tends to eat 'meals on the move'. She is not overweight and does not smoke.

Her indigestion is probably heartburn which is usually short term and self-limiting. It might help if she unties any tight belts or removes tight clothing (she has been out with friends so may well be wearing her 'best clothes' and wearing 'support garments'). She could also help relieve the symptoms by improving her posture and not leaning over the children but bending from the knees to reach their level. Suitable treatment would be an antacid, perhaps an alginate 'rafting' antacid such as Gaviscon. She should also be advised to see her doctor if there is no real improvement after a week.

Example 8.7

A mother is asking for advice about her four-year-old daughter who has recently had problems 'going to the toilet'. She started school, mornings only, about two months ago but is now attending all day.

First you need to check that the mother actually means constipation, which she does. The stools have been hard and pellet-like and the child seems to strain. She has been like this for a week to ten days. The child has no other medical conditions and takes no medication. On questioning you find that the child does not like going to school and cries every day. She is a picky eater and does not like school dinners.

Example 8.7 Continued

The problem appears to be constipation aggravated by emotional and dietary issues. It should improve as the child settles into school and if she is encouraged to eat a diet increased in fibre, wholemeal bread instead of cereals, with more fruit and vegetables. If the new diet is accepted there should be an improvement in symptoms. The mother should be advised to take the child to the doctor if there is no improvement after two weeks.

Example 8.8

A young mother who has recently had a baby complains of difficulty when 'using the toilet'. She tells you that she passes motions every 2–3 days and it is painful. Her stools are hard and she strains. She has been suffering like this for about two weeks. She has an itchy bottom and there is often blood on the toilet paper. There is no obvious blood on the stools. She is not pregnant or breast-feeding but she is not eating properly only having 'snatched meals' and little sleep because of the new baby.

The young woman is likely to have haemorrhoids associated with constipation. Advice on increasing fibre intake, cereals, pulses, fruit and vegetables etc. should be given. You could also suggest a laxative such as senna for short term use. Explain that the bleeding seems to be coming from haemorrhoids made worse by the constipation. Reassure her that it is a common occurrence after childbirth and suggest a cream or ointment to help with the haemorrhoids. Also stress the importance of hygiene and suggest the use of moist toilet tissues.

She should notice an improvement within one to two weeks. If not, she should make an appointment with her GP.

Example 8.9

An elderly woman aged about 70 years requests a bottle of liquid paraffin. A pharmacy assistant tells you that she bought a bottle last week. The woman has also asked the assistant whether there was a 'pick me up' she could suggest.

When asked, the woman explains that she used to go to the toilet every day ('regular as clockwork') until about three weeks ago and now she hardly ever seems to go. She tells you she has had a colicky pain with this constipation and she feels tired all the time. She looks very pale and thin. When asked about her weight she tells you that her friends say she has lost a lot of weight. She takes some water tablets for her heart trouble but apart from 'old age' she is fit and well.

The symptoms suggest that there is a possibility of colon cancer and therefore she needs to make an urgent appointment with her doctor. You can achieve this without alarming the patient by suggesting that the liquid paraffin she has been using is not really suitable for long-term use and that the doctor will be able to prescribe something more suitable.

Example 8.10

A young woman (about 18 years) asks if you have something for a foot problem.

First, you need to confirm that it is the woman that has the problem. It is. The symptoms are inflammation between the toes and peeling of the skin; the skin feels 'soft' between the toes. She is generally in good health, she is not pregnant nor is she diabetic but she does suffer from dysmenorrhoea for which she takes ibuprofen. Her toenails are not affected, nor are any other parts of her foot. She has no pain and her feet look and feel quite normal, just terrible itching between the toes. She has had the problem for about two weeks and last week her friend suggested she tried Mycil powder which seemed to do the trick for 3–4 days but then it came back again.

The symptoms indicate a fungal infection such as athlete's foot. The best suggestion would be to try a cream (one of the imidazoles) and stress that it will take time to cure the condition. The cream should be used regularly and the powder she had used on her feet should be used to dust the inside of shoes to help kill the fungus. Foot hygiene is also important and ensuring the feet are well dried after bathing is essential. Care should be taken as the fungal infection can be spread to other parts of the body so she should keep a separate towel for feet. It will also help if cotton socks and leather or canvas shoes are worn rather than those made of synthetic materials as this will allow the feet to breathe. It is also advisable not to wear the same pair of shoes on consecutive days; the shoes should be allowed to dry out completely from foot sweat etc. to make them less fungus friendly. If there is no improvement after two weeks the woman should see her GP.

Example 8.11

A woman in her mid-20s asks for a good painkiller.

The medication is for her for painful periods. She is diabetic and uses Actrapid and Mixtard insulin. She has tried ibuprofen 400 mg tds but it only seems to have a slight effect. The pain normally starts the day before her period and lasts for two or three days. It has been getting worse over the last five months and now the bleeding is very severe with 'flooding'.

The pain clearly seems to be related to periods and as there is worsening of the symptoms, with severe menorrhagia, the patient should be advised to see her GP.

Example 8.12

A woman in her mid-30s asks for a good treatment for diarrhoea.

You discover that the medication is for her husband not herself. He is aged 35 years. They have recently returned home from a holiday in India. He has no other illness and takes no medication. His wife has given him Dioralyte sachets for the past four days. He has frequent diarrhoea with colicky griping pains

Example 8.12 Continued

in the centre of his tummy. He has not been sick and there is no blood or mucus evident in his motions. He has been running a temperature.

In view of his recent trip abroad and the length of time the diarrhoea has persisted consultation with his GP should be advised. Holiday tummy is normally self-limiting and usually clears up within three days.

Example 8.13

A woman in her 40s asks what you can recommend for cystitis.

The treatment is for the woman herself. She has sharp pain on passing urine, a burning sensation and feels as though she needs to go to the toilet all the time. She has no weight loss, loin pain or discharge. There is no blood in the urine. The symptoms started the previous evening and she has never had anything like this before. She has tried taking cranberry juice as recommended by her friend but this does not seem to have helped. She has also stopped drinking because it is so uncomfortable when she goes to the toilet. The woman is also taking atenolol for blood pressure.

You should advise the patient that cystitis is quite common among women but it is important to drink plenty of fluids to ensure the bladder is flushed thoroughly. Offer a potassium-based proprietary cystitis treatment such as Cystopurin. Advise the patient about the importance of wiping herself from front to back after visiting the toilet and that wearing loose clothing and cotton underwear is sometimes helpful.

You should also suggest that after this bout has cleared she ensures she drinks plenty of water and tries to urinate at least once every 3 hours as woman who often hold their urine for long periods of time tend to have more urinary infections. It is important to try to empty the bladder fully and this is best achieved by sitting back on the toilet rather than leaning forward in a 'reading' position. Advise her to see her doctor if the cystitis does not clear up with the over-the-counter remedy.

Example 8.14

A woman in her mid-30s complains of a 'personal itch' and asks if you can recommend something for her to save her going to see the doctor.

She is a regular customer and you remember that she brought in a prescription for clotrimazole pessaries about four weeks ago. When you ask her about this she tells you that it worked and got rid of the problem but that it has come back again. She tells you that she is fed up with having thrush as she has had several attacks over the last six months. She is not taking any other medication and the only other problem she has is a terrible thirst; she is drinking so much now she often has to get up in the night to go to the toilet.

You explain to her that because the thrush keeps recurring it would be best to see the doctor. It could be recurring because her husband was not treated, which would explain why the last treatment has not

Example 8.14 Continued

'worked'. Also, because she is so thirsty the doctor may want to check her urine to see if this is a cause of the infection. Advise her to make an appointment and to take a urine sample with her. You could also offer her a blood test to check her sugar levels (if you felt that her reaction would be appropriate) but as there is a possibility of diabetes it is imperative she sees her GP to check this out.

Example 8.15

A woman in her mid-20s asks for some HC45 cream. Her neighbour has told her it 'works wonders for insect bites'.

On questioning you discover the cream is for her four-year-old daughter who has been bitten in the garden. She has itchy red lumps on her legs which are suggestive of insect bites. The child is not taking any medication and has no other medical conditions.

HC45 is not suitable as the child is under ten years old. This must be explained to the mother and an alternative offered such as calamine cream/lotion or a topical antihistamine such as Anthisan. Alternatively, an oral antihistamine such as Phenergan could be suggested, but it will make the child drowsy.

Example 8.16

A young girl, approximately 16 years old, wearing very fashionable clothes and lots of costume jewellery wants to buy some hydrocortisone cream she has seen recommended in her magazine.

She wants the cream to treat a rash on her arm. It is red and itchy and is under her watch strap. She has recently taken a course of antibiotics; she is not taking any other medication and has no other medical conditions. She is not pregnant.

The rash is a typical sign of allergic contact dermatitis. Suggest that she stops wearing the watch and offer her some hydrocortisone cream 1%. Advise her to apply it thinly twice a day and use it for one week maximum. If after one week she sees no improvement, she should make an appointment to see her GP.

Example 8.17

A man in his early 20s wants to buy some Betnovate cream for eczema. He has heard that you can now buy steroid creams from the chemist.

The cream is for his personal use. You explain that Betnovate cannot be supplied without a prescription. You ask him why he needs Betnovate and he explains that he has a red, itchy rash behind his knees, on his arms, behind his ears and he has just got a little patch on the side of his face by his ear. He uses

Example 8.17 Continued

a Ventolin inhaler when he gets short of breath and he remembers he had eczema as a child and thought he had used Betnovate.

Refer him to the doctor as steroid creams that are available for over-the-counter purchase are not recommended for use on the face. In addition as this could become an ongoing condition the use of the steroid cream would be best monitored by a doctor.

Example 8.18

A young woman in her late teens (a student) is complaining of headaches and wants to buy some Nurofen that she has seen advertised on the television.

The tablets are for her. She gets headaches particularly when revising and it stops her concentrating. The headaches are not very severe and she has used paracetamol in the past but wondered if Nurofen would be better. She has an inhaler ('it's for wheezing') but rarely uses it. She used to have quite a lot of chest trouble as a child but it is very rare now.

Explain to her that Nurofen would not really be suitable for her because of her history of chest problems. She may well be sensitive to ibuprofen, the ingredient in Nurofen. Also tell her that aspirin could cause her problems and that paracetamol is the best treatment for her. You could also check whether or not she has seen an optometrist for an eye test recently. She may also get some relief from the headaches if she had regular breaks, preferably taking a walk outside to clear her head.

Example 8.19

A man comes in to the pharmacy and wants you to recommend something for a tickly cough. He has tried a couple of different cough mixtures but it just seems to be coming back.

He has had the cough for a month or so. It is really irritating but he does not have any phlegm. He is a smoker but had never had any problems with his chest. He has never had asthma or anything similar. He does take blood pressure tablets. The doctor changed him onto enalapril a couple of months ago.

You need to explain that the cough could be a side-effect of the enalapril and if he returns to his GP he may consider altering his medication. It might also be an opportunity to try to persuade him to attempt to give up smoking.

Example 8.20

A customer wants some eye drops as she has been getting bouts of itchy eyes and a runny nose.

Her eyes are red and itchy and she has a runny nose and keeps sneezing. The symptoms have lasted

Example 8.20 Continued

two weeks and now in desperation she has come to see if there is anything she can use to clear it up. Further details include the fact that she has suffered from hayfever in the past but it is not the right season for that. She admits the symptoms are very similar. On further probing she admits she has a new kitten.

Sodium cromoglicate eye drops should help to relieve the symptoms and perhaps a systemic non-drowsy antihistamine such as loratadine would also help, but the real problem is the source of the allergen (i.e. the kitten) and if the problem continues serious consideration should be given to re-homing the animal.

Explaining is one of a pharmacist's most frequently used skills and lies at the heart of pharmacy practice. It is basically an informative function but also has an educational role with regard to public health. The area will continue to expand as pharmacists engage in new roles, such as medicines use reviews (MURs), pharmacist-led clinics, pharmacist prescribing, etc. If pharmacists and pharmacy technicians are to maximise their potential roles it is essential that their communication skills are maintained to provide positive health benefits to patients.

8.6 Explaining and educating patients to improve concordance

It has been estimated that around half of patients do not take their medicines as intended. To try to improve on this, the trend now is for a prescriber and patient to come to joint decisions regarding their treatment and for the pharmacist, doctor and patient to become members of the same team.

Using a multidisciplinary team means that it is often easier to address the problems that cause lack of compliance (a patient is said to be compliant with their prescribed therapy if they take their medication as advised). Often the pharmacist is seen as more accessible to the patient and therefore in the best position to improve the chances of a patient complying with a medication regimen. If patients understand why they are taking a medicine and the benefits for them they are more likely to be happy to continue treatment.

When a pharmacist conducts a medicines use review (MUR), it is an ideal opportunity to find out exactly what the patient is doing with their medication and how they are complying with the regimen. By empowering the patient by giving them more involvement in decision making, you allow the patient to decide themselves whether or not to take a medication. Because of the openness of the exchange, their reasons for not taking a medication can be rationally discussed and a joint decision to comply with the current dosage regimen (or if necessary an amended regimen) obtained. This is termed concordance.

Compliance and concordance can be affected by the patient's perceived benefit or lack of benefit from the therapy. It can also be affected by the reason for the instigation of medication. A heart attack would be a frightening experience and brings the idea of mortality to the patient's mind and therefore, at least to begin with, the importance of taking their medication will be a priority. But with the passage of time and if no further events happen, encouragement to continue a long-term treatment may be needed. Educating patients about their conditions, particularly if they are 'symptom free' conditions such as hypertension (high blood pressure), may improve compliance. Explaining the damaging effect to the body organs of high blood pressure and the effects it can have on life expectancy can be sufficiently motivating to the patient so that they take part in the decision to take medication and understand the necessity for it.

In order to make compliance easier for a patient it is often better to develop a routine. For example while the kettle is boiling for the first cup of tea of the day get into the habit of taking the first dose of medication. With complex dosage regimens a pill organiser or monitored dosage system may be of value (see Figure 9.22). These are usually seven-day organisers with a compartment for each day that is then split into sections that equate to breakfast, lunch, evening meal and bedtime. Although they have their disadvantages – some medicines cannot be placed in these containers (for example, soluble tablets), they need re-filling weekly, and there is no guarantee that medication has actually been taken if it is missing from the device as it may have fallen on the floor and been lost – they are helpful if the non-compliance is unintentional and a result of forgetfulness.

Similarly when completing an MUR you may find that a patient is not fully compliant because of problems of manual dexterity, either due to inflammatory conditions such as arthritis or neurological disease such as Parkinson's disease. These types of problems can make even the simplest packaging an obstacle to taking the medicine. It is often said that grandma asks the grandchildren to open her child-resistant containers.

Side-effects or the concern about side-effects listed in patient information leaflets can also be a barrier to patient compliance. What patients perceive is the probability of a side-effect listed and what the terminology used actually means is often at variance. According to European Union guidelines, the terms recommended to convey the likelihood of side-effects are as listed in Table 8.2, but most patients tend to overestimate the risks, leading to non-compliance. This is why it is important to explain the risks in the pharmacy.

Pharmacists can play a major part in patient compliance by talking to patients when they are

Table 8.2 The recommended phrases to be used when conveying the likelihood of side-effects

Definition	European recommendation	Patient perception
Very rare	less than a 0.01% likelihood	4%
Rare	0.01–0.1%	8%
Uncommon	0.1–1%	18%
Common	1–10%	45%
Very common	More than 10% risk	65%

Taken from *MeReC Extra*, November 2002, Issue 7.

first prescribed an item, giving the patient another opportunity to raise any concerns and to have an open discussion to allay their fears. Pharmacists are also in an ideal position to review compliance with long-term medication. Often by observation and checking with the patient dosage regimens, pharmacists are able to recognise that a patient has an existing compliance problem. Once the problem is identified it may be addressed and coping strategies or managing strategies may be employed as outlined above. Pharmacists and pharmacy technicians are often the last link in the prescribing chain and if patients are to obtain the best from their medication it is up to the pharmacist to ensure compliance.

8.6.1 Case studies

Consider the following scenarios and how you could address the problems.

Example 8.21

At a recent 'well man' check-up at his local surgery, Mr Chris James was discovered to have hypertension. He was prescribed a beta blocker. Over the next two months Mr James collected his repeat prescriptions from the doctor and had them dispensed at your pharmacy. Today he has arrived at your pharmacy with a prescription for some antibiotics and a painkiller for an ear infection. You notice from

Example 8.21 Continued

your patient medication records that his next repeat for his beta blocker is two weeks overdue. What could you do in this situation?

Pharmacist: Hi Mr James, I've got your antibiotics and painkillers ready for you, but before I explain about those I'm a bit concerned as I noticed that you haven't had a repeat for your blood pressure tablets – unless you took your prescription somewhere else.

Patient: No I haven't gone elsewhere but I have been feeling a lot better lately and I'm not sure I need to keep taking those tablets anyway.

Pharmacist: So you don't really think you need these tablets? Why's that?

Patient: Well the tablets made me feel tired and dizzy, and as you know I am a lorry driver so I need to be alert.

Pharmacist: Have you mentioned the problem of side-effects to your GP?

Patient: No since I've cut down on taking them I feel much better and so I didn't think I needed to bother the doctor.

Pharmacist: When did you have your blood pressure checked last?

Patient: Well I haven't had it checked lately, because I've been feeling a lot better, I've been feeling fine.

The pharmacist in this scenario could now offer to take the blood pressure of the patient and if it is a high reading, reinforce the message that continuing with the medication is desirable and that he should return to his GP for further supplies of his medication or if the side-effects are too intrusive, to consult with the doctor concerning alternative medication. The pharmacist could also use this opportunity to suggest that the patient self-monitors his blood pressure and keeps a record of the readings either by purchasing a home blood pressure monitor or calling into the pharmacy periodically for a blood pressure check. Mr James is more likely to be compliant if he realises his non-compliance causes his blood pressure to rise again.

 Example 8.22

Mrs Jean Akhurst is a 46-year-old woman who works in the local solicitors office. She has a history of hypertension, arthritis, mild heart failure and frequent urinary tract infections. She has a repeat prescription for hormone replacement therapy (HRT), her ACE inhibitor which she takes each morning, her anti-inflammatory which she takes three times a day and also a prescription for some antibiotics which she will need to take four times a day. The pharmacist decides to check that she knows what her tablets are for and when to take them. During this discussion it becomes apparent that she takes them when she remembers.

How might the pharmacist have identified that there may be a compliance problem with Mrs Akhurst? What coping strategies could the pharmacist suggest to solve the non-compliance problem?

It may be obvious from the patient medication record (PMR) that Mrs Akhurst is having repeats of items that are staggered and do not suggest that she is compliant with all her medication. The recurrence of infections may also suggest that she is not completing the courses of antibiotics prescribed for her. You could try and find out if she has tried any strategies to help her remember to take her medication or alternatively you could suggest she tries a monitored dosage system which might prompt her to take the medication. Encourage her to complete the course of antibiotics to prevent further recurrences of the infections.

Example 8.23

An older patient, Mrs Carmella Bianca, has recently moved to this country to live with her daughter following the death of her husband. She has very little English but whenever she comes into your pharmacy you practise your 'holiday Italian' with her. She has been taking oral diabetic therapy, but today she brings in a prescription for insulin and needles. She does not seem her happy bubbly self. What could be the possible cause of her anxiety and how could you help to reassure her?

Pharmacist: Hello Carmella, what's troubling you today?

Patient: The doctor has given me injections; do you think I need them?

Pharmacist: It sounds as though you are not sure that the doctor has prescribed the right medicine for you.

Patient: I don't feel ill enough to need injections.

Pharmacist: You really seem concerned about using injections for your insulin. Have you had to have lots of injections before?

Patient: No, but my husband had lots of injections before he died.

By what she is saying, Carmella is showing concerns that the injections mean that she is seriously ill. Perhaps she sees this as the long slippery slope to death.

The pharmacist now has a chance to alter the way Carmella thinks of injections. The rapport between the patient and the pharmacist can help the patient have more confidence in the change of medication if it is explained and approved of by someone she trusts.

Pharmacist: Carmella, diabetes is a serious illness but it can be controlled by the injections. I have many patients older than you who use insulin injections and they are doing fine. A lot of patients who begin on tablets have to transfer to injections; it should be easier for you to control your blood sugar levels with the insulin.

In this scenario you may also like to consider the use of her daughter as an interpreter, but only with Carmella's approval because of issues of patient confidentiality.

8.7 Written communication

When patients are counselled verbally their understanding at the time of the explanation can be checked, but the length of time the information is retained can vary from patient to patient. In the pharmacy we provide two forms of written communication to patients: the labels on dispensed medicines and the patient information leaflets contained in both prescribed medicines and over-the-counter sales. The labels should clearly convey the instructions from the prescriber to the patient and have been covered in earlier chapters of this book (see Section 3.3.5 for NHS community prescriptions, Section 4.3.4 for NHS hospital prescriptions and Section 5.1.4 for private prescriptions). Cautionary or advisory labels are also covered as outlined in Appendix 9 of the *British National Formulary.*

Pharmacists may also add further cautions with regard to certain formulations. These include pharmaceutical cautions, such as 'For external use only', 'Not to be taken', 'Shake the bottle', storage conditions, such as 'Store in fridge' for items needing to be stored below room temperature, and discard dates for items which should be discarded after a particular date (e.g. reconstituted antibiotic mixtures or eye drops after opening).

The written word is no replacement for verbal communication. Many patients prefer to be told in person about their medication and often seem to feel that the purpose of the patient information leaflet is to highlight every side-effect ever noted. After all, they probably do not have the expertise or knowledge to sort out which side-effect is serious and which are very likely or very unusual.

Some information leaflets include pictograms describing how a product should be used. These can be valuable, for example, when trying to explain the use of eye drops, pessaries, suppositories, inhalers, etc. There are also many leaflets available from the internet (for example, www.medicines.org.uk), where patient information leaflets may be down loaded in large print versions and audio versions. Alternative Braille versions may also be available. Soon downloads will be available for MP3 players. In addition there are links on this web page to medicine guides designed to help patients to understand how to use their medication, such as multi-media pages showing the use of inhalers.

There is a mass of information available to us and the general public and our purpose as pharmacists is to provide the best, unbiased information possible and to ensure that the information is communicated to the patient in an understandable format.

8.8 Communication with other healthcare professionals

While most of the day-to-day communication will be with patients, there will also be times when pharmacists and pharmacy technicians communicate with prescribers and other healthcare professionals.

Communication with other healthcare professions will include both verbal and written communication. For example, patient referral forms would be a form of written communication from the pharmacist to the prescriber. These forms concern information that the pharmacist may have obtained:

- as a result of a 'responding to symptoms' interview with a patient
- as a result of tests perfomed in the pharmacy
- as an information provide to the GP, for example when medicines have been supplied

to a patient following an emergency request from the patient.

In community pharmacy the most common form of contact with a GP is by telephone concerning a prescription that has been received in the pharmacy. As pharmacists we are problem solving all the time, so if there is a problem with a prescription we will normally try to resolve it without resorting to contacting the prescriber. However in certain cases contact with the prescriber will be required.

It is important to prepare for the consultation, as quite often you will be interrupting a busy surgery. There are two main issues: the patient and the drug. Before speaking to the prescriber you need to obtain the complete picture and formulate plans. References need to be checked, such as the *British National Formulary*, summary of product characteristics, other drug information, etc. You also need full information with regard to the patient, name, address, age, most of which will be available from the prescription. The NHS number (or equivalent) for the patient should also be available.

Using the references available to you (do not forget that the patient may also be a valuable information source) you need to formulate a plan. If there is a problem regarding the supply of a drug, for example, a manufacturer's delay or something similar, you need to be able to suggest alternative therapy, and it would be best to suggest an item that is stocked by the pharmacy and therefore easily obtainable.

When you contact a prescriber, introduce yourself, identify the patient and describe your concern (always have a pen and paper with you so that you can jot down information you want to give and any information you receive from the prescriber). The prescriber may suggest a plan of action or may expect you to have already formulated a plan which you could share and modify if necessary. Together you should reach a conclusion and then you need to confirm that you have understood the prescriber's intentions correctly, summarise what you have heard and repeat the information back to the prescriber for confirmation; the strength, dosage and frequency of the medication are particularly important.

All the time *listen* to the information being

given to you. Remember you are speaking to another healthcare professional. Treat them with the respect they deserve, being ever mindful of how you would like to be treated if someone was querying something you had done.

Consider the following examples. These case studies highlight that often the problems we encounter as pharmacists are not of our own making and our role seems to be one of a negotiator.

Example 8.24

Mr Jones brings in his prescription to your pharmacy, he wants to wait for it as he has a bus to catch and 'it won't take long it's only tablets'. You look at the prescription and see that it is for diclofenac 100 mg tds.

You need to check that the prescription is legal and the dose is safe and suitable for the patient (i.e. it can be dispensed). You notice that the dose is outside the normal dosage recommendations for diclofenac. From the patient medication record it appears that Mr Jones has not had diclofenac before, but you do go out and ask him.

Mr Jones states that he has not had this medication before but asks if you could please be quick as he has a bus to catch. It is important to get this medicine because his consultant has suggested it.

You telephone the surgery as the dose is too high but the phone is engaged.

What are you going to say to Mr Jones to placate him and ensure he uses your pharmacy again?

Explain to Mr Jones that there is a query regarding the dose of his tablets. At no point should you suggest that the prescriber has prescribed an overdose; you must not destroy the patient's confidence in the prescriber. Explain that the telephone is engaged and you will try again as soon as possible. You could offer to deliver the medication to him later in the day after the problem has been sorted out with the doctor. (At this point Mr Jones might be uncharitably thinking how could you know better than a consultant!)

What are you going to say to the GP when you get through on the telephone? What could be the alternatives?

When you get through to the doctor she says 'the consultant said to prescribe diclofenac tds'. Once again we never use the word 'overdose'. Suggest to the doctor that normally if diclofenac is prescribed tds it would be 25 mg or 50 mg tds, the 100 mg preparations are modified release that are designed to give a constant blood level of drug over a period of time and therefore in this case it would be a once daily dose of diclofenac MR 100. Alternatively if the tds dosage was required, the strength of tablet should be 25 mg or 50 mg depending on the severity of the condition. The maximum recommended dose is 150 mg daily in divided doses.

The doctor confirms that Mr Jones is in quite severe pain as he has had recent orthopaedic surgery (knee joint replacement) and therefore she feels the intention of the prescriber would be the 50 mg tds, giving an opportunity to reduce the dose to 25 mg if it is not well tolerated. You confirm that she requires 50 mg tds and arrange to send the prescription to the surgery to be amended.

Mr Jones is still waiting and is getting irate as his bus is due at any moment and mentions loudly to the staff that he has never seen such a slow pharmacist.

You dispense the medicine as arranged with the GP and go out to advise Mr Jones about his treatment, the dose change and how to take it, etc. You explain that while it may seem that his prescription was only tablets, each prescription has to be clinically checked and should there appear to be an unusual dose it is a pharmacist's obligation to discuss it with the prescriber. In this instance there had been some

Example 8.24 Continued

ambiguity in the directions from the consultant to Mr Jones' GP, but after consultation with the GP the problem had been resolved and Mr Jones should find that these tablets should definitely ease his knee pain and hopefully this will be a short course of treatment for him during his recovery. You apologise for the delay but explain that your patients are important to you and you want to be sure that they receive the best possible care. He complains that he has missed his bus now, but admits there will be another one in 10 minutes. You could then offer to let him sit in the warm shop until the bus is due.

Consider how you would have tackled this communication exercise. Tact and diplomacy are certainly required!

Example 8.25

You are presented with a prescription for Mrs Smith for warfarin 3 mg daily and cimetidine 400 mg bd.

On performing the clinical check you see that in Appendix 1 of the *British National Formulary* there is an interaction between warfarin and cimetidine: the cimetidine enhances the anticoagulant effect of the warfarin. Has the patient had this treatment before? It is not on her patient medication record, so it is best to check with the patient first.

Mrs Smith is not waiting for her prescription. It is her next door neighbour who has brought in the prescription as Mrs Smith is not feeling very well this morning. On questioning, the neighbour tells you that she thinks she has been on the blood thinning tablets some time but it is her stomach that is playing up now and she thinks that the doctor has given her something new to try.

Explain that you need to check some details with the doctor so you need to ring the surgery. Perhaps she has some more shopping to do? She could pop back and collect the prescription just before she goes home rather than wait.

Before ringing the GP to query the interaction you decide to obtain more information by consulting *Stockley's Drug Interactions*. Here you find that the interaction between warfarin and cimetidine can cause severe bleeding, but in some patients there is no problem at all. Ranitidine and nizatidine seem to be the preferred alternative H_2 receptor antagonists, but even with these bleeding has occurred with a small number of patients.

When you ring the surgery you discover Mrs Smith's doctor is away for the next two days.

The surgery receptionist asks if you would like to speak to another doctor. What are you going to do?

- Is it imperative that she has the cimetidine now or could she wait two days before starting treatment, which would allow you to speak to the original prescriber?
- Will another doctor help you with your problem?
- Should the patient be asked to return to the surgery for a consultation with another GP?

You speak to another GP in the surgery who consults Mrs Smith's notes and cannot see what you are worried about. It appears that in the notes the doctor has arranged for Mrs Smith to come in for a blood test to check her prothrombin times in two days' time, therefore the GP feels that the cimetidine should not cause a problem.

Example 8.25 Continued

Mrs Smith's neighbour returns from shopping and asks if you have sorted out that surgery 'they're always getting things wrong'. You explain that you have a good relationship with the surgery and they were happy to help, even though Mrs Smith's doctor was away. You also tell her that they have been very helpful and you are sorry she feels she has had problems with the surgery before and hope this will go some way to improving her impression of the surgery. Remember that details of your conversation cannot be shared with Mrs Smith's neighbour because of confidentiality issues. You give the neighbour Mrs Smith's medication and ask her to remind Mrs Smith that it is important she keeps her clinic appointment arranged by her GP. Advise the neighbour that if Mrs Smith has any questions she should feel free to phone you at the pharmacy and you will be happy to help.

Example 8.26

Mrs Brown, a regular patient, brings in an NHS prescription from Mr Drillett the local dentist. He has ordered co-amoxiclav 375 mg tablets 1 tds.

While checking the prescription you realise that while clinically acceptable, the prescriber has ordered an item that a dentist is not allowed to prescribe on an NHS prescription (see the *Drug Tariff* Part XVIIA) (see Section 3.2.2). What do you do?

A suitable alternative for a dental infection would be amoxicillin capsules 250 mg/500 mg tds. Alternatively the dentist could give Mrs Brown a private prescription.

You ring the dental surgery and speak to Mr Drillett, carefully explaining that the co-amoxiclav is not allowable on NHS dental prescription. He asks for an alternative. You explain that as co-amoxiclav is amoxicillin 250 mg combined with clavulanic acid 125 mg, and while it is recommended for severe dental infections it is normally reserved for amoxicillin-resistant infections. A first line treatment for dental infections would be amoxicillin 250 mg 8 hourly.

Mr Drillett thanks you for calling and decides to change the medication to amoxicillin 500 mg 8 hourly. He offers to bring a new prescription into the pharmacy later that day.

You explain to Mrs Brown that she now has capsules rather than tablets and that you have agreed the change with the dentist. Mrs Brown wants to know what was wrong with what was on her prescription already. You explain that dentists are only permitted to prescribe certain drugs on NHS prescriptions. As Mr Drillett has a large private practice the restrictions had slipped his mind. However he has chosen an alternative that is allowed on the NHS and this course of antibiotics should clear up her dental infection.

Mrs Brown asks if these capsules are as good as the tablets and wants to know why private patients get better treatment than NHS patients. You explain that the list drawn up by the Government's advisors covers a range of medications that they feel a dentist is likely to need to treat patients effectively. The antibiotic listed, amoxicillin, is the first line antibiotic for dental infections and by giving you the high dose Mr Drillett is ensuring that even the most severe infection should clear up. There is no clinical evidence to show that the co-amoxiclav would be any more effective than the amoxicillin. You explain that if she takes the course of medication as prescribed, the infection should be cleared by the end of the course. Very occasionally a second course of treatment may be required and if she feels the infection is not improving after four or five days she should see Mr Drillett before this course ends in seven days' time.

Example 8.27

You receive a prescription for Mr John Williams, 3 The Grove, Astonbury from a local doctor, Dr Better. The prescription asks for temazepam tablets 20 mg × 100 1 at night. Also on the prescription is Fortisip 200 mL × 30.

The signature on the prescription does not look genuine and Dr Better rarely prescribes temazepam and most of his prescriptions are computer generated not hand-written like this one. What do you do? Do you speak to the 'patient'?

First you ask the 'patient' to wait while you check the availability of the item. Mr Williams says he realises you will probably need to order his 'drinks' because nowhere keeps enough and that he will pop back in 10 minutes.

You decide that you had better contact the surgery using a telephone in the back of the shop rather than the dispensary telephone. You have the number for Dr Better's surgery and do not use the one on the prescription, which also looks as though it has been changed slightly.

On speaking to the receptionist you discover that Dr Better is on holiday in Italy (the prescription is dated today) and is not expected back at the surgery for another three days. She is quite sure that no one has written a prescription for Mr Williams; in fact she is sure that they have no such patient registered with the practice. You thank her for her help.

What do you do now?

The surgery has confirmed that the prescription is a fraud. You should retain the prescription and telephone the local police station to report an attempted prescription fraud. You also need to inform the local PCT (or equivalent) telling them the details on the prescription:

- the type and serial number on the prescription
- patient details on the prescription
- details of the medication and the dose (quite often unrelated items are added to prescriptions to try to make the prescription appear more 'genuine')
- doctor and surgery details as printed on the prescription
- a detailed description of the person presenting the prescription
- how the prescription was forged or altered.

Where possible, fax a copy of the prescription to the PCT.

Mr Williams comes back for his medication and when it is not ready he wants his prescription back. You explain that you have ordered both items for him and they will be in later (when the police will have arrived, you hope) or explain that Dr Better has asked you to keep the prescription for him as he cannot believe he accidentally ordered 100 temazepam tablets. By now the person presenting a forged prescription realises that the 'game is up' and can usually be seen running down the high street at quite a speed. When challenged, it is rare for a forger to stand his ground. Most will run as they fear arrest by the police.

8.9 Chapter summary

This chapter has covered the basics of patient communication. It is important that pharmacists and pharmacy technicians are familiar with both verbal and non-verbal communication and are able to communicate effectively with patients and carers. The next chapter will examine specific counselling points relating to different dosage forms.

9

Patient counselling and communication 2 – Product-specific counselling points

Upon completion of this chapter, you should be able to understand the key counselling points for the following specific dosage forms:

- ear drops and sprays
- eye drops
- eye ointments
- inhalers
- liquid oral dosage forms
- nasal drops
- nasal sprays
- oral powders
- patches
- pessaries and vaginal creams
- suppositories
- tablets and capsules
- topical applications.

The previous chapter (Chapter 8) covered the basics of patient communication, pointing out that pharmacists and pharmacy technicians should be familiar with both verbal and non-verbal communication and able to communicate effectively with patients and carers. This chapter contains specific counselling points relating to the following dosage forms:

- ear drops and sprays (see Section 9.1)
- eye drops (see Section 9.2)
- eye ointments (see Section 9.3)
- inhalers (see Section 9.4)
- liquid oral dosage forms (see Section 9.5)
- nasal drops (see Section 9.6)
- nasal sprays (see Section 9.7)
- oral powders (see Section 9.8)
- patches (see Section 9.9)
- pessaries and vaginal creams (see Section 9.10)
- suppositories (see Section 9.11)
- tablets and capsules (see Section 9.12)
- topical applications (see Section 9.13).

9.1 Ear drops and sprays

Ear drops and sprays are commonly used for the removal of excess ear wax. They are also used for the treatment of otitis externa (inflammation of the ear canal with associated itching and discharge often caused by infections or allergies) and occasionally otitis media.

9.1.1 How to use ear drops and sprays

1. Wash hands with soapy water.
2. Clean and dry the ear gently with a facecloth.
3. If necessary, shake the bottle of drops or spray. Some drops and sprays are suspensions and will need shaking; if applicable, this direction will be on the label.
4. Warm the ear drops or spray by holding the bottle in the hand for a few minutes.
5. Remove the lid.
6. Lie down on side with the affected ear uppermost (or tilt the head to one side).
7. Gently pull the ear lobe upwards and backwards, to straighten the ear canal.
8. Drop the drops or spray into the ear canal.
9. Gently massage just in front of the ear.
10. Stay lying down or with the head tilted for five minutes to allow the medication to run down the ear canal.
11. Return to the upright position and wipe away any excess medication.
12. Repeat if necessary in the other ear.
13. Replace the lid.

9.1.2 Tips when using ear drops and sprays

- The most comfortable position for instillation of ear drops and sprays is lying down.
- Often it is easier if the drops or sprays are not self-administered.
- Do not to scratch or poke the ear canal with fingers, cotton buds, hair grips, etc. as this may further irritate the ear canal and in the case of excess wax, may push the wax and dirt further into the ear. The ear cleans itself and the wax will fall out of the ear as flakes or small crusts from time to time.
- Do not plug the ear with cotton wool.
- Try not to let soap or shampoo get into your ear when showering or washing hair as this may further irritate the ear canal.

- Swimming is not advised while receiving treatment for ear problems. Tightly fitting swimming caps covering the ears should be used if swimming is unavoidable.
- Discard any remaining ears drops four weeks after opening.

Key point 9.1

When using ear drops and sprays:

- The most comfortable position for instillation of ear drops and sprays is lying down.
- Often it is easier if the drops or sprays are not self-administered.
- Do not to scratch or poke the ear canal with fingers, cotton buds, hair grips, etc.
- Do not plug the ear with cotton wool.
- Try not to let soap or shampoo get into your ear.
- Swimming is not advised while receiving treatment for ear problems.
- Discard any remaining ears drops four weeks after opening.

9.1.3 Special points for consideration with children and babies

Babies and small children may wriggle and try to put up their hands to their head to prevent ear drops being instilled. This can be minimised if the child is wrapped tightly in a blanket, making them feel secure, with the arms tucked out of the way.

Older children will not find the process too distressing and generally will cooperate. The main difference when administering ear drops or spray to a child is that the ear lobe needs only to be pulled backwards to open the ear canal.

9.2 Eye drops

The importance of advice to patients with regard to the use of eye drops cannot be underestimated, particularly concerning glaucoma patients where failure to use eye drops correctly can result in blindness.

9.2.1 How to use eye drops

1. Wash hands with soapy water.
2. If necessary, clean the eyes with boiled and cooled water and a tissue (one tissue for each eye) to remove any discharge or remaining wateriness (do not use cotton wool as it may leave fibres behind that may irritate the eye).
3. Shake the bottle of drops if necessary. Some eye drops are suspensions and will need shaking; if applicable, this direction will be on the label.
4. Remove the cap from the bottle.
5. Either sit down or lie down and tilt the head backwards so that you are looking at the ceiling.
6. Gently pull down the lower eyelid with a finger to make a pocket between the eye and the lower lid.

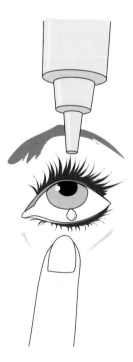

Figure 9.1 The position of the dropper bottle during administration of a dose.

7. Look upwards.
8. Rest the dropper bottle on the forehead above the eye (see Figure 9.1).
9. Squeeze one drop inside the lower eyelid (do not allow the dropper tip to touch the eye).
10. Close the eye and gently blot away any excess drops on a clean tissue.
11. Apply slight pressure to the inner corner of the eye for about 30 seconds. This will prevent the drops running down the tear duct and into the back of the throat, avoiding any unpleasant after taste and also minimising any absorption into the body, reducing the risk of possible side-effects.
12. Replace the cap on the bottle.
13. Remember to discard any remaining drops four weeks after opening.

9.2.2 Tips when using eye drops

- Some patients find it difficult to decide whether or not the drop has actually gone into the eye. If the drops are stored in the refrigerator (not the freezer) it will be easier to detect that the cold drop has actually entered the eye. Patients who regularly use this method also find the cold drops soothing.
- If drops are to be used on a long-term regular basis it may be best to establish a routine to aid compliance. For example if drops are to be used night and morning, the patient could keep the drops next to their toothbrush so that use of the drops is associated with brushing teeth and therefore a reminder is set.
- If more than one type of eye drop is to be used, wait at least 5–10 minutes after putting in the first drop before using the second. This prevents the first drop being washed away by the second before it has time to work. Similarly if using drops and ointment, use the drops first then wait 5 minutes before applying the eye ointment.
- The order in which to use drops is determined by the effect of the drops or their formulation. If one drop causes stinging it should be used last so that the tears produced as a result do not wash out the second drop.

If the eye drops are a suspension or a long-acting preparation these should be used last as any drop put in afterwards could interfere with their action.

- While using eye drops it is often advised that soft contact lenses should not be worn because some drugs and preservatives can accumulate in the soft contact lenses which could potentially harm the eye. This can be prevented if the lenses are removed prior to addition of the drops and not replaced for at least 15 minutes after the drops have been used. For each type of eye drop, it is usually a good idea to check with the manufacturer's recommendations as to whether it would be possible for the patient to continue to use contact lenses.

Key point 9.2

When using eye drops:

- If the drops are stored in the refrigerator it will be easier to detect that the cold drop has actually entered the eye.
- If drops are to be used on a long-term regular basis it may be best to establish a routine to aid compliance.
- If more than one type of eye drop is to be used, wait at least 5–10 minutes after putting in the first drop before using the second.
- The order in which to use drops is determined by the effect of the drops or their formulation.
- While using eye drops it is often advised that soft contact lenses should not be worn.

9.2.3 Special points for consideration with children and babies

Babies and small children may wriggle and try to put up their hands to their eyes to prevent eye drops being instilled. This can be minimised if the child is wrapped tightly in a blanket, making them feel secure, with the arms tucked out of the way.

With older children, an explanation of what is to be done along with a demonstration on their favourite doll or teddy bear may help. Lie the child down on the bed or settee, tilt the head back slightly and proceed with the general method of eye drop use.

As a last resort, if a child refuses to cooperate drops can be administered by lying the child down with the eyes closed. Place a drop onto the closed eye in the corner near to the nose. When the child opens the eye the drop will then bathe the eye.

9.2.4 Use of preservative-free drops in single-use containers

Some patients are allergic to the preservatives included in multi-dose eye drop preparations. Because of this, single unit dose eye drops which are preservative-free have been developed. The application of the drops is the same as with multi-dose drops. Each unit is complete in itself. The cap needs to be removed, usually by snapping it off prior to use, and it is important to discard any remaining drops in the single-use phial and not 'save' them for later use as they are preservative-free and therefore there is a greater risk of microbial contamination.

9.2.5 Compliance aids

Opticare produce eye drop dispensers that make instilling eye drops easier. These eye drop dispensers hold the plastic eye dropper bottles used by manufacturers and make them easier to squeeze, with only slight pressure needed to dispense a single drop. For patients with impaired manual dexterity or arthritis the Opticare Arthro model has extended arms, making the process of squeezing the bottle effortless.

Both styles of eye drop dispenser are fitted with an orbit-shaped eye piece designed to ensure that the drop goes into the eye rather than down the cheek. The design of the eye piece also ensures that the bottle cannot touch the eye, preventing contamination. These compliance aids can be prescribed on the NHS.

9.3 Eye ointments

The procedure for using an eye ointment is very similar to that for instilling eye drops (see Section 9.2). Some patients find eye ointments easier to use than drops. One disadvantage of eye ointments is that transient blurred vision is likely to occur, but providing the patient allows for this and refrains from driving or operating machinery until the vision clears the use of eye ointment will not cause too much inconvenience. In addition it is common to use drops during the day and then use eye ointment in the evening or at night upon retiring when the blurring of vision will be less inconvenient.

9.3.1 How to use eye ointment

1. Wash hands with soapy water.
2. Clean your eye if necessary (as with eye drops; see Section 9.2.1)
3. Sit in front of a mirror.
4. Remove the cap from the eye ointment tube.

Applying the ointment (see Figure 9.2):

5. Gently pull down the lower eyelid, forming a pocket between the lid and the eye.
6. Hold the tube above the eye without touching it.

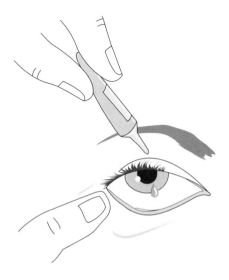

Figure 9.2   The application of eye ointment.

7. Gently squeeze the tube and place about 1 cm of ointment into the pocket, starting from nearest the nose to the outer edge.
8. Twist the wrist to break the strip of ointment from the tube.
9. Close the eye and blink to help spread the eye ointment over the eyeball. Body temperature will help to melt the ointment so that it will spread over the surface of the eye.
10. Vision will be blurred for a few moments. Keep blinking and the vision will clear.
11. Wipe away excess ointment using a clean tissue.
12. Replace the cap of the tube.
13. Remember to discard any remaining ointment four weeks after opening.

9.3.2 Tips when using eye ointments

- To improve the flow of the eye ointment, warm the container in the hands prior to use.
- If using eye drops and eye ointment, use the drops first then the eye ointment 5 minutes later.
- If using two types of eye ointment, apply the first, then wait 10 minutes before applying the second.
- Make sure the tip of the ointment tube does not come in contact with the eye or eye lashes or any other surface.
- Generally, when using eye ointment the use of contact lenses is not recommended.

9.3.3 Special points for consideration with children and babies

When applying eye ointment to a child it is best to either wrap the child tightly in a blanket to minimise wriggling or ask someone else to hold the child. If the child is cooperative, either tilt the child's head back or lie the child flat on its back. Then continue as above. If the child refuses to blink, the ointment can be distributed by gently massaging the lower lid. Anecdotally, some parents have found that they can successfully apply the ointment while a baby is sleeping and find this is the easiest method.

9.4 Inhalers

Inhalers are designed to help medication to be delivered directly into the lungs, where it will act mainly on the lung tissue and systemic effects will be minimised. The doses employed in inhalers are significantly lower than those used in oral medication, so the incidence of side-effects will be reduced. There are a number of different types of inhaler available:

- metered dose inhalers (MDIs) also called aerosol inhalers (see Section 9.4.1)
- metered dose inhalers used with spacer attachment (see Section 9.4.2)
- dry powder inhalers:
  - turbohalers (see Section 9.4.3).
  - accuhalers (see Section 9.4.4).
- breath-actuated inhalers such as Easi-Breathe (see Section 9.4.5).

9.4.1 Metered dose inhalers

Figure 9.3 shows an example of a metered dose inhaler.

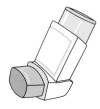

Figure 9.3   An example of a metered dose inhaler.

How to use a metered dose inhaler

1. Remove the cap covering the mouthpiece and check that there is no fluff or dirt in the mouthpiece.
2. Shake the inhaler.
3. If the inhaler is new or has not been used for some time it will need to be tested. To test: Hold the inhaler away from body. Press the top of the aerosol canister once. A fine mist should be puffed into the air. The inhaler is now ready to use.
4. Tilt head back slightly.
5. Breathe out gently.
6. Place the mouthpiece in the mouth between the teeth (do not bite). Close lips around the mouthpiece.
7. Start to breathe in slowly through the mouth, at the same time press down on the inhaler to release the medicine in to the lungs.
8. Hold breath for between 5 and 10 seconds, then breathe out slowly.
9. If a second dose is required, wait approximately 30 seconds and repeat the process.
10. Replace the cap and if the inhaler is a corticosteroid inhaler, rinse the mouth out with water.

Tips for use of a metered dose inhaler

- Practice using the inhaler in front of a mirror to ensure inhalation technique is correct (only when a dose is required!). If mist comes from the top of the inhaler or the sides of the mouth the technique is poor and another dose will be required.
- For patients with arthritis or stiff hands, the inhaler can be held with both hands rather than one hand.
- Use of a spacer device will make the inhaler easier to use successfully (see Section 9.4.2).
- To keep the inhaler clean, remove the canister from the plastic mouthpiece and wash in warm water twice a week. Allow to dry naturally overnight and then reinsert the metal canister the following morning.
- It is important to try to keep track of the amount of medicine left in the inhaler in order to ensure a constant supply. If the dose used is constant (e.g. two puffs twice a day), work out how long your inhaler will last by dividing the number of puffs used into the number of puffs in the inhaler. In the example here four puffs would be used each day, if the inhaler contained 200 doses the inhaler could be expected to last 50 days. Arrange to reorder the item about a week before it will run out. If the inhaler is a reliever and only used infrequently it is advisable to have two inhalers to begin with and when the first inhaler is empty and the second brought into use, a replacement spare inhaler should be

ordered, ensuring availability of the reliever inhaler when it is needed most.

- If more than one type of inhaled medication is taken it is important to take them in the correct order. Bronchodilating inhalers are used first to help open the airways. These are followed by corticosteroid inhalers. This ensures that the airways are open when the corticosteroid is administered, allowing as much of the dose as possible to be absorbed.

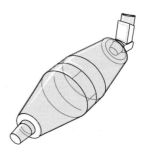

Figure 9.4   A metered dose inhaler attached to a spacer device.

Key point 9.3

When using metered dose inhalers:

- Practice the use of the inhaler in front of a mirror to ensure inhalation technique is correct.
- For patients with arthritis or stiff hands, the inhaler can be held with both hands rather than one hand.
- Use of a spacer device will make the inhaler easier to use successfully.
- To keep inhaler clean, remove the canister from the plastic mouthpiece and wash in warm water twice a week.
- It is important to try to keep track of the amount of medicine left in the inhaler in order to ensure a constant supply.
- If more than one type of inhaled medication is taken it is important to take them in the correct order.

---

placed in the patient's mouth. Alternatively, a mouthpiece can be replaced with a mask which fits over the patient's mouth and nose (see Figure 9.5).

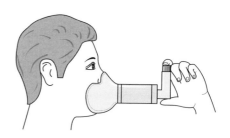

Figure 9.5   A metered dose inhaler attached to a spacer device with a mask.

Special points for consideration with children and babies

Children under the age of 12 years generally cannot use this type of inhaler successfully unless it has a spacer device (see Section 9.4.2).

9.4.2 Metered dose inhalers used with spacer attachment

Figure 9.4 shows a metered dose inhaler attached to a spacer device. The metered dose inhaler is attached to one end of the spacer and the other end contains a mouthpiece which is

How to use a metered dose inhaler with the aid of a spacer device

Different types of spacer device are available for use with metered dose inhalers but all work in basically the same manner. The spacer usually consists of two parts that slot together with a mouthpiece at one end and an opening for an inhaler at the other. There is a one-way valve which ensures that when a dose of the inhaler is expressed into the spacer the drug is stored in what is basically a holding device. This makes it easier to use a metered dose inhaler successfully as the two actions (pressing down on the metered dose inhaler and inhaling the medication) can be separated into two separate events.

1. First assemble the spacer device if necessary as directed by the manufacturer (with or without a face mask).
2. Remove the cap from the inhaler and insert the mouthpiece of the inhaler into the opening at the end of the spacer.
3. Hold the spacer and inhaler together and shake.
4. Breathe out.
5. Put the spacer mouthpiece in the mouth and seal with the lips.
6. Press the inhaler once and then breathe in and out four or five times.
7. Further doses may be taken waiting a few seconds between puffs.
8. Separate the spacer and inhaler. Replace the inhaler cap and store until next dose.

Tips for use of a spacer

- If more than a single dose is required, do one puff at a time.
- Start breathing in as soon as possible after releasing a puff into the spacer.
- Remember to shake the inhaler and spacer between puffs.
- Static charge can build up on spacer devices and this will attract particles of the drug, providing less drug for inhalation. This can be kept to a minimum by washing the spacer occasionally with warm soapy water. The spacer should be left to dry without wiping it.
- Check regularly that the valve opens and closes with each breath.
- Spacers should be replaced every 12 months, especially if they are used daily.

Key point 9.4

When using spacers:

- If more than a single dose is required, do one puff at a time.
- Start breathing in as soon as possible after releasing a puff into the spacer.
- Remember to shake the inhaler and spacer between puffs.

$\rightarrow$

- Static charge can build up on spacer devices and this will attract particles of the drug, providing less drug for inhalation.
- Check regularly that the valve opens and closes with each breath.
- Spacers should be replaced every 12 months, especially if they are used daily.

Special points for consideration with children and babies

A spacer is suitable for use with children and babies. The device gives the child more time to inhale the medication. Instead of fitting a mouthpiece the spacer may be fitted with a mask that will fit snugly around the child's or baby's mouth. Masks are usually used with children under three years old. Children can be encouraged to use the spacer by allowing them to familiarise themselves with it, perhaps decorating it with stickers and playing counting games when inhaling.

The spacer mask can be alarming to young babies and generally a positive smiling parent can cuddle the baby and allay fears. Stroke the baby's cheek with the mask prior to use so that the baby becomes familiar with the device. Often the spacer and mask can be used successfully when the baby is asleep. It is important that if a corticosteroid inhaler is used, the area of the child's face covered by the mask is wiped after use.

9.4.3 Turbohalers

Figure 9.6 shows an example of a Turbohaler.

How to use a Turbohaler

A Turbohaler is a dry powder inhaler. To load it prior to use:

1. Unscrew the cover and remove it.
2. Hold the Turbohaler upright with one hand and with the other twist the grip in one direction as far as it will go.

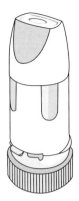

Figure 9.6   An example of a Turbohaler.

3. Now twist back as far as it will go – a click should be heard, showing the inhaler is primed and ready for use.
4. Breathe out gently.
5. Place the mouthpiece between the lips and breathe in through the mouth as deeply and as hard as possible.
6. Remove the inhaler from the mouth and breathe out slowly.
7. Replace the cover.
8. Repeat the above steps if more than one puff is required.

Tips for use of a Turbohaler

- One advantage with this type of inhaler is that there is an indicator on the side showing how many doses are left in the inhaler. When approximately 20 doses are left a red mark appears to prompt the patient to order a new inhaler.
- Never wash the Turbohaler – if water or other fluid gets into the inhaler it may prevent it from working properly. The outside of the mouthpiece should be cleaned using a dry tissue.
- If you accidentally drop or shake the inhaler after it has been primed, the dose will be lost. The inhaler will need to be re-primed for use.
- Some Turbohalers have no taste and patients changed onto these inhalers from metered dose inhalers need reassurance that they have inhaled a dose as they do not get the sensation of the dose hitting the back of the throat.

- Patients with poor manual dexterity can obtain a 'winged' attachment for the Turbohaler to make it easier to twist.

> **Key point 9.5**
>
> When using Turbohalers:
>
> - When approximately 20 doses are left a red mark appears to prompt the patient to order a new inhaler.
> - Never wash the Turbohaler as if water or other fluid gets into the inhaler it may prevent it from working properly.
> - If you accidentally drop or shake the inhaler after it has been primed the dose will be lost.
> - Some Turbohalers have no taste and patients changed onto these inhalers from metered dose inhalers need reassurance that they have inhaled a dose as they do not get the sensation of the dose hitting the back of the throat.
> - Patients with poor manual dexterity can obtain a 'winged' attachment for the Turbohaler to make it easier to twist.

Special points for consideration with children and babies

Turbohalers are suitable for children over the age of six years. There may be problems with some patients as they need good inspiratory flow. A whistle attachment is available for Turbohalers which will demonstrate whether or not the child has sufficient inspiratory flow to successfully use a Turbohaler.

9.4.4 Accuhalers

Figure 9.7 shows an example of an Accuhaler.

How to use an Accuhaler

1. With the Accuhaler mouthpiece facing you, slide the lever away until it clicks. This will have loaded a dose ready for inhalation and

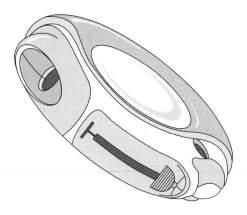

Figure 9.7   An example of an Accuhaler.

the Accuhaler will move the dose counter on.

2. Hold the Accuhaler flat and breathe out away from the inhaler.
3. Seal lips around the Accuhaler mouthpiece and inhale deeply.
4. Remove inhaler from the mouth and hold breath as long as is comfortable.
5. Slide the thumb grip back towards you to close the inhaler.
6. For further doses repeat above steps.

Tips for use of an Accuhaler

• The Accuhaler requires no maintenance or refilling.

Key point 9.6

When using Accuhalers:

• The Accuhaler requires no maintenance or refilling.
• A counter on the Accuhaler counts down from 60 to 0 to show how many doses are left in the inhaler.
• Accuhalers are not suitable for very young or old patients, someone having a severe attack or people unable to generate enough airflow to deposit medicine in the lungs.

• A counter on the Accuhaler counts down from 60 to 0 to show how many doses are left in the inhaler. The last five numbers are in red to show the inhaler is very nearly empty.
• Accuhalers are not suitable for very young or old patients, or if having a severe attack or people unable to generate enough airflow to deposit medicine in the lungs.

Special points for consideration with children and babies

Accuhalers are suitable for children over eight years, and some 5- to 7-year-olds may be able to use them. These products are often licensed for younger children four years and above but in practice they are difficult to use and not generally used in this age group.

9.4.5 Easi-Breathe inhalers

Figure 9.8 shows an example of an Easi-Breathe inhaler.

How to use Easi-Breathe inhalers

1. Shake the inhaler.
2. Hold the inhaler upright and open the cap.

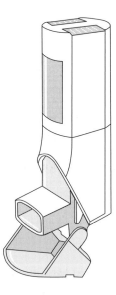

Figure 9.8   An example of an Easi-Breathe inhaler.

3. Breathe out, away from the inhaler.
4. Put the mouthpiece in the mouth, seal lips around the mouthpiece.
5. Breathe in steadily through the mouthpiece.
6. Hold breath for about ten seconds.
7. Keeping the inhaler upright, close the cap.
8. For further doses repeat the above steps.

Tips for using Easi-Breathe inhalers

* Ensure that the air holes in the top of the inhaler are not covered or blocked by the hand holding the inhaler.
* These inhalers are not suitable for use with spacer devices.
* They are suitable for patients who have difficulty with metered dose inhalers as less co-ordination is required.

Key point 9.7

When using Easi-Breathe inhalers:

* Ensure that the air holes in the top of the inhaler are not covered or blocked by the hand holding the inhaler.
* These inhalers are not suitable for use with spacer devices.
* They are suitable for patients who have difficulty with metered dose inhalers as less coordination is required.

Special points for consideration with children and babies

Easi-Breathe inhalers are suitable for children over eight years, and some 5- to 7-year-olds may be able to use them. These products are often licensed for younger children but in practice are difficult to use and not generally used for patients under eight.

9.5 Liquid oral dosage forms

The oral route of administration is the preferred route in the UK, with tablets and capsules being the most common dosage forms (see Section

9.12). However in certain cases liquids are required, particularly where a patient has swallowing difficulties or is a young child.

There are various types of liquid medicines including:

* Solutions: These include elixirs, syrups, linctuses and simple solutions, traditionally termed 'mixtures'.
* Suspensions: In this type of medicine insoluble solids are suspended in the vehicle rather than dissolved in it. Suspensions are also often termed 'mixtures'. Because the solid is likely to separate and aggregate at the bottom of the container, it is important that the medicine is shaken prior to pouring a dose to ensure even distribution of the active ingredients.
* Emulsions: These are essentially mixtures of oil and water which are rendered homogeneous by the addition of an emulsifying agent. There can be some separation or 'creaming' of the two phases (as in milk) hence the reason it is important to shake the bottle before taking a dose.

In order to measure an accurate dose a standard measuring spoon is provided with any liquid medication. The standard spoon size is 5 mL (see Figure 9.9).

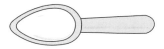

Figure 9.9 A standard 5-mL measuring spoon.

It is important that a standard size spoon is used as a household teaspoon can vary quite considerably from 2 mL to 10 mL with the average teaspoon holding 3.5 mL. If the dose to

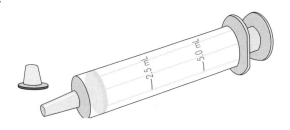

Figure 9.10 An oral syringe.

be administered is less than 5 mL or is to be administered to a small child or baby, an oral syringe is used (see Figure 9.10).

If a large dose is required, medicine measures are also available (see Figure 9.11), and for small doses a 1-mL oral syringe is available, although it should be noted that both of these types of measure are often not manufactured to official standards and should be used with care.

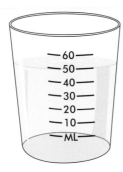

Figure 9.11   A measure for larger volumes of oral liquid.

9.5.1 How to take liquid oral preparations

Taking medicines is a simple procedure. The accurate measuring of the dose is the most important part of the process.

1. Ideally the medicine should be taken while standing or at least sitting upright.
2. Pick up the container with the label against the palm of the hand, to protect the label from staining by any dripping medicine.
3. Shake the bottle (if necessary) and measure the dose onto the spoon.
4. Transfer to the mouth and swallow.
5. If a dose greater than 5 mL is required (e.g. 10 mL, 15 mL), repeat the process the appropriate number of times.
6. Once the dose has been taken, clean the neck of the bottle to help prevent the lid sticking. Then replace the lid.
7. If advised to take the medicine in water, transfer the measured dose to a small glass and add approximately the same amount of water to the measured dose stir and swallow.

9.5.2 Tips when taking oral liquids

It is often a good idea to take the medicine while standing near to a wash hand basin or sink, making it possible to measure the dose and clean away any accidental spillages with ease.

Key point 9.8

When using oral liquids:

*   If possible, take the medicine while standing near to a wash hand basin or sink so that you can measure the dose and clean away any accidental spillages with ease.

9.5.3 Special points for consideration with children

Most medicines for young children are sweetened and flavoured to make them more palatable.

1. Measure the dose to be administered (an oral syringe is preferable).
2. Ensure that the child is standing or sitting up at a 45-degree angle to reduce the risk of choking. Never lay the child flat as the medicine may be inhaled rather than swallowed.
3. Give the medicine along the side of the mouth, on the inside of the cheek where there are no bitter taste buds, and squirt a little at a time.
4. Once the medicine is in the mouth, lift the child's chin slightly to encourage swallowing.

Unpleasant tasting medicines may be mixed with more palatable food stuffs such as apple puree, fruit juice, jam or chocolate syrup. This obviously depends on the medicine concerned and the age of the child. If mixing with a drink it is important that all the drink is taken to ensure the full dose is administered. Another way of making the medicine more palatable is by keeping it refrigerated: the chilled medicine is often more acceptable.

9.5.4 Compliance aids

An oral syringe is a compliance aid as it allows for accurate measurement of small doses of liquid medication. The syringe itself is graduated and accompanied by a bung, with a hole in the centre, which fits into the neck of the medicine bottle.

How to use an oral syringe:

1. Shake the bottle of medicine (if required).
2. Remove the lid and insert the bung.
3. Insert the tip of the syringe into the hole in the bung.
4. Invert the bottle.
5. Pull the plunger of the syringe back to the graduation for the dose required.
6. Turn the bottle back upright.
7. Remove the syringe from the bung, holding the barrel of the syringe rather than the plunger.
8. Gently empty the contents of the syringe into the child's mouth, inside the cheek (see Section 9.5.3 above).
9. Remove the syringe from the child's mouth.
10. Remove the bung from the bottle, clean the neck of the bottle if necessary and replace the lid.
11. Wash the bung and syringe in warm water and leave to dry. If you are giving medicine to a baby it is advised that the syringe be passed through bottle sterilising fluid as well.

9.6 Nasal drops

Nasal drops are solutions or suspensions used to produce a local effect on the nose.

9.6.1 How to use nasal drops

1. Gently blow the nose to clear the nostrils.
2. Wash hands.
3. Shake the bottle of drops. Some are suspensions and will need shaking; if applicable, this direction will be on the label.

4. Remove the lid from the bottle. If the lid includes an integral dropper draw some liquid into the dropper.
5. Position the head as shown in Figure 9.12. The easiest way to do this is to lie on a bed with your head hanging over the edge. Bending forward or kneeling is an alternative but maintaining the position for 2 minutes after using the drops is more difficult. Tilting the head back is not a suitable position as the drops will not cover the upper surface of the nostril.
6. Drop the required number of drops into each nostril. The intention is to spread the drop(s) evenly over the surface of the nostril. Do not allow the dropper to touch the nose.
7. Stay in this position for 2 minutes to prevent the drops running out of the nose and down the back of the throat.
8. Replace the lid.

9.6.2 Tips when using nasal drops

- Some patients find it easier to ask someone else to instil the nasal drops.
- The drops will drain to some extent down the back of the throat. Some drops may have an unpleasant taste, but a drink of water will clear this.
- Try not to blow the nose for 20 minutes after the application to allow maximum contact of the drops with the nasal lining.

Key point 9.9

When using nasal drops:

- Some patients find it easier to ask someone else to instil the nasal drops.
- The drops will drain to some extent down the back of the throat. Some drops may have an unpleasant taste; however, a drink of water will clear this.
- Try not to blow the nose for 20 minutes after the application to allow maximum contact of the drops with the nasal lining.

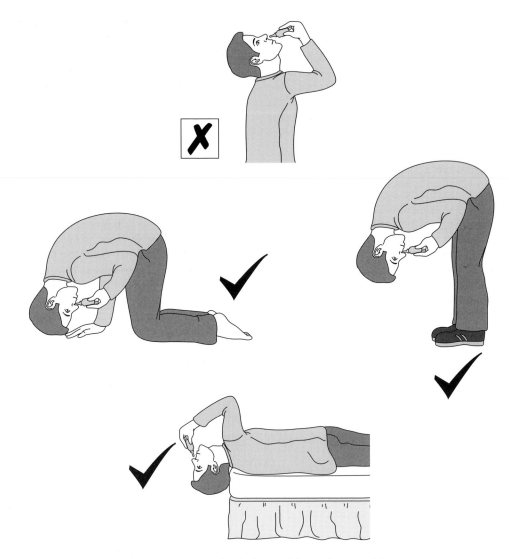

Figure 9.12   The correct (and incorrect) position for the body whilst instilling nasal drops.

9.6.3 Special points to take into consideration with children and babies

If instilling drops into a child's nose, laying the child across an adult's lap with the head hanging down may be the most comfortable position for the child. For small babies or young children, wrapping tightly in a blanket will make them feel secure and reduce wriggling, making instillation of drops easier. Most young children will blow their nose when encouraged, however babies may not be so cooperative. To remove mucus from a baby's nose, tickle the baby's nose with cotton wool. This will make the baby sneeze which in turn should help clear the nose. Children sometimes find the instillation of the drops less distressing if the drops have been warmed slightly by standing the container in warm (not hot) water for a few minutes.

9.7 Nasal sprays

Nasal sprays may be used to treat the nasal lining directly. Examples include:

- decongestant sprays to help clear the nose
- steroid nasal sprays used to reduce the inflammation associated with allergies such as hay fever and rhinitis.

Nasal sprays may also be used to achieve a systemic effect. Intra-nasal drug delivery provides a speedier onset of drug action when compared with oral administration, often with a reduced dosage. Examples include:

- Nicotine nasal sprays: These are the most rapidly acting of all nicotine replacement therapies, offering fast relief for cravings and also easy dose adjustments which can be made by the patient.
- Intranasal sprays designed for rapid relief from the symptoms of migraine.

Currently research is being carried out into the suitability of the nasal route for the administration for drugs for insulin-dependent diabetes and hormone replacement therapy.

9.7.1 How to use nasal sprays

1. Gently blow nose to clear nostrils.
2. Wash hands with soapy water before using the spray.
3. Gently shake the spray. Some are suspensions and will need shaking; if applicable, this direction will be on the label.
4. Remove the cap from the spray.
5. Tilt head slightly forward (look down at feet).
6. Close one nostril; gently press against the side of the nose with one finger.
7. Insert tip of nasal spray into open nostril and slowly breathe in through the open nostril, and while breathing in squeeze the spray to deliver one dose. It is important to keep the spray upright (do not sniff hard as the spray will travel straight to the back of the throat, failing to deposit any medication in the nostril).

8. Remove spray from the nose and breathe out through the mouth. Tilt head backwards for about a minute to prevent the liquid spray running out of the nose.
9. Repeat in other nostril as directed.
10. Replace cap on spray.
11. Try not to blow nose for several minutes after using the spray.

9.7.2 Tips when using nasal sprays

- It may help to 'prime' the nasal spray prior to first using it. This is achieved by spraying the spray into the air (away from the eyes) a few times until a fine mist is produced.
- If two puffs of a nasal spray are to be applied to each nostril, try to aim in a slightly

---

Key point 9.10

When using nasal sprays:

- It may help to 'prime' the nasal spray prior to first using it.
- If two puffs of a nasal spray are to be applied to each nostril, try to aim in a slightly different direction with each spray to cover as much of the lining of the nose as is possible.
- Nasal sprays may cause an unpleasant taste when draining into the throat. A drink of water will help remove the taste.
- If using a decongestant nasal spray, use for one week only, as longer use can result in 'rebound effect'. This increases inflammation of the nose, causing more congestion.
- If using a steroid spray, use regularly. It may take a few days for the effects of the spray to become apparent.
- If a steroid spray is to be used for inflammation and the nasal passages are blocked, the use of a decongestant nasal spray prior to the first uses of the steroid spray can clear the nostrils, ensuring that the steroid spray is delivered to the nasal lining.

different direction with each spray to cover as much of the lining of the nose as possible.

- Nasal sprays may cause an unpleasant taste when draining into the throat. A drink of water will help remove the taste.
- If using a decongestant nasal spray, use for one week only, as longer use can result in 'rebound effect'. This increases inflammation of the nose, causing more congestion.
- If using a steroid spray, use regularly. It may take a few days for the effects of the spray to become apparent. Patients must also be reminded that it may be necessary to use their spray even when the symptoms have cleared, to prevent recurrence.
- If a steroid spray is to be used for inflammation and the nasal passages are blocked, the use of a decongestant nasal spray prior to the first uses of the steroid spray can clear the nostrils, ensuring that the steroid spray is delivered to the nasal lining.

9.7.3 Special points for consideration with children

Nasal sprays are generally not used in children under six years of age because of the problems of coordination encountered and the relative ease with which nasal drops may be used (see Section 9.6).

9.8 Oral powders

Powders for oral use can either be bulk powders or unit dose powders. Bulk powders are usually restricted to less potent medicines intended for symptomatic relief of minor ailments, for example, indigestion. The dose taken is usually measured with a 5-mL spoon, stirred into a quantity of water and then swallowed. This method of measurement can create considerable problems with regard to expected standards of precision dosage. These powders are formulated on the basis of dose weights, whereas the dose is actually measured by volume. A heaped 5-mL spoonful is considered to be equivalent to 5 g of powder. The dose can vary quite considerably, depending on

the patient's interpretation of 'heaped' and the density of the powders involved.

The advantages of bulk powders are that the dry powders may be more stable than their liquid-based equivalent, and absorption from the gastro-intestinal tract will be quicker than with tablets or capsules.

Individual powders differ from bulk powders only in that the dose is pre-measured and individually wrapped, ensuring accurate repeatable dosing. These individual dose powders have the added advantage that they are light in weight. A problem that can be encountered with powders is the taste, as it is very difficult to mask unpleasant or bitter tastes.

9.8.1 How to take unit dose oral powders

1. Ideally powders should be taken while standing or sitting upright
2. Open the powder carefully on a flat surface then either:
   (a) empty the contents of the sachet directly onto the back of the tongue and swallow with a glass of water or
   (b) empty the contents of the sachet into about a third of a tumbler of water. Stir to disperse and swallow resulting solution/suspension.
3. Do not lie down flat for at least 2 minutes after taking the powder.

9.8.2 Special points for consideration with children

Single dose powders can make changing the drug doses to adjust to the ever changing bodies of children easier. They are also very useful as a specially prepared product for an individual child where only adult formulations are freely available.

Some powders can be mixed with feeds, making this an easy way to administer medicines to babies. However it should be remembered that the taste imparted by the powder may render the feed unacceptable to the baby. In addition, unless the whole of a bottle feed is taken, the entire dose will not be administered to the child.

9.9 Patches

Skin (transdermal) patches have become increasingly popular as a means of administering medication. This is because they can be applied and then left until it is time to remove them. In general they are a sustained-release preparation with the time for delivery varying from 12 hours to one week, meaning that regular dosing during a day is avoided. They are also a very discreet way of administering medication.

Skin patches are adhesive patches which contain a reservoir of the drug to be administered. The drug slowly passes from the patch through the skin and into the bloodstream. They are commonly used in hormone replacement therapy, nicotine replacement therapy, pain relief, relief of symptoms of angina, motion sickness, birth control and in the treatment of attention deficit hyperactivity disorder (ADHD).

9.9.1 How to use patches

1. Freshly wash and dry the area of skin where the patch is to be applied. Do not use talc, oil, moisturisers or creams as this may prevent the patch sticking.
2. Tear open the patch package where indicated (use the fingers rather than scissors to prevent accidental damage to the patch).
3. Remove the protective backing from the patch. Try not to touch the adhesive with fingers.
4. Press the adhesive side of the patch to the prepared skin site firmly. Ensure that there is good skin contact, particularly at the edges of the patch.
5. Wash hands thoroughly with soap and water to remove any possible contamination with medicament.

9.9.2 Special considerations when using patches

*   Hormone replacement patches should be applied below the waist on the buttocks or thighs; NOT on the breasts.
*   Contraceptive patches should be applied to the buttocks, abdomen, upper outer arm or upper torso; NOT on the breasts.

*   Andropatch skin patches containing testosterone should be applied on the back, abdomen, upper arms or thighs. Avoid bony areas such as shoulders and hips that may be subjected to prolonged pressure during sleeping or sitting, as this may cause burn-like reactions of the skin. Do not apply the patches to the scrotum.
*   Glyceryl trinitrate patches for angina should be applied to the chest or upper arm.
*   Nicotine replacement patches should be applied to the chest, upper arm or hip.
*   The site of application for fentanyl patches (an analgesic) depends on the brand of product used. Read the individual patient information leaflet for more details.

9.9.3 Tips when using patches

*   Choose an area of skin that is not hairy, scarred, calloused or broken.
*   Try to choose an area where the patch is unlikely to be rubbed off by tight clothing (for example, avoid the waist).
*   Remove the old patch each time you apply a new one.
*   Try not to reuse the same area to apply patches as this will make irritation more likely.
*   Skin patches should be covered and protected from sunlight. The application of heat may increase the amount of medication absorbed.
*   Make sure the edges of the patch are well sealed with no air pockets. This will ensure that you can bathe, shower or swim without removing the patch. (Not all patches allow this; the patient information leaflet will give guidance as to whether or not the patch will remain in place after bathing, etc.)
*   Problems with the patch 'sticking' may be due to the fact that the skin is too hot when the patch is applied. After washing the skin, dry carefully and allow the skin to cool before applying. This may improve the adhesive properties.
*   If the skin feels sticky once the old patch has been removed this can be cleaned away using baby oil.

Key point 9.11

When using patches:

- Choose a skin area that is not hairy, broken skin, scarred or calloused.
- Try to choose an area where the patch is unlikely to be rubbed off by tight clothing (for example, avoid the waist).
- Remove the old patch each time you apply a new one.
- Try not to reuse the same area to apply patches as this will make irritation more likely.
- Skin patches should be covered and protected from sunlight. The application of heat may increase the amount of medication absorbed.
- Make sure the edges of the patch are well sealed with no air pockets. This will ensure that (for some patches) you can bathe, shower or swim without removing the patch.
- Problems with the patch 'sticking' may be due to the fact that the skin is too hot when the patch is applied. After washing the skin, dry carefully and allow the skin to cool before applying. This may improve the adhesive properties.
- If the skin feels sticky once the old patch has been removed this can be cleaned away using baby oil.

9.9.4 Special points for consideration with children

Skin patches are sometimes used for children for travel sickness or ADHD and occasionally for severe pain. Patches must always be applied by an adult. The disposal of patches is particularly important as there will be some active ingredient in the patch reservoir once it has been removed.

To dispose of a patch, close the patch in on itself, adhesive to adhesive, and wrap in a bag prior to disposal. With the increase in popularity of patches there has also been an increase in the incidence of accidental poisoning. Young children are more susceptible as they tend to have a fascination for stickers and plasters. Patches have been known to occasionally peel off without the wearer's knowledge and can be found stuck to bedding or clothing.

9.10 Pessaries and vaginal creams

Vaginal pessaries and creams are medications directly inserted into the vagina, either with or without the aid of an applicator. Vaginal pessaries and creams are used for a number of purposes:

- oestrogen replacement: to directly supplement the vaginal tissue with oestrogen in post-menopausal women, relieving the vaginal symptoms of the menopause
- contraceptives for pre-menopausal women
- treatment of local infections, the advantage being minimal systemic absorption.

Vaginal pessaries are also used to support a womb prolapse – these pessaries are usually made of PVC or polythene and are inserted and removed by healthcare professionals, not by patients. They are usually checked every three to six months.

9.10.1 How to use pessaries or vaginal cream

1. Wash hands with soapy water before using the pessaries/cream.
2. Remove any external foil or plastic packaging from the pessary and applicator.
3. If an applicator is provided, load the applicator as directed by the manufacturer.
4. Stand with one leg on a chair or lie down with knees bent and legs apart.
5. Press the applicator plunger to insert the pessary or cream into the vagina (see Figure 9.13). If no applicator is provided, insert the pessary as high into the vagina as is comfortable by pushing gently but firmly in an upwards and backwards direction using the middle finger.

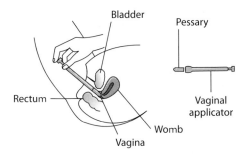

Figure 9.13 How to insert a vaginal pessary.

6. If an applicator is used, wash it ready for next use.
7. Wash hands once more.

9.10.2 Tips when using pessaries/vaginal cream

- If pregnant, do NOT use an applicator to insert pessaries; insert using finger method.
- If using a barrier method of contraception (e.g. latex diaphragm, cap or condoms), it may be damaged and become ineffective with

---

Key point 9.12

When using pessaries or vaginal cream:

- If pregnant, do NOT use an applicator to insert pessaries; insert using finger method.
- If using a barrier method of contraception, it may be damaged and become ineffective with the use of pessaries or cream.
- Pessaries will melt once inserted and therefore with both pessaries and creams there may be a discharge from the vagina.
- Continued use of pessaries or cream for the full length of treatment is necessary, even if the symptoms have disappeared.
- If the treatment coincides with menstruation, the treatment should be continued, but sanitary towels should be worn rather than using tampons.

---

the use of pessaries or cream. Therefore extra precautions should be taken during use and for five days after use (obviously this does not apply to creams or pessaries designed for contraceptive use).

- Pessaries will melt once inserted and therefore with both pessaries and creams there may be a discharge from the vagina. This can be minimised if the application is at night rather than during the day. If used during the day, sanitary towels or panty liners will help to prevent any staining of clothing.
- Continued use of pessaries or cream for the full length of treatment is necessary, even if the symptoms have disappeared.
- If the treatment coincides with menstruation, the treatment should be continued, but sanitary towels should be worn rather than using tampons.

9.11 Suppositories

Suppositories are bullet shaped and intended for insertion into the rectum (back passage). Some have a local action in the rectum and are used to aid the emptying of the bowel; others have a systemic effect and are used as an alternative to oral dosage forms. The rectum has a plentiful blood supply and drugs can easily be absorbed from the rectum for systemic use.

9.11.1 How to use suppositories

1. If possible go to the toilet and empty the bowels.
2. Wash hands.
3. Remove foil or plastic packaging.
4. Warm the suppository in hands to aid insertion.
5. Lie on one side with knees pulled up towards the chest or alternatively squat.
6. Gently but firmly insert the suppository into the rectum with a finger. Insert tapered end first. Push the suppository in as far as possible to prevent it slipping back out. Lower legs and remain still for a few minutes. Clenching buttocks together if neces-

sary to retain the suppository. Unless the suppository is a laxative, avoid emptying the bowels for at least one hour.

7. Wash hands again.

9.11.2 Tips when using suppositories

- Suppositories will melt after insertion and this may cause leakage from the rectum and staining of clothes. This can be minimised by using the suppositories at night.
- If difficulty with insertion is encountered the use of a lubricant gel may help.

Key point 9.13

When using suppositories:

- Suppositories will melt after insertion and this may cause leakage from the rectum and staining of clothes. This can be minimised by using the suppositories at night.
- If difficulty with insertion is encountered the use of a lubricant gel may help.

9.11.3 Special points for consideration with children and babies

Insertion of a suppository can be very distressing to a child and a clear explanation of what is to happen is essential. In addition to encouraging a child to empty the bowel prior to insertion it is helpful if they also empty the bladder as a full bladder may cause extra discomfort.

The easiest position for insertion is to lie the child down on his or her side with knees pulled up. Lubricate the suppository and insert 2–4 cm into the rectum. For a baby, use the little finger to insert; for a child or young person, use the index finger. Then gently hold the child's buttocks together for 5 minutes if possible to prevent expulsion of the suppository. If the suppository is for laxative use ensure that the child has easy access to a toilet or potty. Parents

should be warned that the child may need to go to the toilet several times before the bowel is emptied.

9.12 Tablets and capsules

The oral route of administration is the preferred route for most medications, and tablets and capsules are the most commonly encountered dosage forms in the UK.

In general, the advantage of tablets and capsules over their equivalent liquid preparations is that they are convenient to carry and administer, and as they are unit dose forms the administration of an accurate dose is assured.

9.12.1 Types of tablet

Tablets come in various forms.

Film coated or sugar coated

These coatings are added by manufacturers to mask unpleasant tastes (for example, amiodarone and metronidazole, both of which have a bitter taste) and to make the tablets easier to swallow.

Enteric coated

Enteric-coated tablets are intended to pass through the stomach unbroken and only begin to dissolve when they reach the intestine. The coating may protect the stomach from local damage by the drug (for example, aspirin) or it may protect the drug and ensure that it is released at its intended site of action for a more local effect (for example, bisacodyl). These tablets must be swallowed whole and not crushed or chewed as this would damage the coating and render it ineffective.

Slow-release tablets or 'SR' tablets

These tablets are designed to release their active ingredient slowly over a period of time, usually 12–24 hours. They must be swallowed whole. If chewed or broken in the mouth there is a risk the patient would receive a toxic dose and instead of being absorbed over 12–24 hours, the full day's dose would be absorbed in 1–2 hours. There would also be times during the day when the patient was receiving no medication. These tablets are also known as:

- extended release or 'XL'
- long acting or 'LA'
- modified release or 'MR'
- retard
- slow or slo.

Effervescent, soluble or dispersible tablets

These tablets will dissolve or disperse in water, making them easier to swallow in a quickly prepared liquid form. The onset of action of these tablets may be quicker than their equivalent solid ordinary tablet as the active ingredient may be more readily absorbed from the resultant liquid.

Chewable tablets

These are useful for patients that do not like to swallow tablets whole. They can be chewed and broken down in the mouth before swallowing. Commonly they are sweetened and flavoured to improve their palatability. Common examples include antacid preparations, where the relatively large tablets are still more convenient than the equivalent liquid preparation.

Sublingual or buccal tablets

These are used when it is necessary for the drug to avoid the gastro-intestinal tract and therefore avoid first pass metabolism. They should not be swallowed. Sublingual tablets are designed to dissolve under the tongue and buccal tablets are designed to dissolve in the space between the gum and the cheeks or lip.

9.12.2 Types of capsule

Capsules are also available in two distinct forms: hard gelatin and soft gelatin.

Hard gelatin

These consist of two pieces that clip together. The capsule is filled with the active drug in powder form and any necessary bulking excipient. Controlled-release preparations can be made by giving the capsule itself an enteric coating or making pellets or beads of the active ingredient which are then coated and packaged within the gelatine shell.

Soft gelatin

These are flexible, usually one piece and often contain liquids, for example, fish liver oil capsules. The soft gelatin capsules can be coated to produce modified-release preparations, or enteric resistant coatings can be added to allow for absorption from the intestine.

9.12.3 How to take tablets and capsules

Taking tablets and capsules is generally a simple operation. Special consideration will be given to soluble, sublingual and buccal preparations.

1. Ideally the tablets or capsules should be taken while standing or at least sitting upright.
2. Place the tablet or capsule in the mouth.
3. Swallow with the aid of a glass of water. (Plenty of water ensures that the tablet or capsule reaches the stomach and does not feel that it is 'stuck' in the throat.)
4. Do not lie down flat for at least 2 minutes.

9.12.4 How to take soluble tablets

1. Place the tablet or tablets into a small glassful of water.
2. Stir to dissolve the tablets.
3. Drink the resultant solution.

9.12.5 How to take sublingual tablets

1. Sit down.
2. Take a sip of water to moisten the mouth if it is dry.

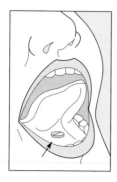

Figure 9.14   Where to place a sublingual tablet.

3. Swallow or spit out the water.
4. Place the tablet under the tongue (see Figure 9.14).
5. Close the mouth and do not swallow until the tablet has dissolved completely. Do not hasten the process by moving the tablet around the mouth with the tongue. Do not chew or swallow the tablet and do not eat drink or smoke while the tablet is dissolving.
6. Do not rinse out the mouth for several minutes after the tablet has dissolved.

9.12.6 How to take buccal tablets

1. Sit down.
2. Take a sip of water to moisten the mouth if it is dry.

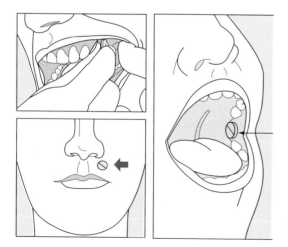

Figure 9.15   Where to place a buccal tablet.

3. Swallow or spit out the water.
4. Place the tablet between the cheek and the upper or lower gum (or alternatively between the upper gum and the lip) (see Figure 9.15).
5. Close the mouth and do not swallow until the tablet has dissolved completely. Do not hasten the process by moving the tablet around the mouth with the tongue. Do not chew or swallow the tablet and do not eat drink or smoke while the tablet is dissolving.
6. Do not rinse out the mouth for several minutes after the tablet has dissolved.

9.12.7 Tips when taking tablets or capsules

*   Some patients find it difficult to swallow tablets and capsules. It may help to put the tablet or capsule in a spoonful of yoghurt or something similar such as porridge or mousse, etc. This is not an option if the medication needs to be taken on an empty stomach or before food.
*   Sugar-coated tablets are generally considered easier to swallow than their film-coated or non-coated equivalents.
*   If patients are having difficulty swallowing tablets or capsules, ensure that they are trying to swallow them one at a time (this may be a problem with patients taking multiple medications at the same time each day).
*   If patients have a number of tablets or capsules to take in a day it may help them to remember to take their medication if the times are linked to daily events such as meal times or brushing teeth, etc.

Key point 9.14

When using tablets or capsules:

*   Some patients find it difficult to swallow tablets and capsules. It may help to put the tablet or capsule in a spoonful of yoghurt or something similar such as

→

porridge or mousse, etc. This is not an option if the medication needs to be taken on an empty stomach or before food.

- Sugar-coated tablets are generally considered easier to swallow than their film-coated or non-coated equivalent.
- If patients are having difficulty swallowing tablets or capsules ensure that they are trying to swallow them one at a time (this may be a problem with patients taking multiple medications at the same time each day).
- If patients have a number of tablets or capsules to take in a day it may help them to remember to take their medication if the times are linked to daily events such as meal times or brushing teeth, etc.

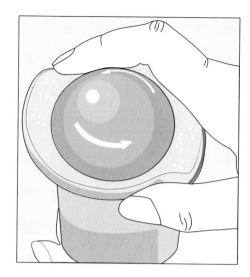

Figure 9.16   Tablet bottle opener.

9.12.8 Special points for consideration with children

In general, preparations intended for babies and young children are in liquid form but occasionally capsules or tablets are given. If tablets or capsules are required to be swallowed whole it is advised that the tablet or capsule is placed on the back of the tongue and the child is allowed to take a drink from an adult's cup or glass so that the tablet or capsule is swallowed along with the drink. Sometimes solid tablets and capsules will be tolerated if mixed into food.

The crushing of tablets and emptying of capsule contents is not recommended unless the patient information leaflet that accompanies the product states that this is a safe practice. For example Slo-Phyllin capsules may be opened and the contents sprinkled onto soft food prior to administration.

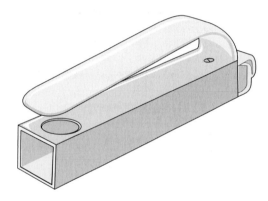

Figure 9.17   Tablet de-blister device.

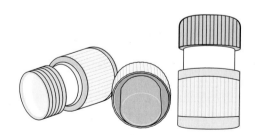

Figure 9.18   Tablet crusher.

9.12.9 Compliance aids

There are many reasons why patients have difficulty when taking tablets. The packaging may be difficult to open, for example child-resistant packaging of tablets is particularly difficult for

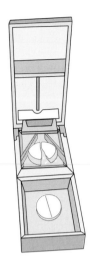

Figure 9.19 Tablet splitter.

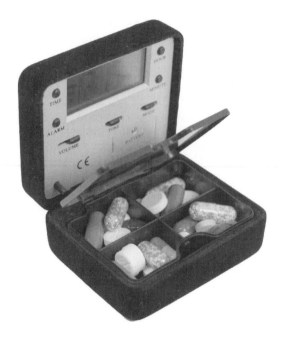

Figure 9.21 Tabtime, an alarmed reminder device.

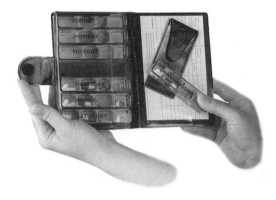

Figure 9.20 Medidos tablet dispenser with seven days of the week and each day split into four compartments, breakfast, lunch, dinner and bedtime. © www.dudley.hunt. co.uk

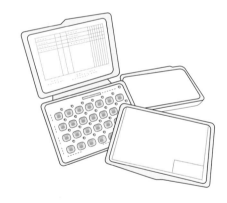

Figure 9.22 Medicines manager system pre-prepared by the pharmacist (including a reminder chart prepared by a pharmacist to help a patient remember when to take their medication).

elderly or disabled patients. Multiple, complex dose regimens and the need to remember when to take the differing medicines, or the size of the dosage form may also cause problems. A number of compliance aids and reminder systems can be purchased (see Figures 9.16–9.22).

9.13 Topical applications

Topical medications are designed for application to the skin (for example, creams, ointments, lotions, etc.) and fall into three main categories (although other uses do exist):

- emollients to treat dry skin
- antibiotic or antiseptic preparations
- steroid preparations designed to reduce inflammation and itch.

Some preparations fit into more than one of these categories. For example, the base of many creams acts as an emollient while the active medication is a steroid or antibiotic. There are also preparations that combine antibiotics and steroids in one formulation.

9.13.1 How to use an emollient cream or ointment

1. Wash area (preferably with an emollient wash) and pat dry gently with a towel (do not rub).
2. Five to ten minutes after washing apply the emollient liberally (the skin will have cooled and the water content of the skin will be highest).
3. Repeat as necessary during the day.

9.13.2 Tips when using emollient creams or ointments

- Avoid putting hands or fingers into large tubs of emollient as this can contaminate the cream or ointment. Take out the required amount with a spatula and replace the lid to prevent contamination.
- Emollients are safe and cannot be overused.
- The emollient may be easier to apply if it has been warmed slightly before application (for example, in an airing cupboard).
- Alternatively the emollient may be placed in a fridge to cool it if there is a problem with itching.
- The emollient may need to be applied more frequently in extreme weather conditions, at least three or four times a day.
- Apply emollients in the direction of hair growth to prevent folliculitis (infected hair follicles).
- Patients often find it more acceptable to use an ointment at night but a cream during the day.
- Continue using the emollient even when the skin feels better.
- An adult can be expected to use up to 500 g of emollient a week (depending on the severity of the dry skin condition); similarly a child will use 500 g every two weeks.

- Emollients can easily be rubbed off hands and feet, particularly in bed when they may damage bedclothes. This can be reduced by wearing cotton gloves after application and by wrapping the feet in cling film and wearing socks.

Key point 9.15

When using emollient creams or ointments:

- Avoid putting hands or fingers into large tubs of emollient as this can contaminate the cream or ointment.
- Emollients are safe and cannot be overused.
- The emollient may be easier to apply if it has been warmed slightly before application (for example, in an airing cupboard).
- Alternatively the emollient may be placed in a fridge to cool it if there is a problem with itching.
- The emollient may need to be applied more frequently in extreme weather conditions; at least three or four times a day.
- Apply emollients in the direction of hair growth to prevent folliculitis (infected hair follicles).
- Patients often find it more acceptable to use an ointment at night but a cream during the day.
- Continue using the emollient even when the skin feels better.
- An adult can be expected to use up to 500 g of emollient a week (depending on the severity of the dry skin condition); similarly a child will use 500 g every two weeks.
- Emollients can easily be rubbed off hands and feet particularly in bed when they may damage bedclothes.

9.13.3 Special points for consideration with children and babies

The problem of dry skin in children and babies is becoming more and more common, possibly due to the extremes of temperature encoutered between our warm, centrally heated homes in winter and cold winds outside, both of which have a drying effect on the skin. The drying effect of central heating can be reduced by using a humidifier or by placing a bowl of water near a radiator.

Children and babies need regular moisturising. The application of moisturising emollient should be applied before any noticeable dry areas of skin can be seen (for example, on the face, where dribbling can cause sore spots). The emollient should be applied in a thin layer and gently stroked into the skin. Vigorous rubbing can damage the skin further and the heat produced can exacerbate itching. In hot weather a lighter emollient may be better as a thick, greasy emollient can make the child hot and itchy. If a thick emollient ointment is used as a soap substitute when bathing the parent must take care as the baby or child can become very slippery.

9.13.4 How to use a steroid cream or ointment

1. Wash hands.
2. Wash area (preferably with an emollient wash) and pat dry gently with a towel (do not rub).
3. Apply the cream or ointment sparingly (thinly) to the affected area.
4. Gently massage the cream or ointment into the skin.
5. After application wash hands again, unless the hands are the area being treated.

9.13.5 Tips when using steroid creams or ointments

- Only apply the cream or ointment to the affected area of skin. Do not use it on normal skin.
- Ointments, although less pleasant to use, are preferable as they remain on the skin longer.
- If other creams or ointments are to be applied to the same area of skin, leave 30 minutes between applications.
- The amount of cream to use is usually described as a number of 'fingertip units'. A

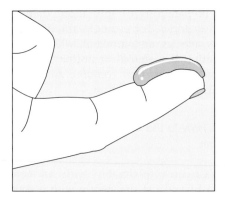

Figure 9.23 A fingertip unit.

fingertip unit is the amount of cream that can be placed from the tip to the first crease of an adult index finger (see Figure 9.23).

The amount of cream to be used for different parts of the body is as follows:

- both sides of one hand – one fingertip unit
- one foot – two fingertip units
- one arm – three fingertip units
- one leg – six fingertip units
- chest and abdomen – seven fingertip units
- back and buttocks – seven fingertip units.

Key point 9.16

When using steroid cream or ointment:

- Only apply the cream or ointment to the affected area of skin. Do not use it on normal skin.
- Ointments, although less pleasant to use, are preferable as they remain on the skin longer.
- If other creams or ointments are to be applied to the same area of skin, leave 30 minutes between applications.

If using a topical corticosteroid cream and an emollient it is important to separate applications by about 20–30 minutes. There is no consensus as to the order these cream should be applied. Steroids may be more effective if

Table 9.1 The number of fingertip units to be applied to different parts of the body for children of different ages

Age	Number of fingertip units				
	Face and neck	Arm and hand	Leg and foot	Trunk (front)	Trunk (back) and buttocks
3–6 months	1	1	1½	1	1½
1–2 years	1½	1½	2	2	3
3–5 years	1½	2	3	3	3½
6–10 years	2	2½	4½	3½	5

applied before the emollient, but it is also argued that if the emollient is applied first, this moisturises the skin thoroughly and prevents the spread of the steroid to other areas of the skin. The advice at present is that it is patient preference that matters and a routine that encourages compliance and is suitable to the patient's lifestyle should be adopted.

9.13.6 Special points for consideration with children and babies

Quantities of steroid cream or ointment to use for a child will still be expressed as adult fingertip units (see Table 9.1). In general, the lowest strength of topical corticosteroid should be prescribed to young children as systemic side-effects such as growth retardation are more commonly seen in children. For this reason it is common for children to have 'steroid holidays' when only emollients are used to control the skin condition and for steroid creams to be reserved for short term use (5–7 days) when flare-ups of the condition occur.

9.14 Chapter summary

Following on from the basics of patient counselling covered in Chapter 8, this chapter has covered the key points relating to the counselling of a variety of different dosage forms. How to use each different dosage form has been described, along with tips to aid use. In all cases, specific points relating to the use of the different dosage forms in babies and children have been described.

It is important that pharmacists and pharmacy technicians are familiar with the points discussed in this chapter to ensure that you can counsel patients and carers effectively in the use of different dosage forms.

10

Poisons and spirits

Upon completion of this chapter, you should be able to:

* understand the legislation relating to the sale or supply of non-medicinal poisons that affect pharmacy, including the Poisons Act 1972 and the Poisons Rules
* understand the legislation relating to the sale or supply of spirits from a pharmacy.

This final chapter provides an overview of the legislation affecting the sale or supply of non-medicinal poisons (see Section 10.1) and spirits (see Section 10.2) from a pharmacy.

10.1 Poisons

The sale of non-medicinal poisons in England, Scotland and Wales is controlled by the Poisons Act 1972, the Poisons Rules 1982 and the Poisons List Order 1982 and amending Orders made to these by statutory instruments. In Northern Ireland, non-medicinal poisons are covered by the Poisons (NI) Order 1976 and the Poisons (NI) Regulations 1983.

The sale of poisons has been controlled since the first Arsenic Act of 1851. This came about as a result of the concerns of the Pharmaceutical Society and doctors at the ease of availability of certain poisons such as arsenic, ergot, nux vom-

ica, opium and oxalic acid and the likelihood of these agents to be used in cases of poisoning. The initial act was only applicable to arsenic and required a register of supply to be kept and the purchaser to sign for their purchase either at the chemist's shop or the hardware shop. The use of arsenic was common and accepted in the nineteenth century, both as a rat poison and cosmetic agent, with some Victorian ladies claiming that arsenic improved their complexion. It was also quite commonly used as a medicinal product and therefore it was also stated that 'non-medicinal' arsenic should be dyed with half an ounce of soot or indigo to ensure that it was easily distinguishable from other white powders and could no longer be 'confused' with flour or sugar, which was a frequent defence of Victorian poisoners.

The problem with the Arsenic Act 1851 was that it only applied to arsenic, and many other toxic substances were easily available without restriction. It also lacked detailed enforcement. Nevertheless, although the Act had its shortcomings, it was significant in that it highlighted the need for proper legislation to cover the sale of poisons.

The Arsenic Act 1851 was superseded by the Pharmacy Act 1868, which limited the sale of 15 defined poisons, including arsenic, cyanide and opium, to registered pharmacists who were obliged as with the Arsenic Act to keep records of the date, the quantity and the purchaser. The legislation was not aimed at the prevention of drug taking 'for pleasure', more at the 'abuse' of the substances, for example the use of opium in the form of laudanum by childminders to keep children passive and the increased number of cases of accidental and intentional poisonings by drugs.

Pharmacists' rights as sellers of poisons were confirmed and extended by the Pharmacy and Poisons Act 1908, which gave a more comprehensive list of poisons; it also gave the police responsibility for enforcing some of the regulations.

The advent of the Pharmacy and Poisons Act 1933 led to further control of supply of poisons. This Act led to the formation of a Poisons Board, responsible for rule making, local authority lists, inspection and enforcement. This legislation was in force until 1968, when the Medicines Act replaced the medicines component of the Pharmacy and Poisons Act, and 1972, when a new Poisons Act replaced the poisons function of the Pharmacy and Poisons Act 1933.

10.1.1 The Poisons Act 1972

A non-medicinal poison is one included in the Poisons List made under the Poisons Act 1972. No matter how toxic or potent a substance may be it will not be termed a poison unless it is included in the Poisons List. Because an item is listed in the Poisons List this does not preclude it from also having medicinal uses. When the substance is sold for medicinal use then the controls applied are those listed in the Medicines Act 1968; it is only when they are sold for non-medicinal purposes that they are subject to the Poisons Act.

An alphabetical list of non-medicinal poisons, including details of the Part (see Section 10.1.1 – The Poisons List) and Schedule(s) (see Section 10.1.2) that apply to each poison can be found in the current edition of *Medicines, Ethics and Practice – A Guide for Pharmacists and Pharmacy Technicians*.

The Poisons Board

The Poisons Board advises the Home Secretary on matters relating to non-medicinal poisons. The Poisons Board consists of at least 16 members, five of whom are appointed by the Royal Pharmaceutical Society of Great Britain and one of whom must be a pharmaceutical manufacturer or wholesaler. The chairman of the board is appointed by the Secretary of State. The purpose of the board is to advise the Secretary of State as to which substances should be included in the Poisons List.

The Poisons List

The Poisons List is the list of substances that are classed as poisons under the Poisons Act and is set out in the Poisons List Order. The list is divided into two parts:

- Part I – These are non-medicinal poisons that may only be sold by persons lawfully conducting a retail pharmacy business. In other words they can only be sold from a registered pharmacy. The sale must be either by the pharmacist or under the supervision of a pharmacist.
- Part II – These are non-medicinal poisons that may only be sold by persons lawfully conducting a retail pharmacy business or a person who is included on a local authority's list of persons entitled to sell non-medicinal poisons in Part II of the list (known as a 'listed seller'). The Part II list contains non-medicinal poisons that are in common use for non-medicinal purposes.

Inclusion on the list of sellers is by application and the local authority can refuse permission if

Key point 10.1

The Poisons List is divided into two parts:

- Part I: These are non-medicinal poisons that may only be sold by persons lawfully conducting a retail pharmacy business.

→

- Part II: These are non-medicinal poisons that may only be sold by persons lawfully conducting a retail pharmacy business or a person (or nominated deputy/deputies) who is included on a local authority's list of persons entitled to sell non-medicinal poisons in Part II of the list.

Table 10.1 Examples of products containing Part II poisons that require a Poisons Register entry

Product	Poison	Use
Clean Sweep	Paraquat	Weed killer
Duratox	Demeton-s-methyl (phosphorous compound)	Insecticide
Gramoxone	Paraquat	Weed killer
Sentry	Aldicarb	Insecticide

they believe a person is unfit. Similarly a person can be deleted from the list for non-payment of a retention fee or following a conviction that would make the person unfit to sell poisons. Each listed seller may nominate one or two deputies who may effect the sale of Schedule 1 poisons (see Section 10.1.2).

Table 10.1 lists examples of products containing Part II poisons that require a poisons register entry (see Section 10.1.2) and Table 10.2 lists examples of products containing Part II

poisons that do not require a poisons register entry.

Enforcement

The function of enforcement is shared between the Royal Pharmaceutical Society of Great Britain (RPSGB) and local authorities. RPSGB inspectors are responsible for enforcement in pharmacies and local authority inspectors are responsible for enforcement at premises not registered with the RPSGB. The local authorities may choose to appoint, with the consent of the RPSGB, the same inspector for non-pharmacy premises. The RPSGB inspector will always be a pharmacist.

If a person is convicted of being in breach of or failing to act in accordance with the requirements of the Poisons Act 1972 or the associated Poisons Rules, they may be liable to a fine of up to £2500 and a further fine of up to £10 for each day the offence continues. In addition, if a person wilfully delays or obstructs an inspector, refuses to allow samples to be taken or fails to give information which they are required to give, they may be fined up to £500 on conviction. It should be noted that the fact that an employee acts without the authority of the employer is not considered to be a defence.

10.1.2 The Poisons Rules

The Poisons Rules are the detailed legislation of the Poisons Act and outline the rules regarding transport and containers, record-keeping and

Table 10.2 Examples of products containing Part II poisons that do not require a Poisons Register entry

Product	Poison	Use
Ataka	Formic acid	Kettle descaler
Brillo Clearway	Sodium Hydroxide	Drain cleaner
Caustic Soda	Sodium Hydroxide	Drain cleaner
Clean Up	48% Phenols	Multi purpose fungicide
Elsan Blue	Formaldehyde	Chemical toilet fluid
Jenolite Bath Stain Remover	Phosphoric Acid	Stain remover
Kleenoff Kay De	Formic acid	Kettle descaler
Scrubbs Cloudy Ammonia	Above 10% Ammonia	Cleaning

storage. The rules ensure the safe distribution and storage of poisons. In addition they may either place additional controls on substances or alternatively may relax some controls where deemed necessary through schedules.

There were originally 12 schedules. Schedules 2, 3, 6 and 7 were deleted by the Poisons Rules Amendment Order in 1985. The functions of the remaining eight schedules are detailed below.

Schedule 1

This is a list of substances to which special restrictions apply with regard to their sale, storage and the keeping of records.

Conditions of sale – knowledge of the purchaser

- The seller must be sure that the purchaser is a person to whom the poison may properly be sold. The purchaser must either be known to be so by the seller or a pharmacist on the premises or the purchaser must produce a certificate stating that he or she is a person who may be supplied.
- The certificate is a declaration made by a householder (see Schedule 10) and if the householder is unknown to the seller it must also be endorsed by a police officer in charge of a police station. Please note that the police endorse the good character of the householder, who may not necessarily be the purchaser. The seller must retain the certificate for two years from the date of supply.

Storage

- Schedule 1 poisons must be stored separately from other items, for example in a cupboard or drawer specifically for that purpose or in a separate part of the premises where customers have no access or on a shelf reserved for poisons storage which has no food stored below it.
- If used in agriculture/horticulture/forestry they should be stored separate from food products (i.e. not in part of the premises where food is kept). If stored in a drawer or

cupboard or on a shelf it must be reserved solely for the storage of poisons.

Labels and containers

The labelling of poisons and the containers used are subject to the CHIP (Chemicals (Hazard Information and Packaging for Supply) Regulations).

Records

The purchaser must sign the completed poisons register as outlined in Schedule 11.

Signed orders apply to sales for purpose of trade, business or profession. The signed order replaces the signature in the poisons register. The order must be given before the sale and state:

- name and address of the purchaser
- nature of trade, business or profession
- purpose for which poison is required
- total quantities of poison to be supplied
- the date (although it is not a legal requirement, the Home Office has indicated that a date should be present on a signed order for a non-medicinal poison).

The seller must be satisfied that the signature is correct, that the person does carry out that occupation and that the poison is reasonably needed for that occupation.

The poisons register must be retained for two years from the last entry/record.

Emergency supply

In an emergency, a Schedule 1 poison may be supplied on an undertaking that a signed order will be supplied within 72 hours. You must be satisfied that:

- there is an emergency
- an order cannot be produced.

It would be prudent to only make an emergency supply to someone known to you personally.

The conditions for sale of Schedule 1 poisons are relaxed in certain circumstances, when 'knowledge of the purchaser by the seller' is interpreted as personal knowledge of the purchaser by the seller where the seller knows that the purchaser is a person to whom the poison may properly be sold. This relaxation is applied to:

- sales of Part II Schedule 1 poisons by listed sellers
- provision of commercial samples of Schedule 1 poisons
- sales of Schedule 1 poisons exempted under Section 4 of the Act (see Section 10.1.3).

Schedule 1 poisons are exempt from the conditions of sale and record-keeping if the poison is to be exported to a purchaser outside the UK, or if the sale is made by a manufacturer or wholesaler to a person who is carrying on a business in the course of which poisons are sold or regularly used in the manufacture of other articles and the seller is satisfied that the purchaser is a person who requires the article for use in his or her business.

Schedule 4

This is a list of substances that are exempt from poison controls. There are two groups:

- Group I consists of articles that contain poisons but are totally exempt from poisons law, for example:
  - adhesives
  - anti-fouling compositions
  - builders materials
  - ceramics
  - cosmetic products
  - distempers
  - electrical valves
  - enamels
  - explosives
  - fillers
  - fireworks
  - fluorescent lamps
  - glazes
  - glue
  - inks
  - lacquer solvents
  - loading materials
  - matches
  - medicated animal feeding stuffs
  - motor fuels & lubricants
  - paints
  - photographic paper

  - pigments
  - plastics
  - propellants
  - rubber
  - varnishes
  - vascular plants and their seeds.
- Group II lists exemptions for certain poisons when they are in specified articles or substances, for example:
  - barium chloride when in fire extinguishers
  - nicotine and its salts when in tobacco in cigarettes
  - phenols in tar either crude or refined
  - sulphuric acid in accumulators.

Schedule 5

Schedule 5 lists Part II poisons that may only be sold by listed sellers in certain forms. Schedule 5 is divided into two parts, Parts A and B. In any other circumstances, the sale of Schedule 5 poisons is restricted to pharmacies.

- Part A contains poisons that may only be sold by listed sellers in certain forms, for example:
  - compounds of arsenic in preparations for agricultural, horticultural and forestal insecticides or fungicides
  - barium carbonate in preparations for the destruction of rats or mice.
- Part B contains poisons that may only be sold to those engaged in trade or business of agriculture or horticulture for use in that business, for example:
  - compounds of arsenic, salts of paraquat, phosphorus compounds such as dialifos, parathion, phosphamidon.

Schedule 8

This outlines the detail required in the form for application for inclusion in the local authority's list of sellers of Part II poisons. An example of this form is shown in Figure 10.1.

Schedule 9

This outlines the detail required in the form for the local authority's list of sellers of Part II

Poisons Act 1972

Application for inclusion in the local authority's list of persons entitled to sell non-medicinal poisons included in Part II of the Poisons List.

Name _____

being engaged in the business of

Business

_____

hereby apply to have my name entered in the list kept in pursuance of section 5 of the above Act in respect of the following premises, namely

Address _____

_____

Postcode _____

Telephone _____ Mobile _____

Email address _____

as a person entitled to sell from those premises poisons included in Part II of the Poisons List.

I hereby nominate

Name _____ Name _____

to act as my deputy (deputies) for the sale of non-medicinal poisons in accordance with Rule 10(1) of the Poisons Rules 1978.

Signature _____ Date _____

Figure 10.1 An example of a form for application for inclusion in the local authority's list of sellers of Part II poisons.

poisons. An example of this form is shown in Figure 10.2.

Schedule 10

This outlines the details to be entered on a certificate for the purchase of a poison. An example of this form is shown in Figure 10.3.

Schedule 11

This specifies the details that need to be recorded in the poisons book on sale of a Schedule 1 poison. An example of a page within the poisons book for the sale of a Schedule 1 poison is shown in Figure 10.4.

Full Name	Address of premises	Description of business carried on at the premises	Name of deputy (or deputies) permitted to sell

Figure 10.2   An example of a form for the local authorities list of sellers of Part II poisons.

Schedule 10

CERTIFICATE FOR THE PURCHASE OF A NON-MEDICAL POISON

For the purposes of Section 3(2)(a)(i) of the Poisons Act 1972 I, the undersigned, a Householder occupying (a) _____ hereby certify from my knowledge of (b) _____ of (a) _____ that he is a person to whom (c) _____ may properly be supplied. I further certify that (d) _____ is the signature of the said (b) _____

_____   _____

Signature of householder giving certificate   Date.

(a)   Insert full postal address.
(b)   Insert full name of intending purchaser.
(c)   Insert name of poison.
(d)   Intending purchaser to sign his name here.

Endorsement required by Rule 25 of the Poisons Rules 1982 to be made by a police officer in charge of a police station when, but only when, the householder giving the certificate is not known to the seller of the poison to be a responsible person of good character.

I hereby certify that in so far as is known to the police of the district in which * _____ resides he is a responsible person of good character.

Signature of Police Officer _____   Rank _____
In charge of police station at _____   Date _____

Official Stamp of Police Station

*Insert full name of householder giving this certificate.

Figure 10.3   An example of a certificate for the purchase of a poison.

POISONS ACT 1972

SALE of POISONS

Register

Date	Name and Quantity of Poisons supplied	Name (a) and Address (b) of Purchaser	Business, Trade or Occupation	Purpose for which stated to be required	Date of certificate (if any)	Name and Address of Person giving certificate (if any)	Signature of Purchaser or, where a signed order is permitted by the Poisons rules 1982, the date of the signed order	Reference No.
		a b						
		a b						

Figure 10.4   An example of a page within the poisons book for the sale if a Schedule 1 poison.

Schedule 12

This applies to restrictions of the sale and supply of strychnine and other substances and the forms of authority required for certain of these poisons. Schedule 12 places further controls on some Schedule 1 poisons as listed below:

- fluoroacetic acid and its salts
- sodium and potassium arsenates
- strychnine (since September 2006 this can no longer be sold for killing moles)
- thallium salts
- zinc phosphide.

In addition to any specific restrictions (see below), all of the above may be sold:

- by way of wholesale dealing
- for export outside the UK
- to persons/institutions involved in scientific education or research
- to persons/institutions involved with chemical analysis for purpose of education or research.

The sale of strychnine is now restricted to officers of DEFRA (formerly the Ministry of Agriculture, Fisheries and Food), who can produce a written authority to purchase for killing foxes in an infected area within the meaning of The Rabies (Control) Order 1974. A sample of part of the form for the purchase of strychnine for killing foxes is shown in Figure 10.5.

For the purposes of Rule 12(1) of the Poisons Rules 1982 and paragraph 5 of Part 1 of Schedule 12 thereto I hereby authorise _____ (An officer of [The Ministry of Agriculture, Fisheries and Food] [The Department of Agriculture and Fisheries for Scotland] [the Welsh Office]) to purchase within four weeks of the date hereof _____ of _____ for the purpose of killing foxes (other than foxes held in captivity) in the following infected area (within the meaning of the Rabies (Control) Order 1974) namely the infected area in _____ (locality)

_____

A person authorised by [The Ministry of Agriculture, Fisheries and Food] [The Department of Agriculture and Fisheries for Scotland] [the Welsh Office]

Date _____

Figure 10.5 An example of part of a sample form for the purchase of strychnine for killing foxes (Note: The Ministry of Agriculture, Fisheries and Food has been replaced by DEFRA).

Fluoroacetic acid can only be sold to a person presenting a written certificate issued under Rule 12 authorising use as a rodenticide for:

- use in ships or sewers
- drains in restricted areas wholly enclosed and inaccessible when not in use
- warehouses in restricted dock areas locked when not in use.

Form A is provided by the local authority or port authority for use as above. Form B is provided by DEFRA to pest control businesses for use in the first two instances. Thallium salts are similarly controlled with a certificate for purchase being issued.

10.1.3 Section 4 exemptions

Section 4 of the Poisons Act 1972 list circumstances when poisons may be sold by individuals who are neither non-pharmacists nor listed sellers. Exemptions include:

- wholesale dealing
- export from the UK
- sale to a doctor, dentist or vet for professional purposes
- sale for use in a hospital or similar institution
- sale by wholesale to:
  - a government department
  - for education or research
  - to enable employers to meet any statutory obligation with respect to medical treatment of employees
  - to person requiring the substance for trade business or profession.

10.2 Spirits

10.2.1 Regulations affecting spirits and denatured alcohol

In England and Wales the main legislation controlling sale and supply of alcohol are:

- Customs and Excise Management Act 1979
- Alcohol Liquor Duties Act 1979
- Denatured Alcohol Regulations 2005.

The legislation relating to spirits within Scotland has historically been different and was controlled by the Methylated Spirits (Sale by Retail) (Scotland) Act 1937. Many of the requirements of the 1937 Act were removed by the Deregulated Methylated Spirits (Sale by Retail) (Scotland) Order 1988. However, section 1(2), which prohibits the sale of methylated spirits to any person under the age of 14, still applies. In addition, the Denatured Alcohol Regulations 2005 also apply in Scotland.

10.2.2 Definition of spirits

The term 'spirits' refers to ethyl alcohol and includes all liquor mixed with spirits and all mixtures, compounds or preparations made with spirits. It does not, however, include denatured alcohol.

Duty is payable on all alcohol imported into the UK and excise duty is levied on all alcohol distilled in the UK.

In the UK in order to sell alcohol a Justice's licence is required. This normally applies to public houses, off licences, supermarkets, etc. A pharmacy would need a licence in order to retail an alcoholic tonic wine but does not need a licence in order to supply or manufacture medicines containing alcohol. A pharmacy would also be exempt from the requirement to hold a licence if selling alcohol to a trader for purposes of trade.

Pharmacists are mainly concerned with the dispensing of alcohol. The *Drug Tariff* states:

> Where Alcohol (96%), or Rectified Spirit (Ethanol 90%), or any other of the dilute Ethanols is prescribed as an ingredient of a medicine for internal use, the price of the duty paid to Customs and Excise will be allowed, unless the contractor endorses the prescription form 'rebate claimed.'

In other words the duty we have to pay if we include a spirit in a medicine on an NHS prescription will be returned to us via the reimbursement we receive as stated in the *Drug Tariff*. The use of alcohol in mixtures prepared extemporaneously has declined with the advent of products that can now more effectively control pain. Brompton cocktail, for example, was used to treat pain in terminal cancer patients. It consisted of morphine and cocaine and was made up in a vehicle that consisted of alcohol, syrup and chloroform water. It was common practice to ask the patient which spirit they preferred, for example, whiskey, brandy, gin or rum.

10.2.3 Denatured alcohol

Denatured alcohol is controlled by Alcohol Liquor Duties Act 1979 and Denatured Alcohol Regulations 2005. There are three types of denatured alcohol, but in pharmacy we mainly encounter two types: completely denatured alcohol (CDA), formerly known as mineralised methylated spirits (MMS), and industrial denatured alcohol (IDA), formerly known as industrial methylated spirit (IMS). The third, less commonly encountered denatured alcohol is trade specific denatured alcohol (TSDA). The formulae for these denatured alcohols render them unfit for human consumption (see the current edition of *Medicines, Ethics and Practice – A Guide for Pharmacists and Pharmacy Technicians* for details of formulae for denaturing, or HM Customs and Excise notice 473 (2005)).

In order for a pharmacy to receive IDA or TSDA for sale or use within the pharmacy they must apply to HM Revenue and Customs National Registration Unit in order to gain authority to receive (see Figure 10.6). Authorisation must be obtained before a supply of IDA or TSDA can be made. Once authorisation has been granted, a copy of the authorisation must be sent to the supplier and then a supply may be made.

A community pharmacist is then authorised to dispense IDA on a prescription either alone or as an ingredient for an item for external use only such as a liniment or lotion (this could be for human or animal use). IDA may also be sold by the community pharmacist but only for medical or scientific purposes. Again, the purchaser would need to have authorisation and a copy of this authorisation would need to be in the pharmacist's possession. It should be noted that the supply can only be made for the use indicated on the user's authorisation and no other use. When labelled for a dispensed item the label must clearly state 'For external use only' and also *British National Formulary* caution 15 'Caution flammable: keep away from fire or flames'. In the case of labelling for sale this will be as outlined in the CHIP regulations.

Conditions are attached to the authority to receive IDA or TSDA. These include:

- Storage – an undertaking must be made that the IDA or TSDA will be stored under lock and key and under the pharmacist's personal control or under the control of an authorised deputy.
- Use – this must only be as laid out in the authorisation.
- Supply – only approved formulations of

Application for authorisation to receive and use IDA or TSDA

Application for Authority to receive

Industrial Denatured Alcohol/Trade Specific Denatured Alcohol*

Part A. *I/We (name of company, partnership, proprietor, as appropriate) apply for authority to receive IDA/TSDA* formulation(s)

_____

_____

for use at (address of premises):

_____

_____

Type of business/activity _____

VAT Registration Number _____

Part B The *IDA/TSDA is to be used for the following purpose(s):

_____

Part C (only for requests to use TSDA for a use not previously approved) CDA/IDA is unsuitable because

_____

Part D *My/Our estimated annual requirement is:

*Industrial Denatured Alcohol _____ litres

*Trade Specific Denatured Alcohol _____ litres

Signature _____

Full name _____

Status _____

(proprietor, partner, director, company secretary etc.)

Date _____

Telephone Number _____ Fax Number _____ E-mail address _____

*Delete as necessary

Figure 10.6   Application for authorisation to receive and use IDA or TSDA.

alcohol can be supplied and if this is not on a prescription a written statement from the authorised user must be obtained or in the case of a medical practitioner a written order.

- Close of business – should a business close the authorisation to possess denatured alcohol would be withdrawn. The National Advice Centre of HM Revenue and Customs should be contacted to arrange how stocks should be disposed of and over what period of time. Once the stock has been cleared the National Registration Unit should be informed in order to cancel the authorisation.

When IDA or TSDA is received, a record of the amount of IDA or TSDA received must be made and a copy of the supplier's delivery note must be signed and returned to the supplier and a second copy must be retained on the premises as an additional record of the supply.

The quantity of CDA that can be supplied has no restriction in the UK. There are also no restrictions on its use (it is commonly used in 'meths burners', for example, in fondue sets, etc.). It is supplied free from duty. IDA and TSDA have more restrictions and may be supplied in quantities less than 20 litres only to authorised users, but there is no restriction on the amount that can be supplied to a medical practitioner on a written order.

All records must show the amount of IDA or TSDA received and supplied and any excess or deficiency in the balance must be accounted for, as if it has been found to be supplied for an unauthorised use a demand may be issued by HM Customs and Excise for the duty payable on the alcohol in the missing amount.

10.2.4 Records of IDA and TSDA

Generally, records must be kept as set out in Notice 206 Revenue Traders Accounts and Records. Specifically:

- a stock account of all the spirits received and used
- such other records as are either specified in the letter of authority, or are necessary to establish that the spirits have been put to the authorised use.

Records must also be kept of all the checks carried out on receipts, storage and use of the spirits. Normal business records may be used for these purposes provided there is a clear audit trail from receipt to final disposal. Records must be kept up to date.

In addition:

- Stock accounts should be balanced at the intervals as required by the letter of authority. The physical stock should be checked and the result noted in the account.
- Any apparent discrepancies should be investigated promptly, and any that cannot be resolved should be reported to the local office immediately.

Records must be kept for at least six years.

10.3 Chapter summary

This final chapter has summarised the key points that pharmacists and pharmacy technicians should be aware of surrounding the sale and supply of both poisons and spirits. Many pharmacists in daily practice may not ever supply poisons or spirits; however, it is possible that requests will be made from time to time. Therefore, it is important that pharmacists and pharmacy technicians are familiar with the key points.

Further and more detailed information on the sale and supply of poisons and spirits can be found in the current edition of *Medicines, Ethics and Practice – A Guide for Pharmacists and Pharmacy Technicians* and *Dale and Appelbe's Pharmacy Law and Ethics*.

Answers to exercises

Chapter 1

Exercise 1.1

- To maintain good customer relations (audit questions 1, 6 and 7).
- To ensure the prescription form presented relates to the named patient (audit question 2).
- To ensure safe dispensing (audit questions 2 and 5).
- To ensure details on the reverse of a prescription form are correctly filled out, and any applicable fee is collected (audit questions 3 and 4).
- To ensure effective communication between patient and pharmacist (audit question 6).

Exercise 1.2

A suggested answer can be found in Figure A1.

Exercise 1.3

- To ensure prescription form details are accurately recorded on patient medication record (audit questions 1 and 2).
- To produce labels that meet the legal and professional requirements (audit question 4).
- To minimise the risk of error due to the incorrect selection or the incorrect labelling of prescription items (audit questions 2, 5 and 6).
- To dispense products to a high professional standard in terms of accuracy and appearance (audit questions 3, 7, 8 and 9).

Exercise 1.4

Question 1: A suggested answer can be found in Figure A2.

Question 2:

- To ensure that all legal requirements re prescription handling are met (audit questions 1 and 5).
- To ensure the completed prescription is handed out to the correct person (patient/representative) including items with specific storage requirements (for example, fridge items or items kept in the controlled drugs cupboard) (audit question 2).
- To provide counselling or additional information when necessary or requested (audit question 3).
- To give patients the opportunity to discuss their medication with the pharmacist (audit question 4).
- To inform the patient or their representative if the supply is not complete and items are owing (audit question 6).

Chapter 2

Exercise 2.1

This supply can be treated as the second type of supply in the list of items which would attract multiple prescription charges (different formulations or presentations of the same drug or preparation are prescribed and supplied).

Although the two preparations are for the same drug, as one is a standard tablet formulation and the second is enteric coated, they are

STANDARD OPERATING PROCEDURE – DISPENSING
PROFESSIONAL CHECK (NHS) – Audit

NAME OF AUDITOR: _____   DATE OF AUDIT: _____

AUDIT QUESTION	SATISFACTORY		AREAS OF NON-COMPLIANCE	RECOMMENDATIONS
	YES	NO		
Review resubmissions (i.e. prescription forms returned from the Prescription Pricing Division).				
1. Are any for disallowed items?				
2. Are any for borderline substances?				
3. Are any querying quantity dispensed as it is unclear on the prescription form?				
4. Any prescription forms returned unsigned by the prescriber?				
5. Any prescription forms returned that are out of date?				
6. Are clinical intervention forms being kept?				

REVIEW DATE: _____   REVIEWED BY: _____

Figure A1   An example of an audit form for the audit of prescription form returns from the Prescription Pricing Division (PPD) within a community pharmacy.

treated as different formulations and therefore attract separate prescription charges.

Had the first preparation also been for enteric coated tables, or had the second preparation not been enteric coated, only one prescription charge would be required.

Exercise 2.2

This supply can be treated as the fourth type of supply in the list of items which would attract multiple prescription charges (more than one piece of elastic hosiery is supplied). Therefore, although the prescription is for one pair of stockings, two prescription charges will need to be collected.

Chapter 7

Exercise 7.1

The request is from a practitioner (Dr Jones) with whom you are not familiar. Therefore, you will need to take reasonable steps to ensure that the request is genuine. This is especially important in this case as the item that is being requested is a Schedule 4 controlled drug (see Chapter 6). This may be difficult to do easily as it is Saturday lunchtime. Had it been a request during normal surgery hours, you could contact the practice manager by telephone to verify the status of the locum doctor. However, in this case, that may not be possible. Unless it is pos-

STANDARD OPERATING PROCEDURE – DISPENSING
HANDING OUT PRESCRIPTION ITEMS (NHS) – Audit

NAME OF AUDITOR: _____   DATE OF AUDIT: _____

AUDIT QUESTION	SATISFACTORY		AREAS OF NON-COMPLIANCE	RECOMMENDATIONS
	YES	NO		
1. Was the pharmacist present and able to give advice?				
2. Was the name and address of the patient checked?				
3. Was the patient counselled discreetly				
4. Was the patient offered the opportunity to speak to the pharmacist?				
5. Was the completed prescription form returned to the dispensary for filing?				
6. Was patient suitably advised when an item was owing?				

REVIEW DATE: _____   REVIEWED BY: _____

Figure A2   An example of an audit form for the audit of a standard operating procedure for the handing out of prescription items within a community pharmacy.

sible to verify the status of the locum doctor, the supply should not be made.

There are a number of methods you could use to verify the status of the doctor including looking back through recent prescription forms to find other supplies requested by the same locum practitioner or ringing other local pharmacies to see if they can confirm his identity. Alternatively, the General Medical Council (GMC) has advised that pharmacists can use the out-of-hours automated service (the telephone number is available via the GMC website – www.gmc-uk.org) to check a doctor's registration if the pharmacist has the doctor's GMC registration number.

If you are able to verify the status of the locum doctor, you will then need to know the following:

- the name and address (and if appropriate, the age) of the patient

- the name and address of the practitioner (Dr Jones) (this will be the address at which Dr Jones is working as a locum)
- details of the medication that the practitioner wishes the patient to take, including the name, form, strength, dose and frequency of the medication.

An entry will need to be made in the prescription-only medicines register stating:

- the date on which the emergency supply was made
- the name, quantity and, except where it is apparent from the name, the pharmaceutical form and strength of the medicine (It is also good practice to record the dose of the medication.)
- the name and address of the practitioner
- the name and address of the patient.

Reference number	Details		Cost
7.03 Date of supply	Emergency supply at the request of Dr Jones John Fish 48 Station Road Anytown 14 Diazepam 5 mg tablets 1 PRN Date on prescription form. Date prescription form received.	Dr Jones The Health centre Anytown	Prescription charge (NHS or private) or details of exemption (NHS).

Figure A3 An example of a prescription-only medicines register entry for Exercise 7.1.

A space must be left for (i) the date on the prescription form and (ii) the date the prescription form was received in the pharmacy.

The prescription-only medicines register entry for this supply would appear in the register as illustrated in Figure A3.

The label for this supply would look as follows (we have assumed that the name and address of the pharmacy and the words 'Keep out of the reach and sight of children' are pre-printed on the label):

Diazepam 5 mg Tablets	**14**
Take ONE tablet when required. Warning. May cause drowsiness. If affected do not drive or operate machinery. Avoid alcoholic drink.	
Mr John Fish	Date of dispensing

Exercise 7.2

The request is from a patient with whom you are not familiar. However, this is not an unreasonable request. You will need to interview the patient and ascertain that:

- there is an immediate need for the prescription-only medicine and that the patient is unable to obtain a prescription form for the item
- the item has been previously prescribed by a doctor, community practitioner nurse prescriber, supplementary prescriber, nurse independent prescriber or pharmacist independent prescriber

- the dose and frequency she states she is taking would be appropriate.

You also need to check whether the patient is taking any other medication to enable you to check that the requested emergency supply does not interact with any other medication currently being taken.

It is up to the individual pharmacist as to what evidence that he or she would like to see to verify that the patient has previously been prescribed the item(s) being requested. Suitable evidence would include old medication packaging, including the dispensing label (usual if the patient has run out of medication), or a repeat medication slip (used to request a prescription form for a further supply from the patient's GP). Alternatively, you could obtain details of the patient's usual community pharmacy and contact them by telephone to verify any previous supply via the patient medication record system. In addition, it would be usual to request to see some form of identification so you can verify the identity of the patient.

If you decide to make the supply, an entry will need to be made in the prescription-only medicines register (see Figure A4) stating the following:

- the date on which the emergency supply was made
- the name, quantity and, except where it is apparent from the name, the pharmaceutical form and strength of the medicine. it is also good practice to include the dose and

Reference number	Details	Cost
7.06 Date of supply	Emergency supply at the request of a patient Jane Thompson Dr Ashwin Patel 12 Cottage Lane 25 High Street Torquay Torquay Residing at: 3 The Grove, Anytown 21 Microgynon 30 — 1 OD The patient is visiting relatives on a Saturday afternoon and has forgotten her oral contraceptive.	Cost of drug + % Mark–up + Professional Fee + VAT

Figure A4   An example of a prescription-only medicines register entry for Exercise 7.2.

frequency of the medication and details of the patient's GP's name and address

- the name and address of the patient and her temporary address
- the nature of the emergency (i.e. why the patient requested the prescription-only medicine and why she was unable to obtain a prescription form).

As the request is for an oral contraceptive, a full cycle may be supplied (see Figure A4).

The label for this supply would look as follows (we have assumed that the name and address of the pharmacy and the words 'Keep out of the reach and sight of children' are pre-printed on the label):

Microgynon 30 Tablets	**21**
Take ONE tablet as directed.	
Emergency Supply (7.06)	
Ms Jane Thompson	Date of dispensing

Appendix 1

Commonly encountered qualifications of healthcare professionals

Medical Practitioners (Registering body: General Medical Council, GMC)

MB, BM	Bachelor of Medicine
MD, DM	Doctor of Medicine (a medical higher degree)
ChB, BChir, BS	Bachelor of Surgery
MRCP	Member of the Royal College of Physicians
MRCS	Member of the Royal College of Surgeons

(Note: It is common for a first degree in medicine to include both a medical and a surgical qualification e.g. MB ChB.)

Dentists (Registering body: General Dental Council, GDC)

BDS, BChD	Bachelor of Dental Surgery
LDS	Licentiate in Dental Surgery

Veterinary surgeons (Registering body: Royal College of Veterinary Surgeons, RCVS)

MRCVS	Member of the Royal College of Veterinary Surgeons
FRCVS	Fellow of the Royal College of Veterinary Surgeons

Ophthalmic opticians (Registering body: General Optical Council, GOC)

MCOptom	Member of the College of Optometrists
FCOptom	Fellow of the College of Optometrists
FBOA	Fellowship Diploma of the British Optical Association
DCLP	Diploma in Contact Lens Practice

Nurses (Registering body: Nursing and Midwifery Council, NMC)

RGN	Registered General Nurse
RMN	Registered Mental Nurse (UK)
RN	Registered Nurse
RNMS	Registered Nurse for Mentally Subnormal
SCM	State Certified Midwife

Chiropodists (or Podiatrists) (Registering body: Health Professions Council, HPC)

MChS	Member of the Society of Chiropodists and Podiatrists
FChS	Fellow of the Society of Chiropodists and Podiatrists
FCPods	Fellow of the College of Podiatrists of the Society of Chiropodists and Podiatrists

Appendix 2

Abbreviations commonly used within pharmacy

aa	ana	of each
ac	ante cibum	before food
ad/add	addendus	to be added (up to)
ad lib	ad libitum	as much as desired
alt	alternus	alternate
alt die	alterno die	every other day
amp	ampulla	ampoule
applic	applicetur	let it be applied
aq	aqua	water
aq ad	aquam ad	water up to
aur/aurist	auristillae	ear drops
bd/bid	bis in die	twice a day
BNF		*British National Formulary*
BP		*British Pharmacopoeia*
BPC		*British Pharmaceutical Codex*
c	cum	with
cap	capsula	capsule
cc	cum cibus	with food
co/comp	compositus	compound
collut	collutorium	mouthwash
conc	concentratus	concentrated
corp	corpori	to the body
crem	cremor	cream
d	dies	a day
dd	de die	daily
dil	dilutus	diluted
div	divide	divide
DPF		Dental Practitioners' Formulary
DT		*Drug Tariff*
EP		*European Pharmacopoeia*
et	etand	and
ex aq	ex aqua	in water
ext	extractum	an extract
f/ft/fiat	fiat	let it be made
fort	fortis	strong
freq	frequenter	frequently
ft mist	fiat mistura	let a mixture be made
ft pulv	fiat pulvis	let a powder be made

garg	gargarisma	a gargle
gutt/guttae/gtt	guttae	drops
h	hora	at the hour
hs	hora somni	at the hour of sleep (bedtime)
ic	inter cibos	between meals
inf	infusum	infusion
inh		inhalation/inhaler
irrig	irrigatio	irrigation
liq	liquor	solution
lin	linimentum	liniment
lot	lotio	lotion
m/mane	mane	in the morning
md	more dicto	as directed
mdu	more dicto utendus	use as directed
mist	mistura	mixture
mitt/mitte	mitte	send (quantity to be given)
n/nocte	nocte	at night
n et m	nocte maneque	night and morning
narist	naristillae	nose drops
neb	nebula	spray
np	nomen proprium	the proper name
ocul	oculo	to (for) the eye
oculent/oc	oculentum	an eye ointment
od	omni die	every day
oh	omni hora	every hour
om	omni mane	every morning
on	omni nocte	every night
paa	parti affectae applicandus	apply to the affected part
pc	post cibum	after food
PC		prescriber contacted
PCT		Primary Care Trust
pess	pessus	pessary
pig	pigmentum	a paint
PNC		prescriber not contacted
po	per os	by mouth
ppt	praecipitatus	precipitated
pr	per rectum	rectally
prn	pro re nata	when required
pulv	pulvis	a powder
pv	per vagina	vaginally
qds/qid	quarter die	four times a day
qqh/q4h	quarta quaque hora	every 4 hours
qs	quantum sufficiat	sufficient
R	recipe	take
rep/rept	repetatur	let it be repeated
sig	signa	let it be labelled
solv	solve	dissolve
sos	si opus sit	when necessary
stat	statim	immediately
supp	suppositorium	suppository

syr	syrupus	syrup
tds/tid	ter in die	three times a day
tinct	tinctura	tincture
tuss urg	tussi urgente	when the cough is troublesome
ung	unguentum	ointment
ut dict/ud	ut dictum	as directed
vap	vapor	an inhalation

Bibliography

Appelbe GE, Wingfield J (2005). *Dale and Appelbe's Pharmacy Law and Ethics*, 8th edn. London: The Pharmaceutical Press.

Baxter K (ed.) (2007). *Stockley's Drug Interactions*, 8th edn. London: The Pharmaceutical Press.

British Medical Association and the Royal Pharmaceutical Society of Great Britain (current edition). *British National Formulary*. London: The Pharmaceutical Press (updated every six months).

British Medical Association, the Royal Pharmaceutical Society of Great Britain, the Royal College of Paediatrics and Child Health and the Neonatal and Paediatric Pharmacists Group (current edition). *British National Formulary for Children*. London: The Pharmaceutical Press (updated every year).

Department of Health (2000). *The NHS Plan*. London: The Stationery Office.

Health and Personal Social Services for Northern Ireland (current edition). *Drug Tariff*. Belfast: Central Services Agency (updated monthly).

Marriot JM, Wilson KA, Langley CA, Belcher D (2006). *Pharmaceutical Compounding and Dispensing*. London: The Pharmaceutical Press.

National Health Service in Scotland (current edition). *Scottish Drug Tariff*. Edinburgh: The Scottish Executive Health Department (updated monthly on-line – available via: www.isdscotland.org).

National Health Service, England and Wales (current edition). *Drug Tariff*. London: The Stationery Office (updated monthly).

National Health Services Business Services Authority Prescription Pricing Division website (available via: www.ppa.org.uk).

Royal Pharmaceutical Society of Great Britain (2005). *The Safe and Secure Handling of Medicines: a Team Approach*. London: Royal Pharmaceutical Society of Great Britain.

Royal Pharmaceutical Society of Great Britain (2007). *Code of Ethics for Pharmacists and Pharmacy Technicians*. London: Royal Pharmaceutical Society of Great Britain.

Royal Pharmaceutical Society of Great Britain (2007). *Professional Standards and Guidance for the Sale and Supply of Medicines*. London: Royal Pharmaceutical Society of Great Britain.

Royal Pharmaceutical Society of Great Britain (current edition). *Medicines, Ethics and Practice – A Guide for Pharmacists and Pharmacy Technicians*. London: The Pharmaceutical Press (updated every year).

Index